JEAN CARPER'S
TOTAL NUTRITION GUIDE

JEAN CARPER'S TOTAL NUTRITION GUIDE

JEAN CARPER

BANTAM BOOKS
Toronto • New York • London • Sydney • Auckland

JEAN CARPER'S TOTAL NUTRITION GUIDE
A Bantam Book / April 1987

Library of Congress Cataloging-in-Publication Data

Carper, Jean.
  Jean Carper's Total nutrition guide.

  1. Nutrition. 2. Nutritionally induced diseases.
3. Food—Vitamin content—Tables. 4. Food—Mineral
content—Tables. I. Title. II. Title: Total
nutrition guide.
RA784.C285 1987   613.2   86-47628
ISBN 0-553-34350-5

Published simultaneously in the United States and Canada

PRINTED IN THE UNITED STATES OF AMERICA

MV   0 9 8 7 6 5 4 3 2 1

Acknowledgments

There are many people to thank for making this book possible. First is Jeffrey Straathof who performed all of the computer work for the nutrient charts. Among those at the U. S. Department of Agriculture's Nutrition Monitoring Division who were so unfailingly available to answer questions are: Brucy Gray, chief, Survey Statistics; Dr. Frank Hepburn, chief, Nutrient Data Research; Grace Matthews and Dr. John Weihrauch, Nutrient Data Research. I am also grateful to the staff of the Food and Nutrition Information Center at the National Agriculture Library which was a prime source of information, as well as to Kate Alfriend, USDA information specialist, for her efficient and cheerful professionalism in producing vital information.

Numerous authorities read all or parts of the book in manuscript and made invaluable suggestions for greater clarity and accuracy in their areas of expertise. I especially want to thank Bonnie Liebman, Center for Science in the Public Interest, for her comments on the entire manuscript; Dr. Walter Mertz, director of the USDA's Human Nutrition Research Center in Beltsville, Maryland, for his comments on the iron chapter; Dr. C.E. Bodwell, chief of USDA's Energy and Protein Nutrition Laboratory, for his comments on the protein chapter; Dr. Sheldon Reiser, chief of the USDA's Carbohydrate Nutrition Laboratory, for comments on the carbohydrate chapter; Dr. John Erdman, professor of food science at the University of Illinois, for comments on the niacin and vitamin A chapters; Dr. Barbara Harland, associate professor, Human Nutrition and Food, School of Human Ecology, Howard University, for comments on chapters on fiber and zinc; Dr. James Smith, director of the USDA's Vitamin and Mineral Research Laboratories, for his comments on potassium and vitamin C chapters; Dr. Daphne Roe, professor of nutrition at Cornell University, for her comments on drug-nutrient interactions; Dr. Burton Altura, professor of physiology, State University of New York, Health Science Center at Brooklyn, and president of the American Society for Magnesium Research, for his comments on the magnesium chapter; Dr. Richard Rivlin, professor of medicine, Cornell University Medical College, for his comments on riboflavin; Dr. Victor

Herbert, Veterans Administration Medical Center, Bronx, for his comments on vitamin B_{12} and folacin; and Dr. Robert Reynolds, USDA's Vitamin and Mineral Nutrition Laboratory, for his comments on vitamin B_6.

None of these people, of course, are responsible for the contents of the book or opinions of the author. Nor does their reviewing the manuscript necessarily constitute an endorsement of the ideas or facts contained within. However, their thoughts and expertise were enormously helpful in clarifying controversies and guaranteeing factual accuracy.

And a fond thanks to my agent, Raphael Sagalyn, for seeing the merits of this book; to his colleague Ann Sleeper, for her invaluable comments on the manuscript; to my friend Thea Flaum for her enthusiasm and editorial input; to my friend Joan Levin for research assistance at times of deadline crises; and to my editor, Grace Bechtold, for her long-time editorial contribution and support.

Contents

<u>Introduction</u>

It is becoming critically important to know what nutrients are in the foods you eat because both deficiencies and excesses of certain nutrients are rampant. If you are female, you need to know you are at high risk of deficiencies in iron and calcium. If you are male, you are probably eating far too much fat and protein and not enough complex carbohydrates. If you are on a low-calorie diet, the chances of robbing your body of vital trace minerals skyrocket. If you are older, it is particularly essential to eat high-nutrient foods, for the aging process often lessens your ability to utilize nutrients. If you smoke, drink alcohol, exercise heavily, or take birth control pills or certain other medications, you are at risk of nutrient deficiencies of various types.

What This Book Tells You

- Which foods will give you the nutrients you need
- How to get the most nutrients for the fewest calories
- How to spot nutritional deficiencies: the common signs and symptoms
- Your chances of being nutritionally deficient
- How nutritional deficiencies and excesses affect your health
- How unsuspected food, nutrient and drug interactions can benefit or destroy your diet
- Possible hazards of specific nutrients
- How to prepare foods to get the most nutrients
- The recommended dietary allowances

In other words, this is the most comprehensive, authoritative single source of information on nutrients—what they are, where they are, and how you can best use them to improve your health.

The New Nutrition "Bible"

The source of inspiration for this book was a desire to make available to everyone the massive amount of nutrient information compiled by that most formidable reservoir of nutrient research and analysis in the world, the U.S. Department of Agriculture. The USDA's nutrient database is widely respected and consulted by experts worldwide—the food industry as well as consumer experts and working nutritionists—as the most comprehensive and solid information available on the nutritional values of foods.

For years, the USDA has packaged its information on nutrient content in what it calls *Handbook 8,* a publication accepted widely as the nation's Bible on the subject. About ten years ago, the USDA, recognizing that much of the information on the nutritional values of foods was out-of-date, began releasing a massive update of *Handbook 8.*

Gradually, the government's new analysis has been put out in volumes of print and on computer tape and disc. But until now this vital information has remained inaccessible to most Americans. The printed volumes are intimidating in their size and technical layouts, and the amount of information is overwhelming.

To give consumers this vital information, we have extracted the pertinent information from the USDA's vast nutrient database and transformed it into easy-to-read charts, listing twenty-one critical nutritional elements for over twenty-five hundred foods.

A Quick Guide to All the Nutrients

The first part of this book is a guide to interpreting the significance of the information in the charts. You will find a complete profile of the major nutritional elements in the charts with advice on getting enough of each one but not too much. These are: protein, carbohydrates, fat, cholesterol, dietary fiber, vitamin A, vitamin C, thiamin, riboflavin, niacin, vitamin B_6, vitamin B_{12}, folacin (folic acid), sodium, calcium, iron, potassium, zinc, and magnesium.

Each section answers the following questions: Who are likely targets for deficiencies or excesses? What are the deficiency symptoms? What are the possible effects on my health of a deficiency or excess? Where do I find the nutrient in the food supply? How much do I absorb? What affects the body's utilization of the nutrient? How do other foods, drugs, and nutrients interact? What is a toxic dose? What are the daily recommended dietary allowances? Which foods are the best sources of the nutrient? Which foods are the best sources for the fewest calories?

After that you will find "minichapters" on four nutrients not contained in the back-of-the-book charts: copper, vitamin E, chromium, and sele-nium, which are commanding increased attention from researchers.

Much of the book is presented in a kind of shorthand with charts, boxes, and lists to make it quickly accessible without extensive reading—a handbook of ready reference.

Now, some personal opinions and a broad sweep of vital information to guide you on your way.

Your Nutritional Risks at a Glance

Here, based on average figures and surveys of nutrient intake, is a rundown of the general risks of under- or overnutrition and special needs at various stages of life and under special circumstances.

• *Infants*. Normal infants have surprisingly low risks of deficiencies whether reared on breast milk, cow's milk, or iron-fortified formula. Breast milk is usually considered best for numerous reasons, including better absorption of many nutrients, such as iron. Of course, this as-sumes that the mother is well nourished. The breast milk from severely malnourished mothers will be deficient, promoting deficiencies in the infant. Nursing mothers need higher intakes of almost all nutrients.

• *Children*. Boys and girls between the ages one and five are apt to have deficient iron intakes. Age one is particularly critical. Another source of trouble: too little B_6, especially after age three. Too much fat in the diet is a hazard after age two. However, do not restrict fat or cholesterol in the diets of infants (under age two); fat restrictions could impair early development.

• *Adolescents*. Girls are at extremely high risk of deficiencies in iron and calcium. Both sexes are likely to eat too little magnesium; also B_6, especially females. Too little vitamin C can be a problem for both sexes. Excessive fat, protein, and sodium intake is likely, along with too little fiber.

• *Women*. Because women eat fewer calories than men, they have much more difficulty getting adequate amounts of nutrients. Calcium deficiency is almost a certainty for women of all ages. Iron is a major problem for women of menstruating age. Women of all ages are at high risk for vitamin B_6 deficiencies (only 8 percent consume 100 percent of recommended levels). Vitamin A and vitamin C intakes may be low, especially among young adult women. Magnesium and copper are also problem nutrients for many women. Women eat too much protein, fat (about the same percentage of calories as men), and sodium, and too little fiber.

• *Pregnant women*. Nutritional requirements rise dramatically during pregnancy. You need about 300 extra calories per day, or 80,000 calories total, to nourish a fetus. That includes 65 percent more protein; 100 percent more folacin and vitamin D; 50 percent more calcium and magnesium; 33 percent more vitamin C; 25 percent more vitamin A, vitamin E, and zinc; and so much more iron that the National Academy of Sciences recommends iron supplements. Also, your sodium intake will rise; experts do not recommend salt restriction for pregnant women.

Pregnant women are often low in thiamin intakes; about half do not get enough, according to one survey. Folacin and zinc deficits are of grave concern during pregnancy because a lack can promote miscarriages and possibly birth defects. One study found that 25 percent of pregnant women have symptoms of anemia caused by folacin-deficiency.

• *Men.* Men consume an average of 50 percent more calories than women, thus they are less likely to have deficient intakes in general. Some possible problems: vitamin B_6, magnesium, copper, and vitamin A. On the other hand, they, like women, eat far more fat, sodium, and protein than needed. And too little fiber.

• *Elderly.* Aging creates vulnerabilities to certain deficiencies for two reasons: elderly people tend to eat fewer calories, and the aging process can alter the body's ability to utilize nutrients. A lack of B vitamins is a special hazard. One survey found that about 25 percent of elderly people have marginal thiamin deficiencies. Most elderly females take in only half of the recommended levels of B_6. Riboflavin is another potential problem. A loss of the ability to absorb B_{12} can occur with age. Other potential deficiencies: folacin, niacin, vitamin C, vitamin D, calcium, zinc, magnesium, and copper.

• *Alcoholics and heavy drinkers.* It is truly astonishing to see, even on the basis of limited research, how destructive alcohol is to nutrients in the body. Alcohol not only has a direct effect in blocking the absorption or utilization of several vitamins and minerals, but its chronic use can change the body's metabolism of nutrients, bringing on malnutrition. Alcoholics also replace food with alcohol. Particularly dangerous are alcohol-induced folacin and thiamin deficiencies that can lead to progressive and irreversible damage to the central nervous system.

Chronic drinkers are likely to be deficient in vitamins A, C, D, thiamin, riboflavin, B_6, B_{12}, calcium, zinc, iron, magnesium, and copper.

• *Dieters on low-calorie diets.* When you restrict calories, you necessarily restrict intake of nutrients and risk vitamin and mineral deficiencies. Dr. Paul A. LaChance, a leading nutritional expert at Rutgers University, analyzed the nutrient intakes in ten popular weight-loss diets and found most of them deficient in thiamin, riboflavin, vitamin B_6, vitamin B_{12}, calcium, iron, zinc, and magnesium. The most nutritionally sound diets, according to the analysis, were Audrey Eyton's F-Plan Diet (although too low in B_{12} and calcium) and the Pritikin 1200 diet (lacking in B_{12} and zinc).

Dieters should take great pains to eat "nutrient dense" foods to avoid squandering calories on poor nutrition. Some may need a general vitamin-mineral supplement providing roughly 100 percent or less of the RDAs. Dr. Walter Mertz, director of the USDA's Human Nutrition Research Center in Beltsville, Maryland, recommends such a supplement for people who get fewer than 1500 calories per day.

• *Vegetarians*. The diets of vegetarians may be as good or better than the diets of meat eaters, but vegetarians must take special precautions. Iron can be a problem even for vegetarians who eat eggs and milk (lacto-ovo vegetarians), especially females. It is more difficult for the body to absorb iron from vegetables, grains, and beans than from meat, chicken, and fish.

Strict vegetarians who eat neither meat, eggs, or milk (vegans) risk B_{12} deficiencies because B_{12} comes only from animal products. Further, the first sign of B_{12} deficiency—a particular type of anemia—may be masked by high intakes of folacin from vegetables. A vegan diet may work for adults who have stores of B_{12}, but youngsters who are raised from infancy on vegan diets with no vitamin B_{12} supplementation risk severe growth retardation and developmental damage. Diets of vegan children are also likely to be deficient in calories, calcium, zinc, and vitamin D.

On the other hand, there is evidence that vegetarians in general have lower rates of chronic diseases such as heart disease and cancer. Eating less meat and more vegetables, beans and grains makes sense for most Americans.

A Short Nutrient Dictionary

The macronutrients—protein, carbohydrates, and dietary fat—are the sources of energy without which life can not go on. Fiber is a constituent of plant foods and has no nutritional value of its own, but it is important for the proper functioning of the body. Vitamins, minerals, and trace elements are the micronutrients, substances usually needed by the body in small amounts. They cannot be manufactured by the body; they must be regularly supplied from outside sources. Such nutrients are labeled "essential." Currently, there are over 40 substances recognized as essential for human nutrition.

Vitamins are categorized as either fat soluble or water soluble. Fat-soluble vitamins—A, D, E, and K—are oily and need the body's natural emulsifiers to dissolve them so that they can be absorbed. These vitamins can then be stored in fatty tissues and drawn upon as needed. Because excess intakes are stored, these vitamins can build up in the body to toxic doses.

Water-soluble vitamins are easily absorbed into the bloodstream, circulate in body fluids, and are not stored in substantial amounts for long periods. The body does provide for small "reserves" of these nutrients to be drawn upon. Beyond that, when a cell's threshold or saturation point is reached, the vitamins are generally flushed out in the urine. Because of this safeguard, water-soluble vitamins have been traditionally considered safe even in outrageously high megadoses. New evidence shows this is not true and that there are some dangers. Water-soluble vitamins are vitamin C and the B vitamins—thiamin, riboflavin, niacin, B_6, folacin, B_{12}, pantothenic acid and biotin. The B vitamins are also sometimes referred to as the B complex vitamins, because they were once thought to be a single vitamin. When it was discovered that they had quite different functions, they were labeled a "complex" of several nutrients and distinguished as B_1, B_2, etc.

Minerals are basic elements that come from the soil and cannot be made by living organisms. Necessary in fairly large amounts are calcium, phosphorus, and magnesium. Then there are the so-called trace elements, essential to the body in minute amounts—copper, iron, zinc, manganese, fluoride, chromium, and selenium, to name a few. Both sodium and potassium are considered electrolytes—minerals necessary to maintain cellular water balance and electrochemical reactions in cells.

The RDAs: How Much Is Enough?

A scientific body, the National Academy of Sciences Committee on Dietary Allowances of the Food and Nutrition Board, periodically surveys the latest medical-nutritional research and decides how much of a particular nutrient the *average* American needs. Then experts boost that figure by around 30 percent to help insure that almost everyone, even those with unusually high nutrient needs, is covered. These figures are called *recommended dietary allowances* or RDAs. They are the nation's most respected guidelines to good nutrition and they roughly indicate whether you are getting too much or too little of a certain nutrient. The pertinent RDAs are listed in each chapter on specific nutrients. (The so-called U.S. RDAs found on nutritional labels are a slightly modified version of the National Academy's RDAs.)

Although most people believe they must get 100 percent of the RDAs, lest they be malnourished, that is not true. The vast majority of Americans do not need to consume 100 percent of the RDAs, according to the RDA committee. Most nutritionists start to worry only when a person eats less than two-thirds of the RDAs. Even so, low intakes do not necessarily mean deficiencies. Only biochemical tests such as blood tests on individuals can determine true bodily deficiencies.

Here's what you should remember about the RDAs:

The RDAs are an excellent guide to approximately how much of which nutrients you should consume based on the latest research. But the figures are not iron-clad for each individual; the RDAs imply a *range* of nutritional acceptability designed to protect the population as a whole. *The RDAs are recommendations, not requirements.*

The RDAs are deliberately set high to accommodate the individual differences of an entire population.

If you don't regularly eat the maximum RDAs, you will not necessarily be malnourished. That depends on a person's particular genetic makeup and biological circumstances.

The RDAs apply to *healthy* populations. People who have inherited metabolic disorders, infections, chronic diseases, and use medications may have special needs beyond the RDAs.

It is not necessarily dangerous to consume two to three times more than the RDAs; many people do in foods and/or supplements. Megadoses (ten times or more the RDAs) can be hazardous.

The RDAs are not permanent. They are subject to change and controversy. As new scientific information appears, the recommended allowances may go up or down. For example, a National Institutes of Health expert committee on osteoporosis recently attacked the calcium RDA as woefully inadequate. They declared: "The RDA for calcium is evidently too low, particularly for postmenopausal women, and may well be too low in elderly men." The National Academy delayed publishing its 1985 updated RDAs because it was unable to agree on suggested changes for several nutrients.

Even though the RDAs are not a perfect fit for each individual, they are the best over-all guidelines to make sure you are well nourished.

What to Do If You Suspect You Are Deficient

The unequivocal message of this book is: if you suspect you are not getting enough nutrients in general or in specific, make it up by eating better foods that have more nutrients and fewer calories. *A good diet, not pills, is the ultimate solution to poor nutrition.* The extensive charts on the nutritional contents of foods in the second part of this book were designed to help you make the right choices.

Admittedly, in special circumstances, supplements may be necessary—for example, iron and calcium tablets for women, especially those on low-calorie diets. Extra vitamins and minerals are routinely prescribed during pregnancy. Additionally, most experts, including the National Academy of Sciences, do not object to daily vitamin-mineral supplements in doses that do not exceed the recommended dietary allowances (RDAs). In fact, there is good reason to consider such low vitamin-mineral doses "health insurance." However, the routine ingestion by healthy people of megadoses of supplements (ten times or more of the RDAs) is not guaranteed to protect health and can be dangerous.

If you believe you are suffering from a deficiency that may need therapeutic attention, consult a physician. Reliable tests, generally blood analyses, can detect most nutrient deficiencies.

Important: Do not depend on hair analysis to determine your nutritional status. These tests are notoriously unreliable and are generally unrelated to nutritional health, as proved by an investigation published in the *Journal of the American Medical Association*. Researchers sent hair samples taken from two healthy teenagers to thirteen laboratories for analysis. The results varied so much as to be totally meaningless. One lab even came up with wildly differing figures on an *identical* sample of hair sent at different times. "Unscientific, economically wasteful and unduly frightening to clients," is how the article branded nutritional hair analysis. Depending on this phony procedure to turn up a serious deficiency that needs medical attention is also quite risky.

One more caution: Deficient intakes or nonoptimal intakes of nutrients do not necessarily mean you have biological deficiencies. Because of individual biochemistry (that may somehow compensate for deficient intakes) it is impossible to tell whether a person is biologically deficient except by medical tests.

Food Is In,
Megadoses of Nutrients Are Out

Megadoses of nutrients are no substitute for food. You cannot take a magic pill that will neutralize a bad diet. It is becoming increasingly apparent that we know very little about the complexities of food and precisely which constituents of food may combat various diseases. It is true that supplements can correct vitamin and mineral *deficiencies,* but there is no documented evidence that vitamin supplements make healthy people healthier. In some cases, there is evidence that therapeutic megadoses of vitamins and minerals for specific diseases may be of benefit, but such doses are to be viewed as drugs and used with medical supervision.

On the other hand, experts increasingly worry about side effects of high doses of nutrients, which are abnormal in food.

Few people realize that such high doses pose serious dangers by upsetting the balance of other nutrients. For example, megadoses of folic acid can mask a deficiency of vitamin B_{12}, which could expose the user to serious and irreversible neurological damage. High amounts of folic acid can also cause zinc deficiencies, which in pregnant women can be alarming, possibly leading to birth defects. Megadoses of vitamin C knock out B_{12} and can raise blood cholesterol. Too much vitamin E blocks the metabolism of vitamin A. High doses of zinc or copper can zap the immune system, creating severe anemia. And on and on. Scientists are just beginning to explore the potential impact of concentrated nutrients on the body and on other nutrients.

Experts once thought that excessive amounts of water-soluble vitamins were harmlessly flushed out of the body. Although this is generally the case, there is now evidence that toxic amounts can remain behind. For example, huge doses of vitamin B_6 (1,000 times the RDA) have produced neurological disorders.

Moreover, there's evidence that the pills may do little good. If you are faithfully plying your child with doses of vitamin and mineral pills to keep him or her healthy, consider this conclusion of several enlightening studies: children who take supplements have the same biological nutritional status as youngsters who don't.

It is not sensible to try to buck up an otherwise nutritionally lacking diet with pills that contain extraordinary doses of chemical concoctions of specific nutrients. Food, on the other hand, carries with it mysterious baggage full of known and unknown nutritional elements; nutrition is a young science, and a multitude of food's secrets are undoubtedly yet to be discovered. Getting nutrients from foods instead of pills, provides a wide range of macro- as well as micronutrients that are very complicated and have vast, ill-understood effects on human life.

The trend these days is away from megadoses of vitamins and minerals to save your life and toward a new appreciation of the health-giving abilities and complexity of nutrients in foods. The challenge is to learn how to eat the right foods to get the most healthful benefits.

Interactions:
How to Make the Most of What You Eat

Once upon a time, scientists believed that what you ate in food was what your body got. No longer. It now pays to know not only what is in food but how other factors work to accentuate or diminish the nutritional value. A new, intriguing subject of inquiry is how interactions among foods, nutrients, and drugs affect the biological availability of various nutrients. Scientists now know that such interactions can substantially cancel out or enhance the effects of certain nutrients. You can eat all the spinach you want in attempts to get more calcium, but your efforts will be to little avail. Spinach, rich in calcium, also contains agents called oxalates or oxalic acid, which wipe out much of the calcium in the spinach.

Other examples:

One of the best ways to defeat iron deficiency is to add vitamin C to meals rich in iron. A little vitamin C—only a glass of orange juice or a papaya—can boost the absorption of the vegetable-type iron by 200 to 500 percent.

Drinking too much tea can help induce iron-deficiency anemia. Even two mugs of moderately strong tea could impair absorption of iron from vegetable foods eaten at the same meal.

Oysters are the richest of all foods in zinc, but if you eat them with dried beans, tortillas, corn chips, or rye bread (high in fiber and agents called phytates), 65 to 100 percent of the zinc can be rendered unusable by the body.

Regular megadoses of vitamin C (1 gram with each meal) can wipe out enough vitamin B_{12} to cause a serious deficiency.

Raw seafood as found in sushi and sashimi, although rich in thiamin, is not a reliable source because raw fish, notably shellfish, contains the enzyme thiaminase, which deactivates thiamin. Red cabbage and brussels sprouts also contain thiaminase. Cooking destroys the enzyme.

A glass of white wine boosts the absorption of iron from a meal; red wine (containing tannins) inhibits it.

Fruits and vegetables high in potassium may help counteract some of the ill effects of too much sodium, especially in people who are "salt sensitive" and have a genetic predisposition to high blood pressure.

Olive oil helps lower blood cholesterol. Also found in studies to favorably modify blood cholesterol are oat bran, dried beans, yogurt, salmon, grapefruit pulp, bean curd (tofu), garlic, and onions, among other foods.

Alcohol, especially heavy drinking, knocks out numerous nutrients including thiamin, calcium, vitamin D, folacin, and B_{12}. The alcohol found in only two beers, two glasses of wine, or two ounces of distilled liquor can impair absorption of thiamin.

Many medications, including birth control pills, interact to increase or decrease the need for several nutrients.

Thus, it is important to know not only how much of a nutrient is naturally present in a certain food, but ways you can help your body preserve and utilize it.

How to Get the Most Nutrition for the Fewest Calories

The modern secret to good nutrition is to get the most nutritional punch for the fewest calories. Few of us can afford to dissipate our calories on empty or low-nutrient-density foods.

That's why you hear a lot from nutritionists about the concept of nutrient density, which is a measure of the ratio between a food's nutrients and its calories—or energy. Foods with lots of nutrients and few calories are nutrient dense. Foods overloaded with calories and scant in nutrients are nutrient deficient or empty calorie.

Most consumer books tell you only the amounts of a nutrient in a serving. For all of the nutrients we have calculated by computer analysis the nutrient-calorie ratios, and have listed those foods that came out best. Thus, you can easily spot which foods give you the most of each nutrient per calorie. This can be invaluable if you are trying to boost your intake of a particular nutrient—for example, calcium. You can even compare the calcium-calorie ratio of cheeses; the variations are surprising.

For people on low-calorie diets, it is particularly essential to make every calorie count by choosing foods high in nutritional value.

Important: Your best insurance against nutritional deficiencies is to eat foods that are nutrient dense.

Stick Close to Nature

Modern processing sometimes strips fantastic foods of much of their nutritional value, turning them into lifeless, wimpy substances unable to support life. This is particularly true of whole grains; the losses of vitamins and minerals are enormous, and the effects show up in modern populations severely deficient in nutrients such as magnesium. To try to correct that hazard, our flour and many of our cereals are "enriched" (some of the lost nutrients are replaced) or "fortified" (the nutrients are boosted beyond nature's levels). Some breakfast cereals are fortified with vitamins that nature never put there in the first place, like vitamin C; such cereals become in effect morning multivitamin pills, supplying 25 to 100 percent of the RDAs for almost everything.

There is nothing wrong with enriched or fortified foods as long as you know what you are getting and that less-processed, whole-grain cereals carry other nutritional benefits, such as high fiber and low sugar and salt. Cereal fortification often makes second-rate cereals look like nutritional superstars when they are not.

As a rule of thumb, fresh or frozen fruits and vegetables are better than canned. Studies show that canned vegetables usually contain less vitamin C, thiamin, riboflavin, B_6, folacin, and niacin, as well as less iron, magnesium, copper, and potassium, than do equivalent amounts of fresh cooked vegetables. Also, processed vegetables usually contain added sodium, and processed fruits, added sugar.

Many people prefer raw fruits and vegetables, but raw is not always better. Cooking sometimes releases nutrients, and sometimes raw foods contain antivitamins that destroy nutrients in other foods. For example, certain nutrients are more readily released by cooking carrots, dried beans, fish, cabbage, and brussels sprouts.

A Cook's Guide to Nutrients

The shorter the cooking time and the less water used, the greater the nutritional value left.

HERE IS THE GENERAL RULE OF THUMB FOR NUTRIENT RETENTION
Best
    Meats: broil, fry, microwave, roast
    Vegetables: microwave, boil in bag, stir-fry, pressure cook, steam, with little water
        Okay
    Meats: stew, crockpot
    Vegetables: bake
Poor
    Meat: braise, boil
    Vegetables: boil, saucepan with excess water

Certain vitamins are more likely to be damaged by heat, moisture, oxygen, light, or acid.
Most susceptible
    Vitamin C
    Thiamin (B_1)
Moderately susceptible
    Folic acid
    Vitamin B_6
    Riboflavin (B_2)
    Pantothenic acid
    Vitamin B_{12}
    Vitamin A
    Vitamin E
    Vitamin D
Least susceptible
    Niacin

Nutritional Superstars

Because nobody is sure where nature has hidden all the nutrients essential to optimal health, the cardinal rule for good nutrition is to eat a variety of healthful foods. Nevertheless, certain foods stand out as nutritional superstars on the basis of their known nutritional composition. Granted, other foods may contain other chemical agents of great worth that we are only dimly aware of, so you would not want to restrict your choices to the superstars for fear of missing some benefits. With that caveat, here is my list of twenty superstar foods—some of nature's highest-potency nutritional packages. In my mind, they are winners for various reasons, based on current research and nutritional analysis.

Almost all of them are nutrient dense—low in calories and packed full of nutrients. A notable exception is olive oil, which is 100 percent fat, but which has other chemical attributes that make it outstanding among fats in helping to fight heart disease.

TWENTY SUPER-FOODS
Almonds
Apricots, especially dried
Beans, dried
Broccoli
Cabbage
Cantaloupe
Carrots
Collard greens
Liver
Milk (skim)
Oat cereals
Olive oil
Oysters
Potatoes, especially sweet potatoes
Salmon
Soybean curd (tofu)
Sunflower seeds
Tunafish
Wheat bran and wheat germ
Yogurt (nonfat)

RECOMMENDED DIETARY ALLOWANCES

Food and Nutrition Board, National Academy of Sciences—
National Research Council (revised 1980)

Here is a condensed table of the recommended daily dietary allowances for nutrients—vitamins, minerals, trace elements, and electrolytes—discussed in this book.

Age	Protein g	A RE	D mcg	E mg	C mg	Thiamin mg	Ribo-flavin mg	Niacin mg NE
To 6 months	kg × 2.2	420	10	3	35	.3	.4	6
6 months–1 year	kg × 2	400	10	4	35	.5	.6	8
1–3	23	400	10	5	45	.7	.8	9
4–6	30	500	10	6	45	.9	1	11
7–10	34	700	10	7	45	1.2	1.4	16
Males								
11–14	45	1000	10	8	50	1.4	1.6	18
15–18	56	1000	10	10	60	1.4	1.7	18
19–22	56	1000	7.5	10	60	1.5	1.7	19
23–50	56	1000	5	10	60	1.4	1.6	18
51+	56	1000	5	10	60	1.2	1.4	16
Females								
11–14	46	800	10	8	50	1.1	1.3	15
15–18	46	800	10	8	60	1.1	1.3	14
19–22	44	800	7.5	8	60	1.1	1.3	14
23–50	44	800	5	8	60	1	1.2	13
51+	44	800	5	8	60	1	1.2	13
Pregnant	+30	+200	+5	+2	+20	+.4	+.3	+2
Nursing	+20	+400	+5	+3	+40	+.5	+.5	+5

	B_6	Folacin	B_{12}	Calcium	Magnesium	Iron	Zinc
To 6 months	.3	30	.5	360	50	10	3
6 months–1 year	.6	45	1.5	540	70	15	5
1–3	.9	100	2	800	150	15	10
4–6	1.3	200	2.5	800	200	10	10
7–10	1.6	300	3	800	250	10	10
Males							
11–14	1.8	400	3	1200	350	18	15
15–18	2	400	3	1200	400	18	15
19–22	2.2	400	3	800	350	10	15
23–50	2.2	400	3	800	350	10	15
51+	2.2	400	3	800	350	10	15

Age	B₆	Folacin	B₁₂	Calcium	Magnesium	Iron	Zinc
Females							
11–14	1.8	400	3	1200	300	18	15
15–18	2	400	3	1200	300	18	15
19–22	2	400	3	800	300	18	15
23–50	2	400	3	800	300	18	15
51+	2	400	3	800	300	10	15
Pregnant	+.6	+400	+1	+400	+150	*	+5
Nursing	+.5	+100	+1	+400	+150	*	+10

*The increased requirement during pregnancy cannot be met by the iron content of habitual American diets or by the existing iron stores of many women; therefore, the use of 30–60 mg of supplemental iron is recommended. Iron needs during lactation are not substantially different from those of nonpregnant women, but continued supplementation of the mother for two to three months after delivery is advisable in order to replenish stores depleted during pregnancy.

ESTIMATED SAFE AND ADEQUATE
DAILY DIETARY INTAKES*

	Copper mg	Chromium mg	Selenium mg	Sodium mg	Potassium mg
To 6 months	.5–.7	.01–.04	.01–.04	115–350	350–925
6 months–1 year	.7–1	.02–.06	.02–.06	250–750	425–1275
1–3	1–1.5	.02–.08	.02–.08	325–975	550–1650
4–6	1.5–2	.03–.12	.03–.12	450–1350	775–2325
7–10	2–2.5	.05–.2	.05–.2	600–1800	1000–3000
Adolescents (11 and over)	2–3	.05–.2	.05–.2	900–2700	1525–4575
Adults	2–3	.05–.2	.05–.2	1100–3300	1875–5625

Source: National Academy of Sciences, 1980

*Because there is less information on which to base allowances, these figures are not given in the main table of the RDAs and are provided here in the form of ranges of recommended intakes.

Protein
Putting an End to the Myths

Protein is one of the three sources of energy from food (the others are carbohydrates and fat). Each gram of protein provides 4 calories of energy. Proteins are a basic substance of the body, found in every cell. Take away water, and half of your body is made up of protein. It is essential for healthy muscle, bone, cartilage, lymphatic system, blood, and skin. Protein is made up of building blocks called amino acids, which link together in different sequences to form hundreds of different proteins used by the body.

Who Is Deficient?

Virtually nobody. Although protein cannot be stored—you need new supplies daily—Americans still eat about twice as much as needed, more than anyone else in the world. The government's National Health and Nutrition Examination Survey (1980) found that the average American eats 92 grams of protein a day! That is compared with the recommended dietary allowance of 56 grams for adult men and 44 grams for adult women. The most frequent consumers of excess protein are males from ages fifteen to thirty-five.

Even the elderly, a usual subject of nutritional concern, eat an average one and a third times more protein than the RDAs call for. However, the elderly are one group that conceivably could be deficient in protein. Protein deficiencies in this country are rare except in severe cases of malnutrition.

Some Protein Myths

• Protein is good for you; therefore, more is better.
• Protein does not make you fat. (In fact, excess protein is converted by the body into fat. Also most of the high-protein foods we eat—whole milk, meat, cheese—also are high in fat and calories. The extra baggage carried by high-protein foods can sink a diet.)

16

• Extra protein is needed for strenuous exercise. (The consensus is that you don't burn up a lot of extra protein during strenuous activity. Athletes now favor complex carbohydrates over protein as a main source of energy.)

• High-protein weight-loss diets are the best. (Very low-calorie, high-protein diets have been declared dangerous by government authorities and should be undertaken only with the supervision of a physician. Dieters are better off with moderate amounts of low-fat proteins combined with low-fat complex carbohydrates such as pasta and vegetables. Some vegetables are also good sources of protein, especially when combined.) One study even showed that animals got fatter eating high amounts of protein than equal amounts of carbohydrates.

Health Dangers of Excess Protein

For ordinary healthy people, the consequences of excessive protein intake are added pounds, and as some experts point out, "the most expensive urine in the world."

Protein and Kidney Disease

When excess protein is broken down in the body, part is stored as fat; another part is converted to nitrogen and flushed out by the kidneys. That is not a problem for people with healthy kidneys. But increasing evidence shows the danger of overburdening kidneys that are already slightly damaged by disease (even though it may be undetected). That's why people with kidney failure are put on low-protein diets. And low-protein, near-vegetarian diets are now prescribed for people with kidney problems to prevent progression toward end-stage renal disease and the consequent need for dialysis. So do your kidneys and your pocketbook a favor: stop processing all that extra protein your body does not need.

Protein and Heart Disease

There is also growing speculation that too much protein, primarily meat protein, as well as dietary fat, may be implicated in clogged arteries, heart disease, and high blood pressure. The theory, proposed some seventy years ago, has been revived by some researchers who believe it has merit. Most experts still believe, however, that the fat in foods is the main enemy of the cardiovascular system.

Protein and Cancer

Some researchers think protein is implicated also as a cause of cancer, although the case against protein is far less established than that against fat. Additionally, in studies it is difficult to separate fat from protein as the culprit because high-protein and high-fat foods (for example, meat and dairy products) are often one and the same.

Suspected as protein-related are cancers of the breast, uterus, colon, rectum, prostate, pancreas, and kidney. For example, one large Japanese study found that those whose diets were high in meat had a 250 percent higher risk of pancreatic cancer than others. Another Japanese study found prostate cancer higher in meat eaters. Numerous animal studies have found cancer-promoting effects from high intakes of protein and specific amino acids. Generally, low-protein diets (5 percent of calories) seemed to squelch the growth of tumors in animals. Intakes of protein between 20 and 25 percent of calories promoted tumors. Many Americans eat that much; although the average intake is 15 percent of calories. A possible connection between protein and cancer is one more good reason to cut back. Most of the studies on protein implicated *animal,* not vegetable, protein, as a contributor to cancer, although other research indicates that vegetable protein may not be totally innocuous.

Two Types:
Complete and Incomplete Protein

All protein is not created equal. Protein is made up of varying patterns of amino acid molecules. Our bodies require twenty-two different kinds of amino acids to function properly. Nine of these we cannot manufacture and must obtain from food. They are called the *essential* amino acids: histidine, isoleucine, leucine, lysine, methionine, phenylalanine, threonine, tryptophan, and valine.

Certain foods match our demands almost perfectly; they provide all nine essential amino acids in amounts sufficient to meet our bodily needs. Such foods are called "complete protein." As you might guess, these are mainly the animal foods—meat, fish, poultry, eggs, milk, and cheese.

On the other hand, plant foods usually do not possess all nine essential amino acids in sufficient amounts, and are therefore "incomplete protein." Thus, the quality of protein from animals and plants differ in their ability to nourish. Animal protein is high quality; vegetable protein, generally lower quality.

A notable exception: Soy bean protein is also high quality. Among vegetable proteins it is tops and even close to milk protein in fostering the growth of laboratory animals. The soy bean, in fact, is 11 percent protein by cooked weight; a cooked egg is 13 percent protein. Except for infants, soy protein contains all the amino acids in amounts adequate for human needs. Soy protein is found in all kinds of products, such as tofu, bean sprouts, soy nuts, soy flour, soy milk, tempeh (fermented soybeans), and textured vegetable protein. But don't count on getting much soy bean nutrition from so-called tofu frozen desserts. They are generally made up of merely water, fructose, oil, and flavorings with very little tofu.

The good news is, you can turn vegetables into high-quality protein. If you eat certain vegetables together with others or add a little meat, the amino acids form a common pool in your digestive system, and the body treats them as one entity. If, *together*, foods supply reasonable amounts of each of the nine essential amino acids, they can become complete-protein sources. For example, mixing rice and dried beans, a common Latin American dish, produces the same quality of protein as a steak. Combining certain vegetables and/or animal protein is an excellent way to make the most of protein and at the same time avoid high fat and calories.

As a practical matter, if you eat more than one or two plant proteins you usually create a combination of complementary proteins without even trying.

SOME COMBINATIONS THAT PROVIDE COMPLETE PROTEIN
- Legumes (navy beans, pinto beans, lima beans, kidney beans, black beans, chickpeas, soybeans, peanuts, black-eyed peas) with rice, wheat, corn, barley, oats, or sesame seeds
- Cereal with milk
- Macaroni with cheese
- Spaghetti with sauce containing a little ground beef and/or grated cheese

Note: The book *Diet for a Small Planet,* by Frances Moore Lappé, is a superb account of how to mix proteins to get the greatest value.

Eat More Vegetable Protein

Americans eat about the same amount of protein today as in the early 1900s. The big difference: today most of it comes from animals. Then, the biggest single source of protein was from plants. USDA statistics from 1909 through 1913 show that 30 percent of the protein consumed came from meat, fish, and poultry. That jumped to 42 percent in the 1970s. Add dairy products, and Americans now get a staggering 67 percent of protein from animal sources.

Recommendation: Get at least two-thirds of your protein from plants. Typical American diet today: only one-third from plants. Vegetables, grains, and beans are wonderful protein sources, and humans can survive perfectly well, as our prehistoric forefathers did, on little or no animal protein.

RICH SOURCES OF PROTEIN

The most protein by weight regardless of calories

Cheese	Beef
Brewer's yeast	Veal
Soybean products	Lamb
Seafood	Nuts
Milk	Peanut butter
Chicken breast	Pumpkin, squash,
Pork	and watermelon seeds

PROTEIN SUPER-FOODS
THE MOST PROTEIN, FEWEST CALORIES

Here are 50 foods that rate exceptionally high in protein content per calorie. Of the approximately 2,500 foods in this book, these are tops in protein nutrient density; they have the highest protein-calorie ratios, giving you the most protein for the fewest calories.

	Food Rating	Protein-calorie ratio (gm of protein per 100 calories)	Common measure	Gm protein	Calories
1.	Tuna, canned in water	22	3 oz	30	135
2.	Cod, smoked	22	3 oz	20	88
3.	Cod, dried	22	1 oz	8	36
4.	Octopus, smoked	21	3 oz	22	106
5.	Shrimp, canned	21	3 oz	21	99
6.	Sturgeon, smoked	21	3 oz	26	135
7.	Squid, boiled	20	3 oz	16	82
8.	Shrimp, steamed/boiled	20	3 oz	20	102
9.	Lobster, steamed	20	3 oz	16	81
10.	Cottage cheese, dry	20	4 oz	19	96
11.	Pigeonpeas, green, cooked	20	½ c	17	85
12.	Turkey, white meat, wo skin	19	3½ oz	30	157
13.	Crayfish, steamed/boiled	19	3 oz	17	88

Food Rating	Protein-calorie ratio (gm of protein per 100 calories)	Common measure	Gm protein	Calories
14. Trout, smoked	19	3 oz	29	153
15. Roe, herring, fresh	19	1 tbsp	3	18
16. Tuna, raw	19	3 oz	21	113
17. Sweetbreads, braised	19	3 oz	28	143
18. Beef, tripe, pickled	19	3.5 oz	12	62
19. Crab, steamed	19	2 med	17	89
20. Chicken, light meat, roasted	18	3 oz	23	128
21. Goat	18	3 oz	28	177
22. Veal, roasted	18	3 oz	20	123
23. Haddock, baked	18	3 oz	18	102
24. Cottage cheese, lowfat, 1% fat	17	4 oz	14	82
25. Chipped beef, dried	17	1 oz	8	47
26. Beef kidney, simmered	17	3 oz	22	122
27. Perch, fillet, broiled	17	3 oz	19	113
28. Sea bass, broiled	17	3 oz	20	117
29. Whiting, broiled	17	3 oz	16	97
30. Salmon, steamed/poached	17	3 oz	21	126
31. Clams, raw	17	3 oz	11	65
32. Pike, broiled/baked	16	3 oz	18	110
33. Flounder, broiled/baked	16	3 oz	17	101
34. Venison, stewed	16	3 oz	25	153
35. Shrimp, broiled w fat	16	3 oz	19	116
36. Tuna, fresh, broiled	16	3 oz	24	155
37. Carp, smoked	16	1 oz	8	50
38. Ham steak, extra lean	16	3 oz	17	105
39. Veal chop, lean, cooked w bone	16	6.5 oz	28	177
40. Scallops, steamed	15	3 oz	13	85
41. Cottage cheese, lowfat, 2% fat	15	4 oz	15	101
42. Lamb, loin, chop, lean, broiled	15	1 chop	17	116
43. Lamb, leg, lean, roasted	15	3 oz	18	117
44. Scallops, broiled/baked	15	3 oz	16	106
45. Turkey, dark meat, roasted	15	3½ oz	29	187
46. Tuna, canned in oil, drained	15	3 oz	25	167
47. Beef, top loin, lean, good, broiled	15	3 oz	24	162
48. Beef, round, lean, broiled	15	3 oz	24	165
49. Liver, beef, braised	15	3 oz	21	137
50. Yellowtail fish, raw	15	3½ oz	21	138

Source: Author's computer analysis from USDA data

*Excludes baby foods. Includes only foods for which one serving supplies a minimum of approximately 10 percent of the RDA.

RECOMMENDED DAILY DIETARY
ALLOWANCES OF PROTEIN

Age	Grams
1–6 months	2.2 for every kilogram* of body weight
6 months–1 year	2 for every kilogram* of body weight
1–3	23
4–6	30
7–10	34
Males	
11–14	45
15+	56
Females	
11–18	46
19+	44
Pregnant	add 30
Nursing	add 20

Source: National Academy of Sciences, Revised 1980

*about 2.2 lbs.

Carbohydrates
The Good Versus the Bad

(See also Dietary Fiber, p. 62)

Carbohydrates are made up of carbon, hydrogen, and oxygen and are of two types: complex carbohydrates, such as starch found in foods like potatoes, and simple carbohydrates, such as ordinary table sugar and the sugar in fruit. A main function of carbohydrate is to supply energy in the form of blood sugar to keep every part of the body functioning. Each gram of carbohydrate supplies the body with 4 calories of energy.

Who Needs to Worry?

Practically everybody. If you are a typical American you eat only 50 percent as much complex carbohydrate and nearly twice as much refined sugar as you should. The average American downs about 125 pounds of processed sugars every year, along with 50 pounds of natural sugars from fruits and milk. Americans eat about one quarter of their calories in sugar. Only 3 percent of that comes from fruits and vegetables and another 3 percent from lactose, the sugar in milk. The rest—about 18 percent—is refined sugar added to food.

HOW MUCH CARBOHYDRATE SHOULD YOU EAT?

	Percent of calories recommended	Percent of calories, typical American diet
Complex carbohydrates (starches) and naturally occurring sugars (fruits, milk and yogurt)	48	28
Refined and processed sugars (table sugar, sweeteners added to processed foods)	10	18

23

Recommendation: Cut your refined sugar intake in half, and boost your consumption of starchy foods by 50 percent.

How to Tell the Good from the Bad

It may seem strange that the starches (good for us) and the refined sugars (not so good for us) are lumped together under the term *carbohydrates*. It is because all types of carbohydrates are made up of molecules of sugar. Starch is a form of sugar, called a polysaccharide— made up of chains of glucose molecules. All carbohydrate must be broken down in the body by digestive enzymes before it can be absorbed into the bloodstream. Glucose or blood sugar, a single-molecule sugar, is the body's main fuel; it keeps the brain and muscles functioning. If your carbohydrate energy source dries up, the body must run on fat and protein.

The terms *simple* and *complex* are appropriate. Complex carbohydrates are literally more chemically complex than simple sugars. Simple carbohydrates are made up of only one or two sugar molecules (monosaccharides or disaccharides). Complex carbohydrates (the starches) are comprised of multiple sugar molecules—(polysaccharides).

The critical difference: Most complex carbohydrates come with big bonuses of many other nutrients and fiber. The simple sugar sucrose, extracted and refined from plants, is a pure energy source with no or few accompanying nutrients. Sucrose is just another name for refined or table sugar. In other words "empty calories."

CARBOHYDRATES SCORECARD

The Good Guys
Complex carbohydrates (starches)
    Sources: cereals, breads, rice, barley, pasta, pizza, beans, nuts, seeds, vegetables of all types
Fiber (an indigestible complex carbohydrate)
    Sources: fruits, vegetables, grains, dried beans

The Okay Guys
Naturally occurring sugars (fructose and glucose)
    Sources: fruits of all types
Milk sugar (lactose): a simple sugar accounting for 100 percent of the carbohydrate in milk
    Sources: milk, yogurt

The Bad Guys
Simple carbohydrates or refined sugars (sucrose, fructose, dextrose)
Sources: table sugars, candy, cakes, pies, cookies, pastries, soft drinks, fruit drinks, fruit sauces, puddings, dessert toppings, sugar-coated cereals, canned syrupy fruits, and condiments (for example, ketchup)

Let's Hear It for Bread and Potatoes

Since the early part of this century the amount of healthful carbohydrates consumed by Americans has dropped dramatically. In 1910, for example, we ate 300 pounds of flour and cereal per person a year. Today it is less than half that much. Starchy foods used to account for nearly 70 percent of carbohydrates consumed, and sugar only 30 percent. Now, nutrient-rich starches account for less than half of carbohydrates eaten; sugar has taken over. Somehow, potatoes, pasta, and bread were unjustly rejected as fattening. Actually, they are much less fattening than most high-protein and high-fat foods.

Recently, complex carbohydrates have staged an impressive comeback, primarily because of health concerns about chronic diseases related to high-fat, high-sugar diets. Eat more complex carbohydrates. That is the plea from numerous health experts, including cancer, heart, diabetes, and obesity specialists. Following are some reasons why.

Seven Good Reasons to Eat More Starch

• When you eat more complex carbohydrates, you cut back on fatty foods. Complex carbohydrates are almost always low in fat.

• Contrary to popular opinion, carbohydrates are not necessarily fattening. Each gram of carbohydrate supplies 4 calories—the same as protein—and about half as much as fat; 1 fat gram supplies 9 calories.

• Unrefined starchy carbohydrates are filling; they are good foods for those who want to lose weight. Recent studies show that diets high in complex carbohydrates are the most nutritious and effective weight-loss diets. As reported by researcher Dr. Roland Weinsier, director of clinical nutritional sciences at the University of Alabama School of Medicine at Birmingham, in the *Journal of the American Medical Association:* "A large intake of complex carbohydrates, such as unrefined starches, fruits, and vegetables—that are high in bulk and low in energy density—will result in a longer eating time (since the person chews longer), will bring about satiety, and will result in a lower caloric intake."

• Unrefined starchy carbohydrates are high in fiber, which may protect against numerous diseases, including some forms of cancer.

Complex carbohydrates—plant foods (grains, vegetables, fruit, nuts) are the *only* source of fiber in the diet. (See Fiber, p. 62.)

• Complex carbohydrates are "nutrient dense"; that is—unlike "empty calorie" sugars—they contain a high ratio of nutrients per calorie; they pack a large nutritional punch.

• People who eat high amounts of complex carbohydrates, such as vegetarians, often live longer and have lower rates of chronic diseases.

• Complex carbohydrate is the only major food constituent—in contrast to fat, sugar, and protein—that has never been tied to any dangerous health consequences.

The Case Against Sugar

Many bad things have been written about sugar—some true, some not. Generally, in some ways sugar does not seem as villainous as once pronounced; at the same time, evidence mounts that certain types may be even worse than suspected. Here is some of the latest evidence.

The Sugar-Fat Connection

Undeniably, one of the reasons some people become fat is their high consumption of sweets. But the reasons for such overconsumption are complex. Some studies show that both normal-weight and obese people prefer sweetened foods only up to a point, and the critical factor that pushes sugar consumption higher may be the addition of high-fat foods.

Research by Dr. Adam Drewnowski of Rockefeller University and Dr. M. R. C. Greenwood of Vassar College found that both normal and obese subjects lost their taste for sucrose-sweetened milks and creams when the sucrose content rose to 20 percent. Surprisingly, overweight people, expected to prefer sugar, liked it less, the higher its concentration. But there was a catch: when a little sugar was combined with very-high-fat milk, the obese loved it.

The conclusion: Sugar added to high-fat foods encourages the obese to eat more. Whether the preference for sweetened fat is inborn or occurs as a result of the obesity is unknown. In any event, the combination of sugar and fat is a dangerous one for many overweight people.

Sugar That Sticks to the Teeth

There's no question that sugar, especially the sticky type that clings to the teeth, promotes the buildup of bacterial plaque and tooth decay. However, it is not how much sugar you eat, but how frequently you eat it and how tenaciously it sticks to the teeth, that determines how much damage occurs. Thus, chewy caramels are worse than soft drinks that go down quickly.

Cavities can be promoted not only by the refined sugar in candy bars but by the sugar in raisins, in fruit juices, and even in milk. Damage to teeth has resulted from allowing youngsters to suck for long periods of time on bottles filled with apple juice or milk. However, generally the fructose in fruits does less damage to teeth than refined sugar or sucrose. And you get nutrients in fruits that are absent from ordinary sugar. Research shows that sweets consumed between meals do the most damage. Sweets eaten with meals are more likely to be washed away by other foods.

Sugar: Bad for Your Heart?

To what extent sugar acts directly to promote heart disease is highly controversial. Sugar may interact with other nutrients to aggravate risk factors associated with heart disease. In some people, table sugar (sucrose) may aggravate the cholesterol-raising ability of saturated fat and cholesterol in the diet. People who have a high-fat diet and also eat sugar boost their levels of blood cholesterol. Table sugar in high doses has also reduced the ratio of HDL-"good" type cholesterol in the blood, according to research at the U.S. Department of Agriculture.

Sugar also interacts with other nutrients to produce severe copper deficiencies, associated with heart disease, and chromium deficiencies linked to diabetes.

New Danger from Fructose

Fructose is a natural sugar found in fruits, and at such low levels it is wholesome. But at the concentrated doses found in countless processed foods, fructose, experts fear, is a new widespread danger. Cheap, high-fructose corn sweeteners have replaced sugar as the number-one sweetener in the country. High-fructose corn syrups sweeten nondiet Coca-Cola and Pepsi, baked goods, cereals, toppings; anywhere sugar goes, so go the fructose sweeteners.

The switch to high-fructose sweeteners may have alarming consequences. In USDA studies, animals that are deficient in copper (as is most of the U.S. population) developed severe cardiovascular disease when they also ate large amounts of fructose—but not when they ate starches. "We are convinced fructose seriously aggravates copper deficiency, and copper deficiency has a profound damaging effect on the cardiovascular system of animals," says Dr. Sheldon Reiser, head of the USDA's Carbohydrate Nutrition Laboratory in Beltsville, Maryland.

HEALTH CONDITIONS THAT MAY BE LINKED TO SUGAR
Obesity
Dental cavities
Heart disease
Impaired glucose tolerance
Diabetes
Mood swings
Crohn's disease (a recent study found that those who developed
    Crohn's disease—inflammatory bowel disease—had a diet high
    in sugar and low in fruit fibers)

Sugar in the Genes

The sweet tooth goes sour. A sweet tooth seems inborn. The sweeter a solution offered to infants, the harder they will suck to get it and the more they will eat. This is an evolutionary survival mechanism. But there is little evidence that children who eat a lot of sugar grow up to be adults who crave sugar. Animals given free access to sugar as infants lose their taste for it soon after sexual maturation, comparable to puberty in humans, possibly because of changes in the way they metabolize sugar. Although overdosing on sugar by children is detrimental—rotting the teeth and replacing nutritious foods—parents can take some comfort in the fact that youngsters may outgrow the desire for it.

Widespread sugar sensitivity. Perhaps partly for genetic reasons, certain people are extrasensitive to sugar; they exhibit slight abnormalities in the way they metabolize sucrose and fructose. This is no small problem. Studies using strict criteria show that 15 to 20 percent of Americans are supersensitive to sugar—a projected 30 to 50 million people. The problem worsens as people age and gain weight. Smaller government surveys, screening people for nutrition studies, found that about one-third abnormally metabolize sugar. Thus, from 15 to 33 percent of Americans may be supersensitive to sugar.

What is the danger? Researchers note that sugar-sensitive people who continue to load up on sugar suffer greater impairment in their ability to metabolize sugar. The fear is that they may eventually worsen enough to be classified as diabetic. This does not mean that sugar per se can *cause* diabetes, but that it may be one factor promoting the disease in those who are susceptible.

The Blood-Sugar Mystery

Which sends blood sugar higher—sugar or potatoes?

Traditional wisdom has held that pure sugar, the simple carbohydrates, sends blood sugar instantly sky-high, while complex carbohydrates release sugar more slowly. But absolute faith in that belief has been shattered by new research, pioneered by nutritionist Phyllis Crapo at the University of Colorado and Dr. David Jenkins at the University of Toronto. They discovered that it is not a simple question of starches versus sugar.

What matters apparently is the *type* of starch. The scientists fed healthy people a variety of carbohydrate foods and then measured their blood-sugar levels. The surprising results: certain starches like potatoes and rice sent blood sugar higher than did plain table sugar. But that does not mean sugar is okay and starches are dangerous. It simply means that all starches are not created equal. Other starches, like pasta and beans, did not spike blood sugar dramatically. Scientists speculate that certain starchy components found to varying degrees in complex carbohydrates are to blame. New research is trying to unravel that mystery by testing the components of starchy foods.

Who needs to be concerned? Diabetics can use the information to choose starches that do not trigger dramatic blood-sugar surges. But experts warn diabetics not to substitute sugar for complex carbohydrates in the mistaken belief it is more healthful. On the contrary, Dr. James Anderson at the University of Kentucky, finds that many diabetics can successfully control their blood sugar without medication by switching to a high-fiber, low-fat, high complex carbohydrate diet.

Normal people may lose sugar tolerance with age, so it's a good idea to be aware of which starchy foods can cause blood-sugar spurts. Aside from that, unless you have good cause—such as a family history of diabetes—it seems unnecessary to worry about starch-triggered blood-sugar rises, especially when the benefits of a high-complex-carbohydrate diet are so great.

THE FOOD–BLOOD SUGAR INDEX

How some foods rank on the glycemic index
(the higher the index, the faster the rise in blood sugar)

	Percent
Maltose	105
Glucose	100
Parsnips	97
Carrots	92
Honey	87
Potato (instant)	80
Cornflakes	80
Broadbeans	79
Bread, whole-meal	72

	Percent
Bread, white	69
Rice, white	72
Mars bar	68
Shredded wheat	67
Raisins	64
Bananas	62
Sucrose	59
Pastry	59
Peas, frozen	51
Spaghetti	50
Sweet potato	48
Sponge cake	46
Oranges	40
Baked beans	40
Apples (golden delicious)	39
Ice cream	36
Yogurt	36
Chick-peas	36
Milk, whole	34
Milk, skim	32
Lentils	29
Fructose	20
Soya beans	15
Peanuts	13

Source: *American Journal of Clinical Nutrition*, 34:362 1981

The Sugar Blahs, Not the Sugar Blues

Tranquilizers. At one time, it was said that sugar disturbed the brain's chemical balance, inciting hyperactivity, and perhaps anger and violence. Now, as Dr. Richard Wurtman, of the Massachusetts Institute of Technology and one of the world's leading carbohydrate researchers, says, "It was exactly the opposite." Instead, carbohydrates, including sugar, seem to have a calming effect, making a person sleepy. The reason: When you eat carbohydrates, there is an intricate biological process that eventually raises the level of a neurotransmitter in the brain called serotonin. Serotonin acts as a mild tranquilizer. That's why, says Dr. Wurtman, a person who eats a heavy meal of carbohydrates, such as pasta and desserts, feels drowsy a few hours later. One way to stay more alert: eat some protein before or with high-carbohydrate meals.

To date, well-controlled studies have not confirmed that sugar has any relationship to hyperactivity in children.

Antidepressants. Several studies show that carbohydrates may have antidepressive effects. One historian observed that a diet high in carbo-hydrates may be associated with lower rates of suicide in some popula-tions. In winter, it has been noted, some people with seasonal affective disorder (SAD), another name for depression, crave more carbohy-drates, possibly as a way to stave off the winter blues.

Warning: Certain people have the opposite reaction to carbohy-drates. They become more alert. According to Dr. Judith Wurtman, a nutrition researcher at MIT, these are usually people who are over-weight; for some reason, they are stimulated by the intake of sugar. Dr. Wurtman's studies also show that many people with a tendency to gain weight have biological cravings for carbohydrates that can be satisfied by small intakes. If they are not, she says, the urge to binge on sweets takes over.

WHERE WE GET SUGAR IN THE DIET

	Percent
Soft drinks	25
Sweets (table sugar, jams, syrups, gelatin desserts, etc.)	18
Baked goods (cakes, cookies, pies, etc.)	13
Ice cream and other dairy foods	10
Bread and grain products	6
Breakfast cereals	5
Candy	2
Other (fruits, vegetables, meats, poultry, fish, coffee, tea, fats, oils, salad dressing, legumes, nuts, seeds, eggs, alcoholic beverages)	21

Source: Center for Science in the Public Interest

The Honey Myth and Other Tales

That honey is superior to other forms of sugar is a pervasive myth. Honey is mostly a combination of fructose and glucose and is absorbed into the bloodstream even faster than is ordinary table sugar, giving an even greater sugar rush. Once honey is eaten, the body cannot tell the difference between it and other sugars. They are all metabolized in the same fashion. What's more, a tablespoon of honey has 65 calories, compared with 45 calories in a tablespoon of white sugar and 50 calories in a tablespoon of brown sugar.

Further, brown sugar and "raw" or turbinado sugar are less processed than white sugar, but, contrary to popular opinion, they are not nutritionally superior. However, molasses, especially blackstrap molasses, does have some iron.

FOODS RICH IN COMPLEX CARBOHYDRATES

Cereals	Vegetables of all types
Flour	Nuts
Popcorn	Barley
Pretzels	Pizza
Pasta	Seeds
Rice	Legumes
Bread	

SUGAR CONTENT OF READY-TO-EAT CEREALS

Product	Percent dry weight
All-Bran	19.1
Alpha-Bits	37.8
Apple Jacks	52.4
Cap'n Crunch	40.4
Cap'n Crunch's Crunch Berries	44.2
Cap'n Crunch's Peanut Butter Cereal	32.2
Cheerios	3.0
Cocoa Krispies	44.6
Cocoa Pebbles	42.1
Cookie-Crisp (chocolate chip and vanilla wafer)	42.3
Corn Chex	4.5
Corn Flakes (Kellogg)	7.1
Cracklin' Bran	28.6
Fortified Oat Flakes	18.3
40% Bran Flakes (Post)	12.5
Froot Loops	48.9
Frosted Mini-Wheats	26.1
Frosted Rice Krinkles	42.2
Frosted Rice Krispies	38.1
Fruity Pebbles	41.8

Product	Percent dry weight
Golden Grahams	29.4
Grape-Nuts	7.0
Grape-Nuts Flakes	12.9
Heartland Natural Cereal	
with Coconut	22.3
with Raisins	26.0
Honeycomb	37.0
Kix	4.3
Life, plain and with cinnamon	17.9
Lucky Charms	42.4
100% Bran	22.2
100% Natural Cereal	
plain	21.6
with Apples and Cinnamon	25.2
with Raisins and Dates	28.4
Product 19	10.4
Quisp	40.7
Raisin Bran (Kellogg)	29.7
Raisin Bran (Post)	30.3
Rice Chex	5.1
Rice Krispies	8.2
Rice Puffed	.3
Special K	7.6
Sugar Corn Pops	46.5
Sugar Frosted Flakes (Kellogg)	39.2
Sugar Smacks	55.8
Super Sugar Crisp	45.2
Team	15.8
Toasties	5.4
Total	8.2
Wheat Chex	4.5
Wheat Puffed, plain	2.5
Wheat Shredded	.5
Wheaties	8.2

Source: U.S. Department of Agriculture

Dietary Fat
The Number One Nutritional Danger

(See also Cholesterol, p. 55)

Dietary fat is a term used to encompass a variety of different kinds of fat and oils found in foods. Fats are a concentrated source of heat and energy, a source of essential fatty acids that help keep the body alive. Fats also give the body structure, are a carrier of fat-soluble vitamins (A, D, E, and K), and are necessary for many metabolic functions.

Too Much Fat

The chances are you are eating three to five times more fat than your body really needs to function. The average American eats about 83 grams of fat every day. Males consume more; the Health and Nutrition Examination Survey (1976–1980), conducted by the Department of Health and Human Services, found that males between six months and seventy-four years of age consume an average of 98 grams of fat daily. (Men also take in more calories.) Females consume an average of 64 grams of fat per day. Some Americans eat twice that much!

So excessive is Americans' consumption of fat that most experts consider fatty foods the number one nutritional health threat in the nation, leading to high rates of coronary heart disease, stroke, certain types of cancer, and obesity. If you could choose one dietary action to prolong your life, experts say, it should be to eat less fat.

If you're average, you are now eating 35 to 40 percent of your calories in fat. Experts generally agree that should be cut at least to 30 percent. Other authorities urge reducing fat intake to 20 to 25 percent to be even safer. Low-fat enthusiasts like the late Nathan Pritikin favor a diet with only 10 percent fat, similar to the pre–World War II diet in Japan, where heart disease barely existed.

Pritikin's Remarkable Legacy

Although Pritikin's regimen is severe, it is apparently effective. An autopsy on Pritikin revealed arteries that were unclogged and pliable and a cardiovascular system virtually free of any sign of disease—

remarkable in a man of age sixty-nine. Since Dr. Pritikin did not start his low-fat regimen until middle age, when he was diagnosed as having coronary problems, this finding raises the tantalizing prospect that adhering to a very-low-fat diet may help *reverse* as well as prevent arteriosclerosis. There is other proof. Studies done on monkeys have found that damaged arteries can be repaired to some extent when fat intake is drastically reduced. This offers hope that it is never too late to start a low-fat diet.

Some experts believe that cutting down fat to 30 percent of calories may help prevent heart disease, but that much lower fat intake, perhaps as low as 10 percent of calories, may be needed to reverse advanced atherosclerotic disease, when arteries are already partially hardened and clogged with plaque.

MAXIMUM RECOMMENDED FAT
PER DAILY CALORIES

Calories	Calories from fat	Grams of fat	Grams of saturated fat
1000	300	33.3	11
1200	360	40	13
1500	450	50	17
1800	540	60	20
2000	600	66.6	22
2500	750	83	28
3000	900	100	33

Low-Fat Diets for Children, Too

Traditionally, experts advised adults, mainly of middle age, to cut their intake of fat. Now some experts urge even children over age two to restrict fat intake. The theory is that deadly atherosclerosis begins in early childhood. Studies show that children with high blood cholesterol levels are more apt to become adults with high blood cholesterol, auguring heart disease. Says Dr. Robert Levy, former director of the Heart, Lung and Blood Institute and now a professor of medicine at Columbia University: "Atherosclerosis, our major killer, is a silent and secret process that starts in childhood and ends in stroke and heart attack." Dr.Levy and other experts insist that fighting high cholesterol in childhood will save hundreds of thousands of lives in the future.

Warning: Do not put infants under age two on restricted-fat diets. It could damage their growth and development. For example, the American Academy of Pediatrics warns that skim milk is not an appropriate food for an infant.

Fat's Double Identity

Basically, dietary fat is of two types: saturated and unsaturated. Saturated, the type that leads to damaged arteries, is predominate in animal foods—meat and dairy products. That's why experts brand too much fatty beef, cream, and cheese bad for the heart and arteries. The fat from plants, known as oils, is generally unsaturated, and in moderate amounts is beneficial to the cardiovascular system—with two notable exceptions: coconut and palm oil. Both are as highly saturated as animal fats. Palm kernel oil, for example, is twice as saturated as lard!

The way food fats affect the body simply depends on their chemical makeup. Just think of all fats as made up of long chains of so-called fatty acids which are carbon and hydrogen atoms bound together. If the chain has all the hydrogen molecules it can hold, it is called "saturated"; if it could hold more hydrogen molecules, it is called "unsaturated." One more distinction: the unsaturated fats can be either "monounsaturated" or "polyunsaturated." This again is merely a difference in how the atoms in the fatty chains are hooked or bound together. If there is only one so-called double bond in the chain, it is monounsaturated fat; if there are more than one, or many double bonds in the chain, it's polyunsaturated. These fatty acid chains then attach to glycerol to form triglycerides, which is another name for fat.

Since the fat in food contains combinations of types of fatty acid chains, all foods are made up of not just one type of fat, but a combination of saturated, polyunsaturated, and monounsaturated. Beef, for example, has lots of saturated fat, but also much monounsaturated fat. What counts for health is whether the fat in a particular food is *predominately* saturated or unsaturated. Since 50 percent of the fat in butter is saturated, butter is called a highly saturated fatty food. Soybean oil, with 48 percent of the fat polyunsaturated is an unsaturated food.

FOOD FAT PROFILES

Saturated	Fat usually solid at room temperature. One-third or more of the fat is saturated. Examples: beef, pork, lamb, butter, cheese, coconut and palm oils.
Polyunsaturated	Fat liquid or soft at room temperature. One-third or more of fat is polyunsaturated; less than 15 percent is saturated. Examples: corn, safflower, sesame seed, soybean, and sunflower oils, many fish oils, soft margarines.
Monounsaturated	Fat liquid or soft at room temperature. Less than 15 percent of the fat is saturated and less than one-third of the fat is polyunsaturated. Examples: Olive and peanut oils, certain margarines and vegetable shortenings.

Hydrogenation: Some foods are "hydrogenated," or partly hardened, by infusions of more hydrogen atoms; for example, margarine is made by hydrogenating liquid oils. The more hydrogenated, generally the harder and more saturated the fat. Even so, most margarines are predominately polyunsaturated or monounsaturated.

DO YOU EAT TOO MUCH FAT?

Recommendations: No More Than—
   Total fat: 30 percent of calories
   Saturated fat: 10 percent of calories
   Polyunsaturated fat: 10 percent of calories
   Monounsaturated fat: 10 percent of calories

What You Need to Know about Fats and Health

Fats Are Fattening

Fats are the most fattening of all the energy sources. One gram of fat provides 9 calories, compared with 4 calories for a gram of protein or a gram of carbohydrate. Every fat-gram has more than twice the fatttening potential of a gram of protein or of carbohydrate.

There is even some evidence that, because of the way the body metabolizes dietary fat, it may manufacture more body fat from a calorie of dietary fat than from a calorie of carbohydrate or protein. In animals, for example, increasing the ratio of fat to carbohydrates has caused high rates of obesity. The theory is that any dietary fat not burned as fuel is immediately stored as fat in the body. This is not true of carbohydrates. According to Dr. Jean-Pierre Flatt, professor of biochemistry at the University of Massachusettes Medical Center at Worcester, the main culprit in creating and maintaining obesity is a high-fat diet. Fatty foods mixed with sugar are particularly damaging to weight watchers.

The Cancer-Fat Connection

"Among the dietary factors we examined, a linkage between total fat consumption and colon, breast, and prostate cancer stands out most prominently," said Dr. Clifford Grobstein, chairman of the National Academy of Sciences' Committee on Diet, Nutrition, and Cancer in 1982.

Many researchers believe that a steady diet of fat somehow encourages cancers to grow. Worldwide surveys show more cancer in countries with high-fat diets. High-fat diets fed to laboratory animals induce high rates of cancer. Cancers most strongly linked to a high-fat diet are those of the breast, colon, prostate, ovary, and uterus.

At first it looked as if saturated fats were entirely to blame, and some experts still say saturated fat is the main culprit. But compelling evidence now shows that polyunsaturated fats, too, cause high rates of cancer in laboratory animals—in some cases much higher than those of saturated fats. However, what appears to be crucial is the *ratio* of polyunsaturated fats to total fat in the diet. Too much polyunsaturated fat in a low-fat diet appears to promote certain cancers. Thus, polyunsaturated fats are not entirely safe; experts at the National Institutes of Health advise eating only 10 percent of your calories in polyunsaturated fat as a precaution. As a practical matter, it is unlikely that you can get more than that out of an ordinary diet. Currently, there is little worry about a link between monounsaturated fat and cancer.

Fatty Foods and Heart Disease

Fat launches its biggest attack on the cardiovascular system. Most heart-disease authorities see a definite connection between heart and blood vessel diseases and the type and amount of fat in the diet. Indisputably, those who have high blood-cholesterol levels, generally associated with high fat consumption, are at a higher risk of heart attacks and strokes. More than one hundred years ago, cholesterol was found in "plaque" (dangerous buildups) on the interior wall of arteries. Later research found that in feeding animals, including monkeys, large amounts of fat produced clogged arteries and high blood cholesterol. The antifat campaign gained momentum in 1953 when Dr. Ancel Keys at the University of Minnesota reported that a diet high in saturated fat was associated with high rates of atherosclerosis—clogged, hardened arteries and blood vessels—in *humans.*

Epidemiological studies show that countries with diets rich in fat, notably animal or saturated fat, have higher rates of heart disease. In countries with low-fat diets, and low blood-cholesterol counts, such as Japan, the heart-disease rate is less than half as high as in the United States. The average blood cholesterol for middle-aged men in Japan is 150 mg per deciliter. In the United States it is about 210 mg/dl. (Milligrams of cholesterol per deciliter of blood—mg/dl—is the standard way of measuring blood cholesterol.)

More important, many heart-disease authorities are convinced that *reducing* blood-cholesterol levels lessens the risk of heart attacks. A major study by the National Heart, Lung and Blood Institute found that middle-aged men with high blood-cholesterol levels of over 265 mg/dl had fewer heart attacks when their cholesterol was forced down by pharmaceutical drugs. The study showed that a drop of 1 percent in blood-cholesterol level produced a 2 percent reduction in heart attacks. Therefore, experts say, if you get your blood cholesterol down 10 percent, you cut your risk of heart disease by 20 percent, or one-fifth.

YOUR ARTERIES' WORST ENEMIES

Important: *Dietary saturated fat,* not dietary cholesterol, is the greatest factor in pushing up blood cholesterol and increasing your risk of heart disease. Cutting down on saturated fat is the best way to cause a steady and dramatic drop in blood cholesterol.

The risk of heart disease for adults goes up dramatically the higher the blood cholesterol. The Framingham Heart Study shows that those with 230 mg/dl are twice as likely to have coronary heart disease as those with 180 mg/dl. The risk quadruples if your cholesterol goes over 300. Children, too, have alarmingly high levels of blood cholesterol. The average American child has a blood cholesterol of 155 mg/dl. Ideal for children according to Dr. Charles Glueck, University of Cincinnati heart-disease specialist, is 110 mg/dl.

IS YOUR BLOOD CHOLESTEROL TOO HIGH?

Age	Moderate risk of heart attack	High risk of heart attack
2–19	Over 170 mg/dl	Over 185 mg/dl
20–29	Over 200 mg/dl	Over 220 mg/dl
30–39	Over 220 mg/dl	Over 240 mg/dl
40 and over	Over 240 mg/dl	Over 260 mg/dl

Source: NIH Consensus Conference: 1984

Two Kinds of Blood Cholesterol: Good and Bad

Once doctors thought it was enough to know your total cholesterol count. No longer. It is more complex than that. Authorities now recognize that blood contains both "good" and "bad" types of cholesterol, and how much you have of each type helps to determine your risk of heart disease.

"Good cholesterol" is known as high-density lipoprotein cholesterol or HDL. "Bad cholesterol" is called low-density lipoprotein cholesterol or LDL. Here's why: Globules of waxy cholesterol are transported through the body in water-soluble protein capsules of either high density or low density. The LDLs—the bad type—deposit cholesterol in artery walls, causing buildups of hardened plaque that lead to blood clots and blocked arteries. The HDLs—the beneficial type—act as scavengers, grabbing up cholesterol from the bloodstream and carrying it away from arteries and to the liver, where it is processed and destroyed.

People with more HDL cholesterol circulating in the blood have fewer heart attacks. Generally, women have more HDLs than men, and less heart disease. Men average 45 mg/dl of HDLs; women average levels of 55 mg/dl. However, the HDL range varies with age and is also partly determined by heredity. For example, if you are a forty-five-year-old man with HDL levels of 70, you are in the top 95th percentile—more resistant to heart disease than 95 percent of other men your age. If your HDLs measure 50 at that age, you're average.

Find Out Your HDL Levels

Especially if your blood cholesterol registers high, you should find out how much of your total blood cholesterol is the HDL (beneficial) type. (Simply ask the lab to do an additional blood analysis for HDLs.) Even if you have comparatively low blood cholesterol, you can still be at risk of heart disease if your HDLs are exceedingly low. And vice versa: a high total blood cholesterol may not be dangerous if your good HDL cholesterol levels are high. But such luck is rare. Studies show that people with high blood cholesterol almost always have high counts of the detrimental LDL type. Only a small fraction of the population— around 10 percent, according to one study—are lucky enough to have high total blood cholesterol but with enough good HDLs to make their risk of heart disease less than total cholesterol would indicate.

You can't eat good or bad cholesterol. HDLs or LDLs are not found in foods. However, you can raise your HDLs by diet, exercise, stopping smoking and losing weight.

The Best Predictor of Heart Disease

Even more important than total cholesterol or your HDLs, insist some experts, is the ratio of the two. Dr. William Castelli, head of the famed Framingham Heart Study, calls this ratio of HDL good-type cholesterol to total cholesterol the single best predictor of future heart disease. You arrive at that ratio by dividing the amount of HDLs into the total amount of blood cholesterol. If your total cholesterol is 200 and your HDLs are 45, your ratio is 4.4, about average. Vegetarians, who have extremely low rates of heart disease, have the best cholesterol–HDL ratios—a mere 2.8. If your ratio is above 4.7, according to Dr. Castelli, you should try to get it down, for you are in a category of higher than average risk of heart attack.

CHOLESTEROL–HDL RATIOS AND
RISK OF HEART DISEASE
THE LOWER YOUR RATIO, THE LESS YOUR RISK

Ratio	
2.8	Vegetarians
3.4	Half average risk (Boston Marathon runners)
4.4	Average risk for women
5	Average risk for men
4.6–6.4	Average *victim* of heart disease, women
5.4–6.1	Average *victim* of heart disease, men
7.1	Twice average risk, women
9.6	Twice average risk, men
11	Triple average risk, women
23.4	Triple average risk, men

Source: Framingham Heart Study as reported in *The New York Times*, January 8, 1985

Number One Villain: Saturated Fat

Few experts disagree that the most potent blood-cholesterol raiser is saturated fat in the diet. Classic studies done by Dr. Ancel Keys at the University of Minnesota prove that loading up on saturated fat causes damaging buildups of cholesterol in arteries. Other investigations show that blood cholesterol in both humans and animals generally goes up in direct proportion to increases in the saturation of the fat consumed. Saturated fat primarily raises levels of the detrimental LDL type of cholesterol.

Recommendation: The National Institutes of Health's committee of experts advised consuming no more than 10 percent of calories from saturated fat.

Unsaturated Fats Are Good for the Arteries

Numerous studies show that polyunsaturated fats—the dominant fat in fish and most vegetable oils—corn oil, soybean oil, safflower- and sunflower-seed oils—help lower blood cholesterol. Experts generally recommend increasing your intake of polyunsaturates to help counter the damage from saturated fats. One rule of thumb: a gram of saturated fat raises blood cholesterol twice as much as a gram of polyunsaturated fat lowers it.

Recommendation: Eat 10 percent of your calories in polyunsaturated fat.

TYPES OF FAT IN OILS, LARD, AND BUTTER

1 tbsp	Total fat gm	Saturated fat gm	Monounsaturated fat gm	Polyunsaturated fat gm
Coconut	13.6	11.8	.8	.2
Corn	13.6	1.7	3.3	8
Olive	13.5	1.8	9.9	1.1
Palm	13.6	6.7	5	1.3
Palm kernel	13.6	11.1	1.5	.2
Peanut	13.5	2.3	6.2	4.3
Safflower	13.6	1.2	1.6	10.1
Soybean (partially hydrogenated)	13.6	2	5.9	5.1
Sunflower	13.6	1.4	2.7	8.9
Lard	12.8	5	5.8	1.4
Butter	11.4	7.1	3.3	.4

However, polyunsaturated oils, while lowering total blood cholesterol, may also slightly depress beneficial HDL cholesterol. Therefore, an even better substitute may be monounsaturated oils. Certain monounsaturated oils were once thought to have a neutral effect on blood cholesterol. New evidence shows them to be extremely active in lowering blood cholesterol.

Good News about Olive Oil

For years health authorities have recognized that people living around the Mediterranean Sea, such as the Greeks, have lower rates of heart disease. Now, laboratory evidence may have discovered part of the reason: Such people eat lots of olive oil. Olive oil is a monounsaturated fat. New studies show that monounsaturated fats lower total blood cholesterol, without lowering the good HDLs—thus, leading to a ratio more favorable to lower heart-disease risk. Dr. Virgil Brown, chairman of the American Heart Association's nutrition committee, says, "Such monounsaturates may be as good if not better than polyunsaturates for lowering heart disease risk factors." In other words, eat more olive oil.

An exception: Avoid peanut oil. Peanut oil is considered a monounsaturate—but, for unknown reasons, peanut oil has caused extreme atherosclerosis in laboratory monkeys. Experts do not recommend peanut oil as a safeguard against heart disease.

OILS THAT ARE GOOD FOR YOU
Olive
Soybean
Safflower
Sesame
Sunflower
Corn
Fish oils

The Fabulous Fish Oils:
Fat *for* the Heart

Amazing new research from prestigious scientific centers shows that eating fatty fish—mainly cold-water fish containing a specific kind of fish oil—lowers blood cholesterol and inhibits clotting leading to heart attacks and strokes. Other scattered research claims that the fish oil can also help the joints, reducing pain from arthritis, and ameliorate and help to prevent migraine headaches.

The evidence: Initial clues came from observations of Greenland

Eskimos, who suffer only one-tenth the rates of heart disease as Americans and little cancer, hypertension, arthritis, obesity, and diabetes. The Eskimos' diet is very high in fish. The Japanese, who eat about six times more seafood than we do, also have low risks of heart disease. A highly publicized report in the *New England Journal of Medicine* also found that among a group of men in the Netherlands, those who consumed a little over an ounce of fish a day had a 50 percent lower death rate from heart disease than did those who did not eat fish. There was an inverse relationship between fish consumption and heart-disease deaths: the more fish eaten, the greater the protection.

In another test of high-risk heart-disease patients, Dr. William E. Connor and colleagues at the Oregon Health Sciences University found that components of fish oil (called omega-3 fatty acids) forced down total blood cholesterol by 27 percent, triglycerides down by 64 percent, and markedly reduced the very low density lipoproteins (VLDLs.) Fish oils were two to five times more potent in lowering blood cholesterol than were vegetable oils.

Besides modifying blood cholesterol, fish oils have a potent anticlotting effect on the blood. There may also be other, unknown protective factors in fish besides the oils.

Omega-3: Fish Oil Extraordinaire

Excitement focuses on what are called Omega-3 fatty acids, probably the most unsaturated fat you can eat. From 5 to 40 percent of the fat in seafood is Omega-3 fatty acids. Of particular interest is an omega-3 fatty acid called eicosapentaenoic acid (EPA). Many scientists suspect that the active heart-protective agent in fish is EPA.

Generally, the fattier the fish, the more of the protective omega-3 fatty acids it contains, although even lean fish can have significant benefits. Apparently, only very small quantities of fish oil are needed to benefit the cardiovascular system. The Netherlands researchers conclude that eating only one or two fish dishes a week may help prevent coronary heart disease.

Beneficial effects of fish oils on arthritis and migraine headaches are less well substantiated. But good studies have found that fish oils seem to have anti-inflammatory properties, and one test on humans with rheumatoid arthritis revealed that those who took fish-oil capsules experienced less morning stiffness.

Especially rich in Omega-3 oils are mackerel, salmon, trout, rockfish, herring, whitefish, anchovy, and tuna.

Freshwater lake trout and whitefish may also be contaminated with pesticides and other industrial chemicals such as PCBs (polychlorinated biphenyls) that have health dangers, especially to developing fetuses and small children.

Other Foods That
Combat Fat in the Diet

Recently, experts have discovered that many foods and nutrients can effectively fight cholesterol-caused damage to the arteries and blood vessels, thereby protecting against heart disease. Some examples: Elderly and middle-aged people who ate brewer's yeast, high in chromium, had lower blood cholesterol. Both garlic and onions—raw or in capsule form—reportedly do wonders for blood cholesterol. Dr. Victor Gurewich, a professor of medicine at Tufts University prescribes an onion a day for people with dangerous cholesterol levels. He says that the juice of a single white onion daily can raise good HDL cholesterol levels by 30 percent. Other research shows that high-fiber foods and numerous soybean products, including tofu (bean curd), help lower total blood cholesterol.

Good for Your Blood Cholesterol

Because people react quite differently to various diets and regimens, it is impossible to know which individuals may benefit. According to research, the following have produced a beneficial effect in many instances by lowering total cholesterol or raising protective HDLs.

Oat bran
Dried beans (pinto, garbanzo, navy, etc.)
Barley
Carrots
Grapefruit pulp
Lentils
Olive oil
Garlic
Onions (may raise HDL cholesterol)
Yogurt
Soybean products (bean curd or tofu, soy milk, soy flour)
Brewer's yeast
Fish oils
Magnesium
Chromium (may raise HDL cholesterol)
Vitamin C (may raise HDL cholesterol)
Aerobic exercise (may raise HDLs if consistent—at least a half-hour three times a week)
Weight loss (may raise HDL cholesterol)

DRUGS THAT INADVERTENTLY BENEFIT BLOOD CHOLESTEROL
Estrogen (postmenopausal women on estrogen-replacement therapy typically have very high levels of HDL cholesterol)
Antibiotics

The Right Kind of Fiber

One of the most tested and successful modifiers of blood cholesterol is food fiber. Certain types of food fiber apparently help bind up cholesterol in the body somehow, reducing its prevalence. But only the right kind of fiber will work.

There are two types of fiber—insoluble and soluble. The insoluble, indigestible fiber—so-called roughage—is the type found in cereals like All-Bran. This does *not* lower cholesterol. The second type is water soluble, like pectins and gums found in fruits, vegetables, and oats. This gummy, soluble type of fiber can significantly lower blood cholesterol, both laboratory tests and studies on humans reveal.

Beans and Oat Bran

Especially potent in decreasing blood cholesterol are two high-fiber foods—oat bran and dried beans. Dr. James Anderson, a prominent fiber researcher at the University of Kentucky, found that only four oat-bran muffins daily (1.8 ounces of bran) lowers cholesterol by 10 percent in ordinary young adults. It works even better on middle-aged men with high cholesterol (over 260 mg/dl). Their blood cholesterol fell by an average of 19 percent within a month after eating either a hot bowl of oat-bran cereal or a cup and a half of navy or pinto beans every day. One man's cholesterol fell from 274 to 190; another's dropped from 218 to 167. Oat-bran cereal and dried beans also increase HDL cholesterol by about 20 percent.

Dr. Anderson speculates that foods high in soluble fiber help wash excess cholesterol out of the blood and reduce the liver's production of cholesterol.

Bad for Your Blood Cholesterol

FACTORS THAT MAY RAISE OR DETRIMENTALLY MODIFY BLOOD CHOLESTEROL
Smoking (may depress HDLs)
Heavy coffee drinking (more than 3 cups a day)
Stress (may incite liver to make more cholesterol)
Obesity (may depress HDLs)

How Much Can Diet Lower Blood Cholesterol?

Low-fat diets are expected to reduce blood-cholesterol levels by an average of 15 percent. But, by cutting down on high-fat foods, certain individuals experience much more dramatic drops in blood cholesterol—reductions of one-third or more within a short time. Dr. Ronald Goor, former coordinator of the federal government's National Cholesterol Education Program, says his blood cholesterol fell from 300 to 200 three weeks after starting a moderately low-fat diet.

Diet can be potent even in fighting a genetically caused disease in which blood cholesterol is so astronomically high that it is routinely lowered by drugs. Through a careful diet, one man reduced his blood cholesterol from a life-threatening 426 to a comparatively healthy 246.

Apparently, the greater the fat restriction, the more the reduction. The blood cholesterol of the low-fat guru, Nathan Pritikin, measured 280 mg/dl in 1955, dropped to 210 in 1958, and was a mere 94 when he died in 1985, although some link the low cholesterol to his leukemia.

WHERE WE GET FAT IN THE DIET

	Percent
Meat	28
Dairy, eggs	18
Fats, oils	16
Desserts, snacks	13
Breads, grains, potatoes	11
Poultry, fish	5
Nuts, beans	3
Miscellaneous	6

Source: Department of Health and Human Services, Health and Nutrition Examination Survey (1976–1980)

Important: By far the most fat came from hamburgers and meat loaf (7 percent). Next, hot dogs, ham, and luncheon meats (6.4 percent); whole milk (6 percent); doughnuts, cakes, and cookies (6 percent); and beef steaks and roasts (5.5 percent). And if you wonder why potatoes ranked so high in the chart, it is not because potatoes are inherently fat. Just the opposite; but potatoes are most often consumed as french fries—high in fat.

How to Tell If a Food Is High in Fat

It is not fair to judge high-fat foods by the percentage of fat by weight. If you did, whole milk, which is 3 to 3.7 percent fat, and mostly water, would be a low-fat food. So would a hot dog, which is 30 percent fat. They are not. In fact, more than 50 percent of the calories in whole milk come from fat, as well as 80 percent of the calories in a hot dog, making both high-fat foods. Here is a short-cut to judging the fat values of foods:

Low-fat food
Fewer than 30 percent of calories from fat
Fewer than 5 grams of fat per serving

Moderate-fat food
30–50 percent of calories from fat
6–10 grams of fat per serving

High-fat food
More than 50 percent of calories from fat
More than 10 grams of fat per serving

Simple Ways to Get Saturated Fat Out of Your Diet

• Use skim milk or 1 percent milk. Whole milk is at least 3 percent fat. Using 2 percent milk makes only a slight difference.
• Eat more fish and poultry, less red meat.
• Trim all visible fat off red meats.
• Remove skin from chicken and turkey before eating.
• Eat less sausage, bacon, and processed luncheon meats. Hot dogs are 30 percent fat.
• Use low-fat yogurt and low-fat cheeses.
• Eat less ice cream, butter, and cream. Substitute sherbet or non-dairy frozen desserts, and margarine.
• Watch out for commercial baked goods made with coconut oil, palm oil, or animal shortening.
• Eat fewer foods fried in animal fats.
• Eat more high-fiber vegetables, beans, grains, and fruits.

Beware: "Nondairy" Does Not Mean Free of Saturated Fat

Generally, experts warn against saturated fats in red meats and dairy products. True. But largely overlooked is the fact that the most highly saturated fat dangers are palm and coconut oils that permeate the food supply. Cheap and easy to use, they are often used in processed foods—in baked goods, to fry snack foods, and primarily in nondairy creams and whipped toppings.

Tragically, many people who avoid rich cream and butter, fearful of the saturated fat, fall into a worse trap with so-called nondairy foods full of coconut or palm oil. Check the labels of nondairy products, especially nondairy creamers and whipped toppings, and baked and snack goods for the presence of coconut or palm oils, and avoid them when possible. They are potent enemies of the cardiovascular system.

Saturated Fat in Fast Foods

You will find plenty of saturated fat in fast foods, not only in foods like hamburgers but in all kinds of fried foods. That is because many chains use saturated fats for frying—such as beef tallow, palm oil, or heavily hydrogenated vegetable oils. Adding hydrogen to a vegetable oil—or "hydrogenating" it—makes it more saturated, although beef tallow raises cholesterol more effectively than either heavily or moderately hydrogenated vegetable oils.

The Center for Science in the Public Interest, a Washington, D.C., consumer group, had french fries (and tempura) analyzed from various fast-food restaurants in Boston, Washington, D.C., and Richmond, Virginia, and found that most of them were fried in highly saturated fat. The Center points out that since many restaurants use the same shortening to fry most foods, the same is probably true of chicken parts and nuggets, fish, and other fried foods.

HOW FAST FOODS COMPARED

	Saturated percent	Unsaturated percent
Beef tallow (may be mixed with a little vegetable oil)		
Arby's	56	44
Burger King**	56	44
Big Boy	55	45
Popeye's	55	45
Hardee's	54	46
Wendy's	54	46
McDonald's	52	48
Palm oil		
Howard Johnson's*	56	44

	Saturated percent	Unsaturated percent
Heavily hydrogenated vegetable oil		
D'Lites	36	64
Rustler	35	65
Long John Silver's	33	67
Church's	32	68
Kentucky Fried Chicken	30	70
Red Lobster	29	71
Moderately hydrogenated vegetable oil		
Denny's	21	79
Friendly's	20	80
Papa Gino's	18	82
Safflower oil		
Open Sesame	13	87

Source: Center for Science in the Public Interest

*Howard Johnson's claims to use vegetable oil at about two-thirds of its outlets, and a number of different oils, including palm oil, at the remaining one-third. Some chains use different oils at different outlets. This survey was based on foods obtained from one outlet of each restaurant. The survey was released in November 1985.
**After the study Burger King switched to vegetable oils for frying all foods except french fries.

Some Fat Facts to Notice

• Avocados are high in fat, most of it unsaturated.

• All margarines, salad oils, butter, and lard are 100 percent fat— that is, *all* their calories come from fat.

• Cheeses are extremely high in fat—cream cheese, the worst.

• The lower the grade of beef, the less fatty it is. For example, a prime steak is the fattiest, a choice steak less so, and a "good" grade steak least fatty of all. However, in hamburger much of the fat cooks out. For example, regular raw ground beef contains 30 grams of fat per 4 ounces compared with 19 fat grams in extra lean ground beef. However, after broiling (well done) the extra lean hamburger has 14 grams of fat per 3 ounces and the regular hamburger has 16.5 fat grams. Thus, the regular hamburger ends up with 2.5 more fat grams worth about 22 added calories.

• Vegetables and vegetable oils are generally low in saturated fat. Two notable exceptions: coconut meat and oil and palm oil.

• Extra lean on a label means no more than 5 percent fat. "Lean" and "low fat" foods must contain less than 10 percent fat.

THE 50 FATTIEST FOODS

(Foods with the highest percentage of calories from fat)

	Percent of calories from fat
Butter	100
Shortening, all types	100
Oils, vegetable, all types (olive, peanut, corn, soybean, safflower, sesame, palm, coconut, walnut, etc.)	100
Margarine, all types	100
Olives, green and ripe	98
Meat fat	98
Pine nuts, piñon, dried	97
Cream, fluid, heavy whipping	97
Macadamia nuts	96
Cream, fluid, light whipping	95
Chocolate, bitter or baking	94
Coconut milk	93
Salad dressings, Italian and other types	93
Cream, fluid, medium, 25% fat	92
Pecans	91
Brazil nuts	91
Hazelnuts	91
Cream cheese	90
Cream, light, coffee or table	89
Coconut meat, dried	88
Sour cream	88
Salad dressing, mayonnaise	87
Walnuts, English or Persian	87
Avocados	86
Pâté de foie gras	85
Lamb, rib chops, prime, broiled	85
Sunflower seeds	84
Almonds	84
Sesame butter (tahini)	84
Beef, rib, choice	84
Deviled ham, canned	83
Sausage, Italian	83
Sausage, pork and beef	82
Beef, T-bone steak, choice	82
Luncheon meat, pork and beef chopped	82
Beef, porterhouse steak, choice	82
Bologna	81
Beerwurst (beer salami), beef	81

	Percent of calories from fat
Sausage, Vienna, canned	81
Knockwurst	81
Cheese, Neufchâtel	81
Bockwurst	81
Frankfurters	80
Pepperoni	80
Beef, tongue, smoked	79
Liverwurst, fresh	79
Kielbasa, Kolbassy	79
Peanut butter	78
Club steak, good grade	77
Beef, corned, boneless, uncooked, medium fat	77

Source: Author's computer analysis

SOURCES OF THE FABULOUS FISH OILS

3½ oz, raw	Total fat gm	EPA fatty acids gm	Total Omega-3 fatty acids gm
Anchovy, European	4.8	.5	1.4
Bass, freshwater	2	.1	.3
Bass, striped	2.3	.2	.8
Bluefish	6.5	.4	1.2
Carp	5.6	.2	.7
Catfish, channel	4.3	.1	.3
Cod, Atlantic and Pacific	.7	.1	.2
Eel, European	18.8	.1	.9
Flounder	1	.1	.2
Grouper, red	.8	.2	.2
Haddock	.7	.1	.2
Hake, Pacific and silver	2.6	.2	.4
Halibut, Greenland	13.8	.5	.9
Halibut, Pacific	2.3	.1	.4
Herring, Atlantic	9	.7	1.7
Herring, Pacific	13.9	.1	1.8
Herring, round	4.4	.4	1.3
Mackerel, Atlantic	13.9	.9	2.6
Mackerel, chub	11.5	.9	2.2
Mackerel, Japanese horse	7.8	.5	1.9
Mackerel, king	13	.1	2.2
Mullet	4.4	.5	1.1
Ocean perch	1.6	.1	.2

3½ oz, raw	Total fat gm	EPA fatty acids gm	Total Omega-3 fatty acids gm
Perch, white	2.5	.2	.4
Pike, walleye	1.2	.1	.3
Pompano, Florida	9.5	.2	.6
Rockfish	1.4	.2	.5
Sablefish	15.3	.7	1.5
Salmon, Atlantic	5.4	.3	1.4
Salmon, chinook	10.4	.8	1.5
Salmon, chum	6.6	.4	1.1
Salmon, coho	6	.3	1
Salmon, pink	3.4	.4	1
Salmon, sockeye	8.6	.5	1.3
Seabass, Japanese	1.5	.1	.4
Seatrout, sand and spotted	1.7	.1	.2
Smelt, rainbow	2.6	.3	.8
Smelt, sweet	4.6	.2	.7
Snapper, red	1.2	trace	.2
Sole, European	1.2	trace	.1
Sprat	5.8	.5	1.3
Sturgeon, Atlantic	6	.1	1.5
Sturgeon, common	3.3	.2	.4
Swordfish	2.1	.1	.2
Trout, brook	2.7	.2	.6
Trout, lake	9.7	.5	2
Trout, rainbow	3.4	.1	.6
Tuna, albacore	4.9	.3	1.5
Tuna, bluefin	6.6	.4	1.6
Tuna, skipjack	1.9	.1	.4
Whitefish, lake	6	.3	1.5

Shellfish

Crab, Alaska king, blue, Dungeness	1	.2	.3
Crayfish	1.4	.1	.1
Lobster, European and northern	.9	.1	.2
Shrimp, Atlantic brown or white	1.5	.2	.4
Shrimp, Japanese prawn	2.5	.3	.5
Spiny lobster	1.4	.2	.3

Mollusks

Abalone	1	trace	trace
Clam, hardshell	.6	trace	trace

3½ oz, raw	Total fat gm	EPA fatty acids	Total Omega-3 fatty acids gm
Clam, softshell	2	.2	.4
Conch	2.7	.6	1
Mussel, blue	2.2	.2	.5
Mussel, Mediterranean	1.5	.1	.2
Octopus	1	.1	.2
Oyster, eastern	2.5	.2	.4
Oyster, European	2	.3	.6
Oyster, Pacific	2.3	.4	.6
Periwinkle	3.3	.5	.7
Scallop	.8	.1	.2
Squid, Atlantic	1.2	.1	.4
Squid, short-finned	2	.2	.6
Fish oils			
Codliver oil	100	9	19.2
Herring oil	100	7.1	12
Menhaden oil	100	12.7	21.7
MaxEPA (trademark) fish body oils	100	17.8	29.4
Salmon oil	100	8.8	20.9

Source: U.S. Department of Agriculture

Cholesterol
New Facts, New Controversy

(See also Dietary Fat, p. 34)

Cholesterol is a pearly, fatty, alcohol substance, found in significant amounts only in animals, never in plants. It has no calories. Although cholesterol is the same substance whether it is found in animal foods or circulating in the blood of humans, food cholesterol is usually correctly called "dietary cholesterol," and blood cholesterol "serum" or "plasma" cholesterol.

Cholesterol's importance in food is linked to the suspicion that it can lead to high blood-cholesterol levels and consequently to high rates of heart disease and atherosclerosis. The theory is that by cutting back on high-cholesterol foods, blood-cholesterol levels will decrease, preventing heart and blood-vessel diseases. That is a matter of intense controversy.

Nobody *Needs* Dietary Cholesterol

There is no required daily dose of cholesterol in the diet. Cholesterol is not an essential nutrient. The diet is not even the *main* source of cholesterol in the body. The body, mainly the liver, can manufacture all the cholesterol you need—some 500 to 1,000 mg per day. Nevertheless, the average American takes in through diet another 300 to 500 mg daily. About half of this is absorbed, depending on the individual. The

---

RECOMMENDED *MAXIMUM* INTAKE OF DIETARY CHOLESTEROL

250 to 300 mg per day
for everyone over age two

Typical American now eats
450 to 500 mg per day
—National Institutes of Health advisory panel

---

problem with cholesterol, then, is not deficiency, but possible excess. Americans eat far more cholesterol than they need, or than some experts say is safe.

Who Needs to Worry?

That is the controversial question. Experts disagree over to what extent cholesterol in food raises the blood cholesterol of most Americans. It may seem logical that eating more cholesterol would boost levels of cholesterol in the body, but it is not that simple. Research shows that individual metabolic ways of handling food cholesterol determine whether you need to restrict your intake. In any event, there is widespread confusion in the public's mind about the connection between dietary cholesterol, blood cholesterol, and heart disease.

The trend even among heart experts is to downplay the role of food cholesterol as the primary culprit in atherosclerosis and heart disease. In the hierarchy of heart-disease risks, dietary cholesterol ranks in importance *behind* total fat and saturated fat in the diet, as well as behind smoking, high blood pressure, and obesity.

A Public Misunderstanding

Many people think that dietary cholesterol is synonymous with blood cholesterol, and that all they have to do to lower their blood cholesterol is to eat fewer high-cholesterol foods. "This is a major misconception," says Dr. Ronald Goor, former coordinator of the federal government's National Cholesterol Education Program. "Merely cutting back on dietary cholesterol will generally have an insignificant effect on blood cholesterol." This does not mean you should not worry about high *blood* cholesterol and trying to reduce it by other dietary or lifestyle changes. But relying on success mainly from a diet low in cholesterol probably won't work for most people.

Nevertheless, some authorities label it bad public-health policy to suggest that the threat of high-cholesterol foods is not universal; they fear that no one will pay attention to the warnings—even those who should. They also point out that eating less cholesterol cannot be

---

Important: Although everybody may be threatened by high *blood* cholesterol, only certain individuals may be threatened by high-cholesterol *foods.*

harmful and may be beneficial. Others argue that it is misleading and dangerous to urge everybody to cut back on food cholesterol when only a small percentage of the population may be affected by it.

Bad Eggs in a New Light

Recent studies reveal much individual variation in response to cholesterol in the diet. Years of research at New York's Rockefeller University, under the supervision of Dr. Edward Ahrens, concludes that only certain Americans need worry about high-cholesterol diets. According to Dr. Ahrens, when high loads of dietary cholesterol are dumped into the body, several things might happen, depending on the individual's unique metabolism: 1. The excess cholesterol is metabolized and excreted, leaving blood levels unchanged. 2. The liver compensates for the overload of cholesterol by cutting back its own production of cholesterol, so that excess cholesterol does not get into the blood. 3. The liver does not act as a safeguard; instead, it allows the excess cholesterol to enter the bloodstream and subsequently to be stored in the body, including the blood vessels and coronary arteries. These "storers" of dietary cholesterol, as Dr. Ahrens calls them, are most likely to be damaged by high-cholesterol foods and to benefit from dietary-cholesterol reductions.

In a recent study, Dr. Ahrens found that about 20 percent of men who ate high-cholesterol diets (three eggs daily for three weeks) experienced blood-cholesterol increases of more than 10 percent. The other 14 percent excreted the extra cholesterol. The remaining 66 percent maintained the same blood-cholesterol equilibrium by automatic metabolic changes, such as slowing down liver production of internal cholesterol.

Thus, he argues that most Americans safely cope with overloads of cholesterol in the diet. However, he also warns that some people are "exquisitely sensitive" to food-cholesterol overloads, which send blood cholesterol soaring. These "cholesterol sensitive" people obviously, he says, should watch their food-cholesterol intakes. The problem is that there is no laboratory test to reveal which individuals release dietary cholesterol into their bloodstreams. One way to find out, Dr. Ahrens says: If you have an abnormal blood-cholesterol count, cut back on high-cholesterol foods for six to eight weeks. Then have another blood-cholesterol analysis to see if your cholesterol is down. If it drops by at least 10 to 15 percent, you are probably sensitive to cholesterol in food.

So Why Not Avoid Cholesterol?

Even though you may not be adversely affected by high-cholesterol foods per se, there is still good reason to beware of them. Foods high in cholesterol, notably dairy foods, are apt to be high in saturated fat, which does decidedly raise blood-cholesterol levels in most people. So, by shunning high-cholesterol foods you automatically pass up highly saturated animal fats, cutting calories and helping protect your blood vessels. When you cut down on cholesterol, you usually cut down on calories and fat.

Myths about Seafood and Cholesterol

Unless you have been in space for the last quarter century, you must have heard umpteen times that fish and especially shellfish are dangerous repositories of cholesterol and not suitable for diets of those concerned about heart disease. Wrong. Compelling studies now show that certain seafood, though relatively high in cholesterol or fat, actually protects against heart disease. Scientists observe that Eskimos have low blood cholesterol and one-tenth the heart disease we do, even though their diet is primarily seafood. They are convinced that certain fish oils help lower blood cholesterol and prevent heart disease in other ways. (For more on this, see Dietary Fat, p. 43).

Bad Rap for Shellfish

Scientists even find that shellfish, long considered poison to those on cholesterol-lowering diets, have been seriously maligned. For example, Dr. William Connor and colleagues at the Oregon Health Sciences University fed subjects high amounts of shrimp, crab, and lobster (one pound a day for three weeks). Their blood cholesterol did not go up. Dr. Connor theorizes it may be that beneficial fatty acids in the shellfish neutralize any detrimental effects of the cholesterol.

Further, early calculations of the cholesterol content of seafood turn out to be erroneously high. Oysters were once reported to contain 200

Important: Cholesterol is not found in fruits, vegetables, nuts, or plant foods. Cholesterol is found only in animal foods—meat, poultry, seafood, eggs, and dairy products.

mg of cholesterol per 3 ounces. New methods reveal only 42 mg. Experts now say that fish and shellfish are a legitimate part of the diet for those with heart or blood-vessel disease.

Misleading Food Advertising and Cholesterol

Some corn oils and margarines promote their brands as "cholesterol free," leading consumers to believe that other corn oils and margarines contain cholesterol. Pay no attention to this advertising. No oils, margarines, or shortenings made from vegetable products contain cholesterol, whether they are yellow, white, liquid, semiliquid, or solid. Only fats from animals—namely lard and butter—contain cholesterol. Similarly, peanut butter, although many people are unaware of it, contains no cholesterol. The term *butter* is deceptive. The same goes for almond butter and seed butters such as tahini, and even "butter milk," which is low in cholesterol.

Also, just because a product is labeled "cholesterol free," don't assume it is safe. Some fats, such as coconut and palm oil, contain no cholesterol but are so saturated that they clog the arteries worse than pure lard.

Beware: Hidden Cholesterol

Much cholesterol, like sodium and sugar, is hidden in processed foods, notably baked goods, mainly because of the addition of eggs to pies, cakes, and pastries. Also, servings of dairy products are not as high in cholesterol as many believe. Highest among cheeses are cream and Neufchâtel.

50 FOODS HIGHEST IN CHOLESTEROL
(by common measure)

	Cholesterol (mg)
Brains, pork and beef: 3 oz	2169-1700
Eggs, goose: 1 egg	1227
Eggs, duck: 1 egg	619
Chicken liver: ½ c	440
Beef liver, fried: 3 oz	410
Sweetbreads, cooked: 3 oz	396
Calf liver, fried: 3 oz	372
Fish roe (cod and shad), cooked: 3½ oz	345

	Cholesterol (mg)
Duck, meat/skin: ½	320
Eggs, chicken, yolk: 1 large	272
Coconut cream pie: ⅛ of 9-inch diameter	205
Lamb liver: 1 6-oz slice	197
Squid, cooked: 3 oz	176
Sponge cake: ¹⁄₁₂ of 10-inch diameter	172
Shrimp, boiled: 3 oz	168
Pound cake: ¹⁄₁₀ of loaf	150
Octopus, smoked: 3 oz	145
Veal chop: 1 chop	144
Goat: 3 oz	144
Pie, chiffon, chocolate: ⅛ of 9-inch diameter	138
Cheesecake, chocolate: ¹⁄₁₂ of 9-inch diameter	136
Custard pie: ⅛ of 9 inch diameter	123
Lemon meringue pie: ⅛ of 9-inch diameter	122
Lamb chop, lean/fat: 1 chop	121
Jelly roll: ¹⁄₁₀ of roll	120
Pheasant: ½ breast (4½ oz)	112
Rabbit, domestic: 3¾ oz	111
Liver pâté, chicken: 1 oz	111
Caviar: 2 tbsp.	110
Veal, boneless, cooked: 3 oz	105
Pork, spareribs: 3 oz	103
Cake, carrot: ¹⁄₁₂ of 10-inch diameter	102
Cheesecake: ¹⁄₁₂ of 9-inch diameter	100
Sardines: 3 oz	100
Chocolate cream pie: ⅛ of 9-inch diameter	97
Crab, hardshell, steamed: 2 medium blue	95
Crayfish, boiled/steamed: 3 oz	95
Mackerel, canned, drained: 3 oz	95
Oysters, fried: 3 oz	95
Mackerel, fillet, broiled: 3 oz	94
Pumpkin pie: ⅛ of 9-inch diameter	94
Herring, smoked, kippered: 3 oz	93
German chocolate cake: ¹⁄₁₂ of 8-inch diameter	90
Squirrel: 3 oz	90
Crab, softshell, fried: 1 crab	87
Crab, canned or cooked: 3 oz	86
Banana cream pie: ⅛ of 9-inch diameter	85

	Cholesterol (mg)
Herring, 3 oz	85
Ground beef, ext. lean, well done: 3 oz	84
Chicken, dark meat, stwd: 3 oz	80

Source: Author's computer analysis of USDA data

Dietary Fiber
The Nonnutrient of the Decade

Dietary fiber, or "roughage," is a substance that is found primarily in plant cells and is not completely digested. Food fiber contains few calories and is primarily nonnutritious. It includes substances known as cellulose, lignin, hemicelluloses, pentosans, gums, and pectins. Food fiber provides bulk in the diet, aids elimination, and is vital in thwarting disease processes in ways not fully understood.

Fiber Comeback

Since fiber contributes so slightly to the energy or nutrient requirements of the body, it has long been ignored. No longer. Fiber is now heralded as one of the most important dietary factors of the decade. Too little fiber is one of the scourges of the modern Western diet. If your diet is deficient in fiber, you are cheating yourself of considerable protection against a long list of chronic problems and diseases. And it is highly probable that you are not consuming as much fiber as you need.

How Much Fiber Should You Eat?

Experts have not set recommended levels, but the consensus is that the modern Western diet is alarmingly deficient in dietary fiber. According to the U.S. Department of Agriculture's most recent ten-year National Food Consumption Survey, total dietary fiber intake ranged from 8 to 32 grams a day. Newer research shows the average to be a shocking 11 grams. In contrast, people in third-world countries, with much lower rates of heart disease, diabetes, and similar chronic diseases, consume about four times more fiber—40 to 60 grams daily. Sixty grams may be too much for most Americans. But some authorities advocate at least tripling the adult intake of dietary fiber to about 35 or 40 grams a day. Children need less.

> Warning: Individuals who have digestive diseases should consult their physicians before going on a high-fiber diet. The fiber could aggravate the condition, causing more harm than good.

You Can't Tell Fiber by the Look or the Crunch

Important: *Fiber occurs almost exclusively in plant foods.* Although meats, poultry, and fish may be fibrous, they are not a significant source of dietary fiber. Nor are dairy products such as cheese, eggs, and milk.

You cannot judge which fruits, vegetables, and grains have the most fiber simply by appearance. High-fiber foods are not necessarily coarse in texture. Celery, for example, is mistaken for a high-fiber food simply because it is crunchy and stringy. In fact, peas have four times more fiber. Dietary fiber may actually be invisible to the eye, detectable only through laboratory analyses.

Important: Generally, the less highly processed the food, the more fiber it has. Fresh, raw, unpeeled fruit and vegetables, for example, are high in fiber. Cooking fruits and vegetables, especially to the mushy stage, destroys much fiber. Juices have little or no insoluble fiber; some may, however, have soluble fiber. Similarly, unrefined grains products, such as whole-grain rolled oats, oat groats, and whole wheat bread are good fiber sources. Brown rice beats out white rice in fiber; stone ground corn meal is higher in fiber than degermed corn meal. Breads highest in fiber will list whole wheat, not just wheat flour, as their chief ingredient on the label.

Fiber: Not Just Another Word for Bran

Wheat bran is one of the highest-fiber foods known—about 50 percent fiber. And for years when experts talked about fiber, everybody knew they meant this bran, the laxative fiber. But recent research shows that different types of fiber in grains and vegetables are also as important and have previously unsuspected but critical effects on health.

One for the Digestion, One for the Heart

Think of fiber as coming in two types—either water-soluble or water insoluble. Wheat bran—the outer layer of the whole wheat kernel—is the classic example of insoluble fiber; it is coarse, chewy, and won't dissolve even in hot water. This insoluble fiber is associated with hastening food through the digestive tract; thus, its reputation for promoting "regularity." Although insoluble fiber is primarily concentrated in whole grains, cereals, and breads, smaller amounts are also found in fruits and vegetables, such as raw blackberries, lima beans, and peas. Most complex-carbohydrate foods are mixtures of both types of fiber.

Soluble fiber, recognized more recently, is found primarily in fruits and vegetables (gums and pectin) and in another type of bran—oat bran, the outer shell of the oat kernel. Oat bran, now sold as a cereal, is rich in a gum called beta-glucan, which dissolves easily in water. Soluble fiber is more often associated with reducing the risks of heart disease and diabetes. Soluble fiber apparently has a subtle but powerful impact on the body's metabolism of sugars and fats.

The upshot: It appears that insoluble fiber may help prevent digestive problems such as diverticulosis, constipation, and colon cancer. Soluble fiber works against high blood pressure, glucose intolerance, and high blood cholesterol. It is possible that some of the high-soluble-fiber foods might also have beneficial effects on digestion, but it is as yet unclear.

The best advice: Eat foods high in *both* types of fiber.

MAJOR TYPES OF FOOD FIBER
Cellulose—insoluble, absorbs water, laxative effect
Hemicelluloses—insoluble, absorb water, laxative effect
Gums—soluble, decrease fat absorption, lower blood-cholesterol levels, slow sugar absorption
Mucilages—soluble
Pectin—soluble, decreases fat absorption, lowers blood cholesterol, slows sugar absorption
Lignin—insoluble, absorbs little water, lowers blood cholesterol

Fiber and Cancer

Cancer experts, including the National Cancer Institute and the American Cancer Society, urge people to eat more fiber as well as less fat as protection against colon cancer. Foods high in soluble fiber might also protect against cancer for reasons other than their fiber content. For example, certain fiber-rich vegetables are known to contain chemicals called indoles, which in laboratory animals block the development of several types of cancers; these indoles are found particularly in vegetables of the cruciferous family—broccoli, brussels sprouts, cabbage, and cauliflower. Carrots and other vitamin A-containing fruits and vegetables have been found in epidemiological studies to help ward off lung cancer.

The strongest fiber link, however, is with colon cancer, which kills more than fifty thousand Americans a year. English physician Denis Burkitt first proposed the theory in 1969 after observing that rural Africans have virtually no digestive diseases, particularly colon cancer. He related it to their high-fiber grain and cereal diets.

Later surveys showed that the colon cancer rate in Western countries with low-fiber diets is eight times greater than that of many developing countries with diets rich in grains and vegetables. One worldwide analysis showed that the higher a population's colon-cancer rate, the lower the consumption of cereals. Controlled studies in Scandinavia have shown conclusively that the higher the cancer rate, the lower the fiber intake and higher the fat intake. In northern India, where the diet is high in fiber, colon cancer is virtually unheard of, whereas in southern India, where diets are low in fiber, there is much more colon cancer. Also, in laboratory animals, both wheat bran (insoluble) and fiber from citrus fruits (soluble) protect against chemically induced colon cancer.

High-fiber diets may even protect somewhat against the cancer promotion of high-fat diets. The Finns, for example, who slather butter on their bread and consume lots of high fat cheese have about one-half our rate of colon cancer. However, the bread they use as a vehicle for their fat indulgence is very coarse and high in fiber. Researcher Dr. John Weisburger at the American Health Foundation speculates that the high fiber may help counteract any carcinogenic effects of the fat.

Recommendation: Eat both more fiber and less fat. Doing both is more likely to cut your chances of cancer than doing only one or the other.

HEALTH PROBLEMS THAT MAY BE LINKED TO LOW-FIBER DIETS

Research on animals and/or humans proves or suggests a connection between low-fiber intake and the following diseases:

Constipation
Appendicitis
Colon cancer
Diverticular disease
Spastic colon
Hiatal hernia
Varicose veins
Hemorrhoids (piles)
Coronary heart disease
High blood pressure

Gallstones
Diabetes
Obesity
Ulcerative colitis
Crohn's disease

Fiber and Coronary Heart Disease

There is little question that a high-fiber diet can help lower or favorably modify blood cholesterol. A high-fiber diet can also lower blood pressure, helping prevent strokes as well as heart attacks. A recent study among 556 men in the Baltimore Longitudinal Study of Aging found that fruit fiber was potent in decreasing blood pressure as well as blood cholesterol. Men of all ages who ate the most fruit fiber had the healthiest blood profiles and lowest blood pressure.

Dr. James Anderson, of the University of Kentucky, a leading authority on health and fiber, has also succeeded in getting numerous diabetics off insulin by putting them on high-fiber diets. The fiber apparently helps regulate glucose metabolism. (For more details on Dr. Anderson's research on the impact of fiber on blood cholesterol, see Dietary Fat, p. 46.)

HIGH-FIBER FOODS SHOWN TO HELP FIGHT CARDIOVASCULAR DISEASE

Oat bran	Grapefruit pulp
Dried beans	Lentils
Barley	Sweet potatoes
Apples	Raw green peppers
Carrots	Asparagus
Cucumbers	

HOW FIBER DECREASES ABNORMALLY HIGH BLOOD PRESSURE, CHOLESTEROL, AND BLOOD SUGAR

	Amount of decrease with each gram increase of fruit fiber
Systolic blood pressure	1.2 mm Hg
Diastolic blood pressure	0.7 mm Hg
Fasting glucose (blood sugar)	0.5 mg/dl
2-hour glucose (Oral GTT)	2.0 mg/dl
Blood cholesterol	1.5 mg/dl
Blood triglyceride	3.7 mg/dl

Source: National Institute of Aging,
Gerontology Research Center (Baltimore)

Can Fiber Deplete Other Nutrients?

Is a high-fiber diet dangerous because it ties up certain nutrients in the digestive tract, preventing their full utilization by the body? Unquestionably, a high-fiber diet may interfere with the absorption of protein, fat, and certain vitamins and minerals. But most authorities believe that this is not a major risk to healthy people, although it could affect such high-risk groups for deficiencies as children, pregnant women, and the elderly.

In any case, any possible deleterious effects on the absorption of other nutrients is not nearly as serious as the consequences of a low-fiber or fiber-free diet. Still, you should be aware that fiber in foods can bind or interfere with the absorption of other nutrients, so you can boost intakes if you wish.

Also found in most high-fiber foods are compounds called phytates, which can significantly tie up minerals, making them unavailable to the body. (For a partial list of high-phytate foods, see p. 196.)

FIBER INTERACTIONS

Studies in both humans and animals show that fiber may decrease the absorption of:

Protein

Fat

Vitamin B_6

Vitamin B_{12}, vitamin A, riboflavin

Calcium, zinc, copper, magnesium, iron

Drugs of all types, lessening their pharmaceutical effectiveness

Why So Many Fiber-Food Charts Are Wrong

Pay no attention to charts that list "crude fiber"; the information is meaningless. Until recently, nutritionists measured only cellulose and lignin and called it "crude fiber," overlooking the other types of fiber. Many books, still being sold, report merely crude fiber, an obsolete, inadequate, measurement by today's standards. Crude fiber significantly underestimates the amount of fiber in foods.

Modern, sophisticated methods measure not only "crude fiber" but the other major types of fiber. The sum of the total is called "dietary fiber," which can be up to 38 times higher than crude fiber, according to the Center for Science in the Public Interest.

Some foods still lack proper measurements for dietary fiber. But the USDA is striving to bring its information up-to-date and has added dietary fiber to many of the food-composition charts shown in this book.

HOW TO PUT MORE FIBER IN YOUR DIET

Eat this	Instead of this
Wheat or bran cereals	Highly processed, sugary cereals
Oat bran or oatmeal	Instant oatmeal
Whole-wheat bread	White bread
Brown rice	Instant or polished white rice
Fresh fruits	Fruit juices
Fresh vegetables	Frozen or canned vegetables
Popped corn and nuts	Potato chips and pretzels
Dried beans	Meat protein
Whole-grain flour	White flour
Unpeeled fruits and vegetables	Peeled fruits and vegetables

Warning: Sawdust Fiber

Some manufacturers have added something called alpha cellulose to their bread, creating, they say, a high-fiber, low-calorie bread. Alpha cellulose is, in fact, wood pulp, or highly refined sawdust. And it may not have the same beneficial effect on the body as do natural fibers. This fiber additive is pure cellulose, whereas natural food fibers are combinations of several different types, such as lignin, hemicelluloses, pectin, and cellulose.

Scientists are not sure which of these best prevent cancer and lower blood cholesterol, so to isolate cellulose may not be the wisest choice. In any event, look for the words on the label to be sure of what you are getting. One thing is sure: Although these breads may masquerade as healthful breads, they are not nearly as nutritious as whole-wheat bread, which has real fiber and many more nutrients.

Wrong Cooking Destroys Fiber

The way you cook high-fiber foods may also determine how much of the fiber your body can use. To get the most fiber from dried beans, you should soak them overnight, then cook them slowly at a low temperature. Cooking unsoaked dried beans in boiling water toughens the beans, reducing the release of fiber and other nutrients.

Too Much Fiber

Sudden shifting to a high-fiber diet may cause some discomfort. Extremely high doses have caused impactions (blockages) and ruptures of the bowel wall. Generally, you will adapt to a high-fiber diet, so side effects may be avoided by initiating it gradually. Is there a toxic dose for fiber? Neither government agencies nor scientific bodies have yet determined that. Dr. Barbara Harland, associate professor in the Department of Human Nutrition and Food at Howard University's School of Human Ecology, and a noted authority on fiber, cautions against consuming more than 45 grams of total dietary fiber daily for the average American. Children, being smaller, should consume less.

POSSIBLE SIDE EFFECTS OF A HIGH-FIBER DIET
Gastrointestinal irritation
Flatulence (this can be lessened by *gradually* adopting a high-fiber diet)
Bloating
Nausea, vomiting
Diarrhea
Impaction—a blockage in the lower bowel (due to extremely high amounts of wheat bran)
Rupture of the bowel wall (due to extremely high intakes of wheat bran)

Fiber Supplements

A number of companies make fiber supplements, usually as capsules or as powders to be sprinkled on other foods or dissolved in beverages. These products are a quick, easy way to add more fiber and are undoubtedly better than nothing for people who fail to get enough fiber in foods, or who may need it therapeutically, as prescribed by a physician. However, most people can reach the desired fiber levels without supplements. Also, food carries other vital nutrients, which may or may not be currently recognized. If abused, the high-fiber supplements can be dangerous. When not taken with a lot of water, they have become stuck in the throat, causing rupture of the esophagus. In excess, they can also cause the same side effects as high-fiber foods.

SUPER SOURCES OF SOLUBLE FIBER

(*Note:* Almost all high-fiber foods are also fairly low in calories. So you don't have to worry about adding calories and fat to get high doses of fiber.)

	Grams soluble fiber
Grains	
Oat bran: ⅓ c dry	2
All bran: ⅓ c	1.7
Oatmeal: ¾ c cooked	1.4
Rye bread: 2 slices	.6
Whole-wheat bread: 2 slices	.5
Dried beans and peas	
Black-eyed peas: ½ c cooked	3.7
Kidney beans: ½ c cooked	2.5
Pinto beans: ½ c cooked	2.3
Navy beans: ½ c cooked	2.3
Lentils: ½ c cooked	1.7
Split peas: ½ c cooked	1.7
Vegetables	
Peas: ½ c canned	2.7
Corn: ½ c cooked	1.7
Sweet potato: 1 baked	1.3
Zucchini: ½ c cooked	1.3
Cauliflower: ½ c cooked	1.3
Broccoli: ½ c cooked	.9
Fruits	
Prunes: 4 fruits	1.9
Pear: 1 fruit	1.1
Apple: 1 fruit	.9
Banana: 1 fruit	.8
Orange: 1 fruit	.7

Source: Janet Tietyen, research dietician with Dr. James Anderson, University of Kentucky Medical Center

SUPER SOURCES OF INSOLUBLE FIBER

	Grams total dietary fiber
Grains	
Whole wheat: 1 slice	1.6
Cracked wheat: 1 slice	1.2
Pumpernickel: 1 slice	.9
Barley: 1 oz dry	2.1
Wheat bran: 1 oz (about ¼ c)	11.3
Cereals, 1 oz	
All-Bran	8.5
Bran Buds	7.9
100% Bran	8.4
Bran Chex	4.6
40% Bran (Kellogg)	4
Corn Bran	5.3
Cracklin' Bran	4.3
Fiber One	12
Fruit 'N Fiber	2
Honey Bran	3.2
Raisin Bran (Kellogg)	3
Raisin Bran (Post)	3
Raisin Bran (Ralston-Purina)	3.6
Shredded Wheat (Nabisco)	2.6
Total	2
Wheat Chex	2
40% Bran Flakes (Ralston-Purina)	3.5
40% Bran Flakes (Post)	3.9
Fruits and vegetables	
Dates: 1 oz (about 3 dates)	1.4
Blueberries, raw: ½ c	2.1
Blackberries, raw: ½ c	3.2
Prunes: 1 oz (about 3 prunes)	1
Peas, green, cooked: ½ c	3.1
Lima beans, cooked: ½ c	3.8

Source: U.S. Department of Agriculture

Vitamin A
New Anti-Cancer Agent?

Vitamin A is an essential, fat-soluble vitamin with a key and versatile role in several important bodily processes. It is essential in cell differentiation, vision, immunity, and healthy skin, hair, and mucous membranes (linings of the mouth, stomach, intestines, lungs, uterus, vagina, bladder, eyelids, sinus, et cetera). It is also necessary for proper reproduction, bone growth, and development of teeth. New evidence shows that low vitamin A intake is associated with a higher incidence of certain cancers.

Who Is Deficient?

Your chances of consuming 100 percent of the recommended dietary allowance (RDA) for vitamin A are fifty-fifty. About 30 percent of Americans get less than 70 percent of the RDA. Women generally take in more vitamin A than men. However, studies show that some Americans take in as little as 10 percent of the recommended levels. Most apt to get too little vitamin A: young children and adolescents.

Although overt deficiencies of vitamin A with serious symptoms are rare, new evidence shows that mild deficiencies may subject a person to decreased immunity to infections and resistance to cancer. Therefore, some experts are convinced that everyone should consume the full recommended levels.

Vitamin A: Two Types

Vitamin A comes essentially in two varieties. One is the so-called active or preformed type, called retinol. Found only in animal foods, mainly liver, retinol is instantly available for bodily use. The other type of vitamin A, found in fruits and vegetables (orange and deep-green) is carotene or beta-carotene, also called provitamin A or a precursor to vitamin A. Beta-carotene must be converted by the body into active retinol-type vitamin A before it can be properly utilized.

SYMPTOMS OF VITAMIN A DEFICIENCY
Dry, rough skin
Slow growth
Thickening of bone
"Dry eye"
Night blindness
Increased susceptibility to infections

First Sign: Night Blindness

The first major sign of vitamin A deficiency is night blindness, or the inability to see in low levels of light. This condition is easily prevented and sometimes reversed by adequate vitamin A intake. (Even Hippocrates recommended beef liver to cure night blindness.) A prolonged vitamin A deficiency can destroy eyesight and cause death. Vision destruction from xerophthalmia ("dry eye") caused by vitamin A deficiency is rare in the United States, but mild symptoms do occasionally occur, notably among young children.

However, according to the World Health Organization, half a million children in Africa, Asia, and Latin America are permanently blinded each year by lack of vitamin A. An estimated five to ten million children worldwide suffer from night blindness and other severe symptoms of vitamin A deficiency.

Vitamin A Fights Infections

Although scientists have long suspected that vitamin A is a potent protector of the immune system, startling evidence of vitamin A-connected deaths adds urgent confirmation to that theory. Children in Indonesia with severe vitamin A deficiency, according to a large-scale study, had four to twelve times the death rate of children with adequate vitamin A. Fully 16 percent of the deaths were traced directly to vitamin A deficiency, according to chief investigator Dr. Alfred Sommer, a professor of ophthalmology at Johns Hopkins University.

Dr. Sommer ties the deaths to systemic infections that were allowed to flourish because of changes in the linings of the respiratory, urinary, and gastrointestinal tracts, caused by vitamin A deficiency. Dr. Sommer noted that vitamin A deficiencies can "interfere with normal immune responses." Other studies show that a vitamin A deficiency may suppress the immune system either directly or indirectly.

Anti-Cancer Agent?

The scientific community is in a flurry of excitement over the potential of vitamin A to prevent several kinds of cancer—lung, stomach, larynx, esophagus, bladder, and possibly colon, rectum, and prostate.

Convincing new evidence is accumulating, especially for lung cancer. Scientists at Roswell Park Memorial Institute in Buffalo, New York, found that heavy smokers who also consumed the fewest vitamin A foods had a two and a half times greater risk of lung cancer than smokers who ate lots of foods high in carotene.

Researcher Richard B. Shekelle, at the University of Texas, discovered a direct relationship between the amount of carotene foods eaten and the lung-cancer rate. Men smokers, he studied over a nineteen-year period, who ate the most beta-carotene foods had the lowest lung-cancer rates; the male smokers who ate the least carotene were eight times more likely to develop lung cancer. Dr. Shekelle pointed out that eating only half a cup of carrots a day might help protect against lung cancer—even in smokers. However, the carrot-eating smokers still had a higher rate of lung cancer than nonsmokers.

Although no one understands precisely how vitamin A influences cancer, it is believed that both retinol and beta-carotene may work, but in different ways and on different cancers. Synthetic retinoids (a concentrated variety of retinol vitamin A), when tested in animals and less extensively in humans, have prevented some forms of cancer. Even more powerful, it appears, is beta-carotene. A large-scale study is in progress at Harvard Medical School to test the anticancer effects of 50 mg of beta-carotene daily on twenty-two thousand physicians nationwide. The director of the study, Dr. Charles Hennekens, believes the beta-carotene prevents cancer by acting as an antioxidant in the body to protect cells against breakdown by dangerous roaming "free radicals" —substances thought to contribute to cancer.

DISEASES THAT MAY BE LINKED TO VITAMIN A DEFICIENCIES

Research on animals and/or humans proves or suggests a link between vitamin A deficiences and:

Night blindness

Xerophthalmia (the Greek word for "dry eye"—a common cause of widespread blindness in third-world countries)

Infections

Anemia (iron-deficiency related; in some cases vitamin A is required to correct the anemia)

Certain cancers, mainly lung, larynx, esophagus, stomach, and bladder

A Sweet Potato a Day

One of the fascinating findings is how little vitamin A may be needed for protection against cancer. One serving a day of rich carotene food may do it. Research suggests that a mere 100 percent of the RDA—1,000 REs or retinol equivalents (5,000 IUs or international units)—is protective. In one study the group with the lowest cancer risk ingested about 1,000 REs per day, while the group with the highest risk consumed only half that much. A medium-size sweet potato gives you twice the RDA of vitamin A per day.

Important: Don't boost your vitamin A intake by overdosing on liver. Liver is an excellent source of vitamin A, but it can be poisonous. A report in the *Journal of the American Medical Association* noted severe headaches and other symptoms similar to those of a brain tumor in several men and women who overdosed on liver. Their intakes were 60,000 to 87,000 IUs per day (15,000 to 17,000 REs); one patient ate 340,000 IUs (68,000 REs) per day. Two of the patients bought between 6 and 24 pounds of liver a week.

Vitamin A from beta-carotene foods or supplements is not dangerous, because the beta-carotene is not converted in the body to usable retinol-type vitamin A unless needed. The most beta-carotene can do is give you yellow skin, which goes away when you stop eating too much. Luckily, most of the vitamin A in the diet comes from beta-carotene.

The Body Soaks Up Vitamin A

Remarkably, most people absorb from 60 to 80 percent of the retinol vitamin A in their diets and about 20 to 25 percent of the beta-carotene. The more beta-carotene consumed, the lower the percentage absorbed. The body can store enough vitamin A to last an entire year or more, so even if you stop eating vitamin A, deficiency signs don't show up until the stored vitamin A is depleted.

Although most tissues contain some vitamin A, by far the greatest portion of it—over 90 percent—is stored in the liver. That is true of food animals too, which makes liver a megavitamin A food source. However, if you are deficient in vitamin A, little incoming vitamin A is directed to liver storage; instead, the vitamin A is instantly mobilized and rushed to needy tissues.

You need to eat some fat to absorb vitamin A, but it is virtually impossible with the American diet to eat so little fat as to block absorption of vitamin A. There is no evidence that even extremely low-fat diets jeopardize vitamin A utilization.

Vitamin A Antagonists and Helpers

Animal and/or human studies reveal that the following factors may affect how vitamin A is absorbed or utilized by the body; the extent of the effect depends on many unknowns, and the interaction may be important only if the antagonist or booster is of sufficient magnitude.

FACTORS THAT MAY BLOCK VITAMIN A, INCREASING NEED

Vitamin E megadoses (greater than 600 IUs daily) have interfered with absorption of beta-carotene

High fiber (more than 10 percent of diet)

Stress (Dr. Eli Seifter, Albert Einstein College of Medicine, says that stress can cause the body to lose up to 60 percent of its vitamin A)

Alcohol

FACTORS THAT MAY BOOST UTILIZATION OF VITAMIN A

Dietary fat deficiency (virtually unheard of in the United States)

Protein

Fiber (a little fiber—5 percent in diet—promotes absorption of beta-carotene; too much fiber, on the other hand, prevents absorption)

Lecithin (promotes beta-carotene absorption)

Iron

DRUGS THAT MAY DEPLETE VITAMIN A

Laxatives containing mineral oil

Cholestyramine (blood-cholesterol reducer)

Colchicine (anti-inflammatory agent)

Neomycin (antibiotic)

A New Way of Measuring Vitamin A

At one time, everybody measured vitamin A in food in international units (IUs). But, it is now known that that was imprecise because it did not take into account the conversion of carotene in the body. Now, vitamin A in food is measured in retinol equivalents (REs). The National Academy of Sciences lists the recommended daily allowances for vitamin A in REs, and others are converting their data to this new measurement.

The charts in this book list the vitamin A content of food in the new REs. However, you may still find some old listings and vitamin labels with the IUs. A rule of thumb is that 1 RE equals 10 IUs of beta-carotene (vitamin A from plants) and 3.33 IUs of vitamin A from animal foods. Thus, to get the approximate vitamin A REs for carrots, divide the number of IUs by ten. To do the same for liver, divide by 3.33.

Color Vitamin A Orange

The dozen foods highest in vitamin A (with the exception of liver) are orange or deep green. With good reason. The chemical compound vitamin A is a pale yellow; carotene is deep yellow, almost orange. Then what accounts for the bright green? The chlorophyll, or green pigment, of leafy vegetables simply covers up the orange carotene.

To get the most vitamin A, choose vegetables deepest in orange and green. The deeper-green the leaves of lettuce, the more vitamin A they have. The leafy parts of collard greens, turnip greens, and kale have much more vitamin A than the stems or midribs. Green asparagus has ten times more vitamin A than white asparagus. Romaine lettuce, the dark green kind, has four times more vitamin A than iceberg lettuce. The brighter orange a carrot, the richer in vitamin A. Color is the clue. However, that does not hold true for all fruits. Apricots and peaches are wonderful sources of vitamin A, but pineapples and oranges have modest amounts.

Cooking Cautions

Vitamin A is fairly resistant to damage from heat, water, and long periods of storage. However, it is sensitive to light. And prolonged cooking of green, red, and yellow vegetables causes chemical reactions that can reduce amounts of vitamin A by 15 to 35 percent. On the other hand, moderate cooking of vegetables, such as carrots, actually releases about 25 percent more vitamin A, possibly by breaking down the plant's cellular walls. The same thing, say experts, is probably true of green leafy vegetables like broccoli. (USDA figures assume a *loss* of vitamin A from cooking, thus, the charts in this book show more vitamin A in raw than in cooked carrots.)

Toxicity and Supplements

Too much of a good thing. Some experts are now as worried about vitamin A excess as vitamin A deficiency. Experts fear that publicity about high-powered retinoids (vitamin A–like drugs) to treat acne and possibly prevent cancer has put Americans on a vitamin A binge. "There is growing concern that hypervitaminosis A is becoming a clinical problem of increasing frequency and risk in the United States," Dr. DeWitt S. Goodman, of the Columbia University College of Physicians and Surgeons, recently wrote in the *New England Journal of Medicine*.

Vitamin A is dangerous stuff, because excesses are stored in the fat, primarily the liver, and can cause jaundice and liver damage. Doses of a mere 50,000 IUs daily have caused harm. Children, pregnant women, and adults with liver disease are most susceptible. From 5,000 to 10,000 REs daily is considered the minimum toxic dose, five to ten times the dietary recommended dose.

It is retinol in vitamin A, not the beta-carotene constituent, that apparently produces the toxic effects. The symptoms go away when you stop taking the overdoses.

SYMPTOMS OF VITAMIN A POISONING
Headache
Nausea
Vomiting
Bone pain
Very dry skin
Hair loss
Blurred vision
Skin sores
Itchy eyes
Blood abnormalities
Liver injury
Symptoms imitating a brain tumor

RICH SOURCES OF VITAMIN A

The most vitamin A by weight regardless of calories

Beef and pork liver	Dried apricots
Liverwurst	Winter squash
Carrots	Mangoes
Pumpkins	Collards
Sweet potatoes	Parsley
Dandelion greens	Turnip and beet greens
Spinach	Cantaloupe
Kale	Red peppers

SUPER SOURCES OF CAROTENE

	Mg per 100 g	Mg per serving
Carrots, raw and cooked	12	½ c: 6.6
Dandelion leaves	7.9	½ c: 4.3
Carrots, canned	7.3	½ c sliced: 5.3
Parsley leaves	7.3	10 sprigs: .7
Apricot, dried	4.7	10 halves: 1.6
Sweet potato, cooked	4.6	½ c: 2.7
Spinach, raw	4.2	½ c: 1.2
Kale	4.1	½ c: 2.7
Spinach, canned	3.3	½ c: 3.5
Mango	2.8	½ fruit: 2.8
Carrot juice	2.6	½ c: 3.2
Pumpkin	2	½ c: 2.4
Broccoli, cooked	1.9	½ c: 1.5
Apricot, raw	1.8	1 medium fruit: .6
Muskmelon	1.8	½ fruit: 4.8
Squash, winter	1.4	½ c: 1.4
Endive	1.1	½ c: .3
Tomato	.8	1 medium: .9
Lettuce	.8	10 leaves: .8
Papaya	.6	½ fruit: .9

Source: Calculations based on figures supplied by USDA

VITAMIN A SUPER-FOODS
THE MOST VITAMIN A, THE FEWEST CALORIES

Here are 50 foods that rate exceptionally high in vitamin A content per calorie. Of the approximately 2500 foods in this book, these have the greatest vitamin A nutrient density; that is, they have the best vitamin A-calorie ratios, giving you the most vitamin A for the fewest calories.

	Food Rating	Vitamin A-calorie ratio (RE of Vitamin A per 100 calories)	Common Measure	RE Vitamin A	Calories
1.	Beef, liver, braised	6577	3 oz	9011	137
2.	Carrots, raw	6542	½ c	1547	24
3.	Pumpkin, canned	6488	½ c	2691	41
4.	Carrot juice, canned	6437	½ c	3167	49
5.	Carrots, canned	5987	½ c	1005	17
6.	Carrots, fresh, cooked	5456	½ c	1915	35
7.	Spinach, canned	3817	½ c	939	25
8.	Spinach, fresh, cooked	3561	½ c	737	21

	Food Rating	Vitamin A-calorie ratio (RE of Vitamin A per 100 calories)	Common Measure	RE Vitamin A	Calories
9.	Dandelion greens, fresh, cooked	3545	½ c	608	17
10.	Cress, garden, fresh, cooked	3348	½ c	524	16
11.	Pork, liver, braised	3254	3 oz	4589	141
12.	Chicken, liver, simmered	3129	1 c	6878	220
13.	Spinach, raw	3054	½ c	188	6
14.	Turnip greens, fresh, cooked	2750	½ c	396	14
15.	Liverwurst, fresh	2546	1 oz	2353	93
16.	Peppers, sweet, red	2344	1 veg	422	18
17.	Kale, fresh, cooked	2312	½ c	481	21
18.	Turkey, liver, simmered	2214	1 c	5237	237
19.	Bok choi, fresh, cooked	2142	½ c	218	10
20.	Sweet potato, baked in skin	2118	½ c	2182	103
21.	Beet greens, fresh, cooked	1890	½ c	367	20
22.	Squash, butternut, baked	1750	½ c	714	41
23.	Sausage, liver cheese	1711	1 oz	1489	86
24.	Sweet potato, boiled mashed	1624	½ c	2796	172
25.	Peas and carrots, frozen	1617	½ c	621	38
26.	Collards, fresh, cooked	1586	½ c	211	13
27.	Chicken, giblets, simmered	1417	1 c	3232	228
28.	Amaranth, cooked	1319	½ c	183	14
29.	Braunschweiger, smoked (liver sausage)	1175	1 oz	1196	102
30.	Cantaloupe	920	½ fruit	861	94
31.	Sweet potatoes, in syrup, canned	663	½ c	702	106
32.	Vegetable juice cocktail, canned	616	½ c	142	22
33.	Mangoes	598	1 fruit	809	135
34.	Tomatoes, red, raw	595	1 veg	139	24
35.	Apricots, raw	543	3 fruit	277	
36.	Melon balls, frozen	536	1 c	307	58
37.	Turkey soup, chunky, canned	532	1 c	715	136
38.	Papaya, raw	515	1 fruit	611	117
39.	Chicken soup, chunky, canned	362	1 c	600	167
40.	Apricots, canned in water	495	3 halves	109	22
41.	Apricots, dried	304	10 halves	253	83
42.	Cherries, sour red, raw	256	1 c w pits	132	51
43.	Pâté de foie gras, canned (goose liver pâté)	216	1 oz	285	131
44.	Milk, skim	165	1 c	149	90
45.	Guava, raw	155	1 fruit	71	45

Food Rating	Vitamin A-calorie ratio (RE of Vitamin A per 100 calories)	Common Measure	RE Vitamin A	Calories
Cereals: five with highest vitamin A-calorie ratio				
46. Total	1504	1 oz	1502	100
47. Product 19	1390	1 oz	1502	108
48. All-Bran	532	1 oz	375	71
49. Bran Buds	513	1 oz	375	73
50. Oats, instant	434	1 pkt	455	104

Source: Author's computer analysis from USDA data

*Excludes baby foods. Includes only foods for which one serving supplies a minimum of approximately 10 percent of the RDA.

RECOMMENDED DAILY DIETARY ALLOWANCES OF VITAMIN A

Age	RE
1–6 months	420
6 months–3 years	400
4–6	500
7–10	700
Adult males	1000
Adult females	800
Pregnant	add 200
Nursing	add 400

Source: National Academy of Sciences/National Research Council, Revised 1980

Vitamin C
(Ascorbic acid)
Essential and Plentiful

Vitamin C, also known as ascorbic acid, is a water-soluble essential nutrient. Unlike most animals, humans cannot manufacture their own vitamin C. Vitamin C is critical in producing and maintaining collagen, a kind of basic protein glue that holds the body together, supporting and repairing muscles, bones, teeth, and skin. Vitamin C also helps fight infections and is important in producing hormones that regulate basal metabolic rate and body temperature.

Who Is Deficient?

Very few Americans need to worry about vitamin C deficiency, because our diet is full of it. The average American, of any age and either sex, consumes about one and a half times the recommended dietary allowance (RDA) for vitamin C. Only 15 percent of us eat less than half of the RDA. Experts do worry, though, that some pregnant women and the elderly may not get enough vitamin C. Serious cases of vitamin C–deficient scurvy have recently been reported in medical journals among the elderly who live alone, some of whom are also malnourished alcoholics. There is also some evidence that the elderly and pregnant women require more vitamin C.

SYMPTOMS OF MILD VITAMIN C DEFICIENCY
Easy bruising
Shortness of breath
Bleeding gums
Swollen or painful bone joints
Anemia
Nosebleeds
Digestive problems
Slow wound-healing
Longer-lasting infections

Wide-Ranging Health E

Vitamin C is undoubtedly one of those ʳ
guards health in a multitude of known and unkr
it dramatically boosts the absorption of iron fʳ
wonders in somehow augmenting the immune
deficiencies result in fewer white blood cells
killer agents for the immune system. Lately, much oᵢ ᵗⁱⁱⁱᵥ
has been attributed to the fact that it is an antioxidant; as such, ᵢₜ ᵤₑ
battle in the body with cancer-causing agents and dangerous elements
called free radicals, which participate in chemical reactions that leave
cells damaged and disorganized. Such cell destruction is thought to be
a prelude to cancer.

There is also evidence that people deficient in vitamin C are more
apt to have abnormal blood profiles, including higher cholesterol, pre-
disposing to heart disease. Increasing vitamin C intake has lowered
blood cholesterol and increased "good" HDL-type cholesterol.

Vitamin C and Cancer

Many cancer experts speculate that the widespread availability of
vitamin C in fruits and vegetables has reduced the rates of certain kinds
of cancers—mainly those of the stomach, esophagus, and larynx. The
incidence of stomach cancer has dropped in this century so as to be a
rare threat to Americans. One theory is that vitamin C helps counteract
cancer-causing agents, called nitrosamines, formed in the intestinal
tract by other foods such as cured meats. There have been other
studies showing lower rates of colon cancer in people who eat lots of
cabbage, which is high in vitamin C.

**HEALTH PROBLEMS THAT MAY BE LINKED TO VITAMIN C
DEFICIENCY**

Research on animals and/or humans proves or suggests a connection between vitamin C deficiencies and:

Common colds
Anemia
Atherosclerosis
Asthma
Cancer, especially stomach and esophagus cancers
Infertility in males
Rheumatoid arthritis
Cataracts

Scurvy:
The Classic Vitamin C Disease

Scurvy was that deadly scourge of sailors until 1747, when Dr. James Lind, a naval surgeon, discovered that the juice of lemons, limes, and oranges would cure it. Even so, scurvy has not been completely wiped out. Scurvy is the end stage of severe ascorbic-acid deprivation. In scurvy, muscles waste away, wounds don't heal, bruises appear, gums bleed and deteriorate, and bones develop improperly in children. Scurvy appears only after several months of severe vitamin C inadequacy. A mere 10 mg of vitamin C a day generally prevents scurvy.

A Saturation Point

You are likely to absorb from 80 to 90 percent of the vitamin C in food—high compared with other vitamins and minerals. Megadose vitamin C pills, however, are absorbed less efficiently. Absorption depends on the individual, but body tissues generally become saturated after 100 to 200 mg per day, and the excess vitamin C is flushed away by the kidneys.

Vitamin C Antagonists and Helpers

Animal and/or human studies reveal that the following factors may affect how vitamin C is absorbed or utilized by the body; the extent of the effect depends on many unknowns, and the interaction may be important only if the antagonist or booster is of sufficient magnitude.

FACTORS THAT MAY BLOCK VITAMIN C, INCREASING NEED
Smoking (smokers need about 50 percent more vitamin C than nonsmokers, because smoking somehow speeds up the metabolism of vitamin C)
Infections
Environmental pollutants
Stress (such as surgery, burns, trauma)
Alcohol
Pectin (a fiber in citrus foods)
Erythorbic acid (a food additive)

DRUGS THAT MAY DEPLETE VITAMIN C
Tetracycline
Aspirin in high doses

Vitamin C: Easily Lost, Easily Saved

Vitamin C is the most unstable of all vitamins and minerals. As much as 100 percent can be destroyed by cooking and processing. Fortunately, citrus fruits and tomatoes—excellent sources of vitamin C—retain the vitamin well. Here are some pointers to minimize loss of vitamin C.

Use a sharp blade when trimming, cutting, or shredding vegetables; a dull knife tends to bruise the vegetable tissues, releasing vitamin C.

Wrap cabbage or keep it in the vegetable crisper of the refrigerator, where humidity is high.

Let tomatoes ripen out of the sun at sixty to seventy-five degrees F. Overripe tomatoes lose vitamin C.

Cook vegetables only until tender in small amounts of water in a pan with a tight-fitting lid. Vitamin C leaches into water; the more water, the greater the loss. For example, if the water is four times the volume of the cabbage, you lose about half of the vitamin C. If the water equals about one-third the amount of cabbage, you lose only 10 percent of the vitamin C.

Boil or bake tuber and root vegetables such as carrots and potatoes in their skins; this retains more vitamin C and other nutrients.

Stir-frying vegetables conserves vitamin C.

Reheating or storing cooked vegetables causes loss of vitamin C—one day in the refrigerator can slash the vitamin C in cooked vegetables by 25 percent. Cooked vegetables held in the refrigerator for two or three days have only one-third to one-half the amount of vitamin C.

You get about two-thirds of the vitamin C when you squeeze an orange for its juice as when you eat the orange sections. Orange juice from all sources—fresh, reconstituted, or canned—keeps in the refrigerator for several days without loss of vitamin C.

Freezing fresh fruits causes very little damage to vitamin C.

Microwave cooking of vegetables, especially without added water, saves vitamin C.

Toxicity and Supplements

Clearly, vitamin C is of low toxicity—even in megadoses. Although high doses may not be desirable for various reasons (for example, supplements of vitamin C can destroy B_{12} and reduce absorption of copper), vitamin C does not seem to be toxic in doses up to 5,000 mg per day. And many people have taken much higher doses of vitamin C over long periods with no observable adverse effects.

Since vitamin C is water soluble, amounts in excess of what the body can use are rather rapidly excreted. However, some individuals can't tolerate high doses of vitamin C, and may experience diarrhea and abdominal cramping from as little as 500 mg a day.

POSSIBLE SIDE EFFECTS OF VITAMIN C MEGADOSES

Gastrointestinal disturbances, related to the laxative effect of vitamin C

Diarrhea

Abdominal cramps

Promotion of kidney stones in susceptible persons

Allergic reactions (very rare)

Reduction of copper status in the body

Warning: High doses of vitamin C can alter the results of certain diagnostic tests, including urine and blood tests. For example, large doses of vitamin C can give a false reading on sugar in the urine and on blood in the stool. If you use vitamin C supplements, tell your physician, so that this can be considered when interpreting the results of certain diagnostic tests.

Vitamin C Withdrawal

If you take huge doses of vitamin C and then suddenly stop, you could experience something called "rebound scurvy," temporary scurvylike withdrawal symptoms, while your body readjusts to lower doses. Also, pregnant women taking megadoses of vitamin C have given birth to infants with "rebound scurvy," which was corrected by

---

FOODS RICH IN VITAMIN C

The most vitamin C by weight regardless of calories

Green and red peppers	Peas
Guavas	Cantaloupe
Kiwi fruit	Apple juice
Orange juice	Potatoes
Grapefruit juice	Tomatoes
Papayas	Blackberries
Broccoli	Cherries
Cauliflower	Kale
Cabbage	Tangerines
Strawberries	Brussels sprouts
Oranges	

gradually decreasing amounts of vitamin C supplements. Such cases of vitamin C dependency are rare, but have happened.

Warning: Pregnant women should not take megadoses of any vitamin (including C), mineral, or drug without medical supervision. If you cut down on vitamin C, do it gradually to avoid "rebound scurvy."

VITAMIN C SUPER-FOODS
THE MOST VITAMIN C, THE FEWEST CALORIES

Here are 50 foods that rate exceptionally high in vitamin C content per calorie. Of the approximately 2500 foods in this book, these are tops in vitamin C nutrient density; they have the highest vitamin C-calorie ratios, giving you the most vitamin C for the fewest calories.*

	Food Rating	Vitamin C-calorie ratio (mg of Vitamin C per 100 calories)	Common Measure	Mg Vitamin C	Calories
1.	Acerola (cherry), raw	5242	1 fruit	80	2
2.	Peppers, sweet, red, raw	760	1 pepper	141	18
3.	Peppers, sweet, green or red, cooked	619	1 pepper	81	13
4.	Peppers, hot chili green or red	606	1 pepper	109	18
5.	Peppers, sweet, green, raw	512	1 pepper	95	18
6.	Guavas, raw	360	1 fruit	165	45
7.	Pimientos, canned	352	4 oz	107	30
8.	Bok choi, raw	346	½ c	16	5
9.	Broccoli, raw	333	½ c	41	12
10.	Cauliflower, raw	333	½ c	36	12
11.	Currants, European black, raw	287	½ c	101	36
12.	Kale, raw	240	½ c	41	17
13.	Cauliflower, fresh, cooked	231	½ c	34	15
14.	Broccoli, fresh, cooked	217	½ c	49	23
15.	Cabbage, common, raw	212	½ c	17	8
16.	Amaranth, cooked	196	½ c	27	14
17.	Strawberries, raw	189	1 c	84	45
18.	Lemons, wo peel	183	1 med	31	17
19.	Sauerkraut juice, canned	180	1 c	44	24
20.	Mustard greens, fresh, cooked	169	½ c	18	11
21.	Kiwi fruit	161	1 fruit	74	46
22.	Brussels sprouts, fresh, cooked	159	1 veg	13	8
23.	Papaya, raw	158	1 fruit	188	117
24.	Vegetable juice cocktail, canned	146	½ c	33	22
25.	Turnip greens, fresh, cooked	137	½ c	20	15
26.	Kale, fresh, cooked	128	½ c	27	21

Food Rating	Vitamin C ratio (mg of Vitamin C per 100 calories)	Common Measure	Mg Vitamin C	Calories
27. Grapefruit	108	½ fruit	42	38
28. Cantaloupe	121	½ fruit	113	94
29. Cabbage, common, cooked	116	½ c	18	16
30. Oranges	113	1 fruit	70	62
31. Orange juice, fresh	111	from 1 fruit	43	39
32. Turnip greens, canned	111	½ c	18	17
33. Brussels sprouts, frozen, cooked	109	½ c	36	33
34. Asparagus, fresh, cooked	108	½ c	24	22
35. Tomato juice, canned	108	½ c	22	21
36. Orange juice, chilled or from concentrate	97	4 fl oz	52	56
37. Asparagus, canned	97	½ c	22	24
38. Tomatoes, red, ripe, raw	93	1 veg	22	24
39. Mandarin oranges, canned in juice	92	½ c	42	46
40. Grapefruit, sections, canned in juice	92	½ c	42	46
41. Orange juice, unsweetened, canned	82	4 fl oz	44	52
42. Turnips, raw	78	½ c	14	18
43. Tomato soup, canned	78	1 c	66	86
44. Fruit, mixed, frozen	76	1 c:thawed	187	245

Source: Author's computer analysis from USDA data

*Excludes baby foods. Includes only foods for which one serving supplies a minimum of approximately 10 percent of the RDA.

RECOMMENDED DAILY DIETARY
ALLOWANCES OF VITAMIN C

Age	Milligrams
Birth to 1 year	35
1–10	45
11–14	50
Males and females, over age 14	60
Pregnant	add 20
Nursing	add 40

Source: National Academy of Sciences, Revised 1980

Thiamin
The "Nerve" Vitamin

Thiamin, also called B₁, is an essential vitamin of the B complex family. Thiamin is concentrated in the skeletal muscle, heart, liver, kidneys, and brain. (About 50 percent of it is found in the muscles.) It is essential in the metabolism of carbohydrates, thus is known as an "energy" vitamin. Because it is critical for the transmission of high-frequency impulses in the central nervous system and is vitally linked with the health of the nervous system, it is also called the "nerve" vitamin.

Who Needs to Worry?

In general, a thiamin-poor diet is not common. The U.S. Department of Agriculture's food-consumption survey showed that 55 percent of Americans take in over 100 percent of the recommended dietary allowances, and only 17 percent consume less than 70 percent of the RDAs. Serious thiamin deficits, so grave in the last century, have disappeared mainly because of the enrichment of flour, breads, and cereals.

Nevertheless, surveys show that pockets of the population lack or do not properly metabolize enough thiamin. Pregnant women, the elderly, and primarily heavy drinkers often face thiamin deficiencies. The government's Ten State Nutrition Survey revealed that 45 to 50 percent of all pregnant women take in less than two-thirds of the RDA for thiamin.

The High-Risk Elderly

Especially vulnerable are older people who don't eat enough thiamin or lose their ability to utilize it. A Colorado study of seventy elderly women pinpointed thiamin as the most common nutritional deficiency, confirmed by blood tests. Twenty-five percent of elderly people living at home suffered a thiamin deficiency, according to another study. Several studies show that older women eating low-calorie diets tend to take in less of the RDA than do men. Overall, according to blood samples, an estimated 10 to 20 percent of elderly Americans show biological evidence of thiamin deficiency. Another 25 percent may be marginally deficient with no signs. Older people are more quickly affected by even moderate depletions of thiamin and are slow to respond to increased intakes of thiamin.

Also, in a major study of general psychiatric patients, 53 percent were deficient in either thiamin, riboflavin, or vitamin B_6; the most common deficiency was thiamin. Because thiamin deficiency does have a profound effect on the nervous system, some experts suggest that it may be associated with some forms of mental disorders. Thiamin deficiency can also be mistaken for senile dementia or Alzheimer's disease.

Heavy Drinking: An Added Hazard

Most of the serious symptoms related to thiamin deficiency in all developed countries are related to alcohol consumption. Heavy drinkers get a double whammy; they not only consume less thiamin, but much of it is not absorbed in the body. Apparently, alcohol use, especially over long periods of time, injures the small intestine, impairing the ability to absorb thiamin. One study showed a malabsorption problem in about half of hospitalized alcoholics. Absorption became normal after six weeks of abstaining from alcohol. Biochemical tests on another group of alcoholics showed that 25 percent had a thiamin deficiency.

Consequently, heavy drinkers are the number-one victims of a thiamin-deficiency nerve disease called Wernicke's encephalopathy, or Wernicke-Korsakoff syndrome, both serious disorders. Some alcoholics may also have a genetic defect making them susceptible to the disease.

Early signs: extreme loss of appetite, which only exacerbates the condition; nystagmus (involuntary rapid eye movements); ataxia (loss of balance); and mental disturbances such as anxiety, loss of concentration, loss of short-term memory, depression, and disorientation. Hallucinations and coma may occur unless the disease is reversed by administration of thiamin. Wernicke's disease is considered a medical emergency, requiring injections of thiamin; the earlier the treatment, the greater the chances for improvement. In some cases a chronic memory disorder—Korsakoff's psychosis—persists despite vigorous administration of thiamin.

Thiamin deficiency is such a common consequence of heavy drinking that there have been proposals to fortify alcoholic beverages with thiamin just as we do bread.

Beriberi and Other Damage

Since a thiamin lack is usually accompanied by other B vitamin deficiencies, its particular signs are difficult to spot, and there is evidence from autopsies that serious cases of thiamin deficiency often go overlooked. The end stage of thiamin deficiency is the dread disease called beriberi, once deadly among seamen. Beriberi, still a surprisingly widespread scourge in parts of the world, is extremely rare in the United States, although cases of alcohol-induced beriberi occasionally show up.

Primarily, thiamin deficiency attacks the cardiovascular system and the nervous system, rending its victims weak, mentally disabled, and with permanent heart damage. The severity of the symptoms, of course, depend on how drastic and longstanding the deficiency is. Most symptoms of thiamin deficiency disappear rather quickly after oral intake or injections of thiamin. In a group of women, mild symptoms were gone in one day after a dose of 1.4 mg, a little over the daily recommended amount. Severe deficiencies may require injections of 100 to 200 mg of thiamin.

SYMPTOMS OF THIAMIN DEFICIENCY
Early signs
Loss of appetite
Nausea
Vomiting
Constipation
Painful calf muscles
Depression
Fatigue
Poor eye-hand coordination
Irritability
Headaches
Vague feelings of anxiety, uneasiness, and fear

Advanced signs
(beriberi is the classic end-stage disease from chronic thiamin deficiency; some of its consequences):
Swelling of the limbs
Atrophy of leg muscles, causing difficulty in walking
Emaciation
Mental confusion
Loss of short-term memory
Hallucinations
Heart failure
Coma
Death

HEALTH PROBLEMS THAT MAY BE LINKED TO THIAMIN DEFICIENCY

Research on animals and/or humans proves or suggests a connection between thiamin deficiencies and:

> Beriberi, the classic thiamin-deficiency disease
> Vision problems (Thiamin combined with vitamin A clears up night blindness better than vitamin A alone.)
> Wernicke-Korsakoff syndrome
> Constipation
> Depression
> Anxiety
> Heart damage
> Central nervous system disorders

Thiamin Antagonists and Helpers

Animal and/or human studies reveal that the following factors may affect how thiamin is absorbed or utilized by the body; the extent of the effect depends on many unknowns, and the interaction may be important only if the antagonist or booster is of sufficient magnitude.

FACTORS THAT MAY BOOST UTILIZATION OF THIAMIN

> Vitamin C
> Garlic
> Onions
> Dietary fat

FACTORS THAT MAY BLOCK THIAMIN, INCREASING NEED

> Alcohol (Even the amount of alcohol in two glasses of beer or wine or two shots of whiskey can interfere with the absorption of thiamin taken in at the same time. However, regular heavy drinking is needed to induce malabsorption injury and consequent thiamin deficiency.)
> Coffee, including decaffeinated coffee (In one study, a quart of coffee in a three-hour period reduced the absorption of thiamin by about 45 percent, compared with plain water.)
> Tea, possibly from the tannin in tea leaves or other chemicals (Tea is a potent destroyer of thiamin, although the vitamin is somewhat protected if vitamin C is consumed at the same time as the tea.)
> Sugar and other carbohydrates
> Baking soda
> Betel nuts
> Fermented fish

Thiaminase, an enzyme in some raw fish and raw shellfish. (For this reason, raw fish used for Japanese sushi and sashimi may not be a good source of thiamin. The enzyme is destroyed by cooking.)

Deficiencies in magnesium, B_6, B_{12}, or folacin (Adequate levels of all are needed for proper thiamin functions.)

Smoking

Stress

Cooking

To avoid losses of water-soluble thiamin, cook with as little water as possible, and as quickly as possible. The higher the heat, the greater the loss, although microwaving does not seem to increase losses. Pork roasted at 163 degrees centigrade retains 75 to 100 percent of its original thiamin—much less if the heat is higher.

Also, for some reason, the thiamin in certain foods is more vulnerable to heat destruction. More thiamin is lost from spinach, liver, and lamb than from peas, beans, pork, and carrots.

Important: Adding baking soda, an alkali, to cooking water destroys thiamin (and vitamin C). Washing rice before cooking partly flushes away many nutrients, including thiamin.

Toxicity and Supplements

Thiamin, like other water-soluble vitamins, is considered exceptionally safe on the assumption that excesses will be flushed out of the body. One expert puts the minimum toxic dose at 300 mg, about 200 times the recommended daily allowance.

However, other authorities report side effects from only 10 mg of thiamin per day taken for two and a half weeks, including headache, irritability, insomnia, rapid pulse, and weakness. Injections of thiamin have caused allergic reactions.

FOODS RICH IN THIAMIN

The most thiamin by weight regardless of calories

Wheat germ	Pecans
Pork	Peanuts
Beef	Bacon
Pine nuts	Sausage
Brazil nuts	Beef and lamb kidneys
Ham	Walnuts
Salami	Wheat bran
Hickory nuts	

THIAMIN SUPER-FOODS
THE MOST THIAMIN, THE FEWEST CALORIES

Here are 50 foods that rate exceptionally high in thiamin content per calorie. Of the approximately 2500 foods listed in this book, these have the greatest thiamin nutrient density; that is, they have the highest thiamin-calorie ratios, giving you the most thiamin for the fewest calories.*

	Food Rating	Thiamin-calorie ratio (mg of Thiamin per 100 calories)	Common Measure	Mg Thiamin	Calories
1.	Brewer's yeast	5.5	1 tbsp	1.2	23
2.	Ham, extra lean, roasted or canned	.8	3 oz	.9	116
3.	Luncheon meat, ham, extra lean	.7	2 slices	.5	74
4.	Pork, chop, lean, broiled	.5	1 chop	.8	166
5.	Wheat germ	.5	1 oz	.5	108
6.	Peas and carrots, frozen, cooked	.5	½ c	.2	38
7.	Canadian bacon, cooked	.5	2 slices	.4	86
8.	Luncheon meat, luxury loaf	.5	1 oz	.2	40
9.	Melon balls, frozen	.5	1 c	.3	58
10.	Peas, green, frozen, cooked	.4	½ c	.2	62
11.	Soybean sprouts, cooked	.4	1 c	.2	76
12.	Sunflower seeds	.4	1 oz	.6	162
13.	New England Brand sausage	.4	1 oz	.2	46
14.	Pigeonpeas, green, cooked	.3	½ c	.3	85
15.	Squash, acorn, baked	.3	½ c	.2	57
16.	Pork, loin, lean, braised	.3	1 chop	.5	166
17.	Ham, chopped	.3	1 slice	.2	65

	Food Rating	Thiamin-calorie ratio (mg of Thiamin per 100 calories)	Common Measure	Mg Thiamin	Calories
18.	Peas, green, fresh, cooked	.3	½ c	.2	67
19.	Luncheon meat, minced ham	.3	1 oz	.2	75
20.	Soup, crab, canned	.3	1 c	.2	76
21.	Wild pig, cooked	.3	3 oz	.6	197
22.	Bran, unprocessed	.3	¼ c	.1	31
23.	Soup, green pea, mix	.2	1 c:prep	.2	133
24.	Corn, yellow, fresh, cooked	.2	½ c	.2	89
25.	Pompano, broiled/baked	.2	3 oz	.4	218
26.	Bread, flat, pita	.2	1 small	.2	165
27.	Muffins, English	.2	1 muffin	.2	132
28.	Pike, broiled/baked	.2	3 oz	.2	110
29.	Bread, bran	.2	1 slice	.2	110
30.	Crab, fresh, cooked	.2	2 med blue	.2	89
31.	Oysters, wo shell, raw	.2	3 oz	.1	56
32.	Luncheon meat (Mother's loaf)	.2	1 oz	.2	80
33.	Salami, pork, dry or hard	.2	1 oz	.3	126
34.	Bratwurst, cooked	.2	3 oz	.5	256
35.	Italian sausage, cooked	.2	1 link	.5	268
36.	Brazil nuts	.2	1 oz	.3	186
37.	Soybeans, green, cooked	.2	½ c	.2	127
38.	Sesame butter, tahini	.2	1 oz	.3	169
39.	Pine nuts	.2	1 oz	.2	146
40.	Lamb, liver, broiled	.2	1.6 oz	.2	117
41.	Buckwheat, whole-grain	.2	3½ oz	.6	335
42.	Watermelon, raw	.2	1/16 fruit	.4	152
43.	Beef, kidneys, simmered	.1	3 oz	.2	122
44.	Soybean curd (tofu)	.1	½ c	.1	66
45.	Cowpeas (incl. blackeye), dry, cooked	.1	½ c	.1	89

Cereals: five with highest thiamin-calorie ratio

46.	Total	1.5	1 oz	1.5	100
47.	Product 19	1.4	1 oz	1.5	108
48.	100% Bran	.9	1 oz	.7	76
49.	Puffed wheat, fortified	.7	½ oz	.4	52
50.	Oats, instant	.5	1 pkt	.5	104

Source: Author's computer analysis from USDA data

*Excludes baby foods. Includes only foods for which a serving supplies a minimum of approximately 10 percent of the RDA.

RECOMMENDED DAILY DIETARY ALLOWANCES
OF THIAMIN

Age	Milligrams
Birth–6 months	.3
6 months–1 year	.5
1–3	.7
4–6	.9
7–10	1.2
Males	
11–18	1.4
19–22	1.5
23–50	1.4
51 and over	1.2
Females	
11–22	1.1
23 and over	1
Pregnant	add .4
Nursing	add .5

Source: National Academy of Sciences, Revised 1980

Riboflavin
(Vitamin B₂)

Milk Drinker's Delight

Riboflavin, a water-soluble B vitamin, is essential for growth and repair of tissues and aids in DNA synthesis. It works with other substances to metabolize protein, fats, and carbohydrates; thus, it is critical for the release of energy. Riboflavin is found in every cell of the body.

Who Is Deficient?

Experts are beginning to suspect that riboflavin deficiency is much more extensive than previously thought. Although most Americans eat high amounts of riboflavin-rich foods, which should theoretically prevent deficiencies, biological surveys show some disturbing signs of deficiency, notably in youngsters, especially those in low-income families.

According to the U.S. Department of Agriculture's most recent ten-year food-consumption survey, 66 percent of Americans eat more than 100 percent of the recommended dietary allowances (RDAs) of this B vitamin, making it one of the highest nutrients consumed (along with protein, niacin, and vitamin B_{12}). Only 12 percent of the population consumed less than 70 percent of the RDA. The average American in all age groups takes in the recommended levels.

Nevertheless, children, especially of lower socioeconomic status, show signs of deficiencies. A study of 431 high-school students turned up biological evidence of subnormal riboflavin intakes in 16 percent of the girls and 6 percent of the boys. The deficiency was reversed by half a milligram of riboflavin per day for a week. A major study of 210 white, Hispanic-American, and black teenagers in New York City found biological evidence of riboflavin deficiency in 26 percent of them. In another survey, one out of four of a group of adolescent girls evidenced deficiencies. Surveys among the elderly have shown about one-third lacking in riboflavin.

People who exercise heavily or engage in strenuous physical work, such as construction workers, may need more riboflavin.

Alcoholics often show signs of marginal deficiencies of vitamin B_2.

A Complex Deficiency

A riboflavin deficiency is hard to spot because it is usually linked to a lack of other B vitamins. Foods that are rich in riboflavin are also rich in the complex of B vitamins. Additionally, the lack of riboflavin blocks the metabolism of niacin, folic acid, and B$_6$. If you are deficient in riboflavin, you are likely to be deficient in other B vitamins.

Further, the worse a riboflavin deficiency is, the worse it becomes, because without a good supply of riboflavin you lose the ability to make use of the little you do have. The deficiency feeds upon itself in a vicious circle. According to Dr. Richard Rivlin of Cornell University Medical College, a noted authority on riboflavin, animal studies suggest that "The less you have, the less you are able to utilize. Once the body gets sick, it gets sicker, because it lacks the enzyme for converting riboflavin into its metabolically active form and therefore cannot utilize what little vitamin there is in the diet."

Signs of deficiency appear only after low intakes for many months.

SIGNS OF RIBOFLAVIN DEFICIENCY
Fuchsia or purplish colored tongue
Cracks at the corners of the mouth
Sores and burning of the lips, mouth, and tongue
Itchy inflamed eyelids
Flaky skin around the nose, ears, eyebrows, or hairline
Light sensitivity to the eyes
More advanced signs are anemia and nerve disorders

Health Consequences

Nobody really knows what the subtle consequences of marginal riboflavin deficiencies might be—as one researcher suggested, perhaps nothing more than feeling slighty ill, lackadaisical, mildly anemic, and easily tired. Scientists have been tracking down several leads on more concrete riboflavin-deficiency consequences. Although there are few final conclusions, here is some of the evidence.

The Cataract Connection

For more than half a century, researchers have noted a connection between riboflavin deprivation and cataracts in laboratory animals. Rats, pigs, kittens, salmon, and trout deprived of riboflavin have developed cataracts. And researchers have found the same thing in humans. One study done by physicians at the University of Alabama noted that of a group of patients over age fifty with cataracts, 34 percent had blood deficient in riboflavin. Startlingly, *none* of the patients over age fifty without cataracts had riboflavin-deficient blood. Although this is a lead, experts are still not sure that there is a definite connection.

Birth Defects in Animals

Unquestionably, a lack of riboflavin in pregnant animals causes a variety of severe birth defects, including cleft palate and grossly deformed skeletons. Pregnant women often have low levels of riboflavin. Thus, although it is not certain that riboflavin deficits can cause birth defects in humans, there is sufficient concern that experts warn pregnant women to take in adequate riboflavin to be on the safe side.

If you exercise heavily, you also need more riboflavin than the RDAs call for to stay healthy. Young women put on strenuous jogging programs used up about 16 percent more riboflavin than when they were not exercising.

HEALTH PROBLEMS THAT MAY BE LINKED TO RIBOFLAVIN DEFICIENCY

Research on animals and/or humans proves or suggests a connection between riboflavin deficiencies and:

Cataracts

Birth defects

Anemia (probably as a result of a disturbance in the body's ability to metabolize folacin because of lack of riboflavin)

Riboflavin Antagonists and Helpers

Animal and/or human studies reveal that the following factors may affect how riboflavin is absorbed or utilized by the body; the extent of the effect depends on many unknowns, and the interaction may be important only if the antagonist or booster is of sufficient magnitude.

FACTORS THAT MAY BOOST UTILIZATION OF RIBOFLAVIN

Lactose

Fiber, especially coarse bran

Meals that are large, hot, and contain fat (Studies show that under such conditions, riboflavin remains in the stomach and intestines longer, allowing more time for it to be absorbed.)

FACTORS THAT MAY BLOCK RIBOFLAVIN, INCREASING NEED
Caffeine
Zinc
Iron
Copper
Saccharin
Vitamin C

DRUGS THAT MAY DEPLETE RIBOFLAVIN
Chlorpromazine, thorazine, other phenothiazines (potent antipsychosis tranquilizers)
Tricyclic antidepressants, imipramine, and amitriptyline (Tofranil and Elavil)
Thyroid hormones

The Pill: A Question

At one time experts thought that oral contraceptives destroyed riboflavin, causing deficiencies. More recent studies failed to find riboflavin deficiencies in American women who take the pill and consume adequate levels of riboflavin. Although the issue is still scientifically unsettled, many experts believe that the pill does not directly affect riboflavin in women who are not malnourished in the vitamin in the first place.

Milk: A Quick, Easy Source

One of the best ways to become deficient in riboflavin is to scorn milk and other dairy products. That's where about 35 percent of our riboflavin comes from. The New York City study of youths deficient in riboflavin found that those who drank the least milk had the lowest levels of riboflavin. Those with the highest levels of riboflavin drank three cups of milk a day; those with the lowest levels, a mere cup a week. Black teenagers were especially at risk because they often cannot tolerate the lactose in milk; in those with lactose intolerance, milk causes cramping and diarrhea. People who drink milk seldom lack riboflavin.

Few Cooking Losses

You are not likely to lose much riboflavin in cooking or canning when the juices are saved. It is fairly heat-stable and not very soluble in water. Roast beef and pork retain from 70 to 90 percent of their riboflavin. Perhaps 10 to 30 percent might be lost in cooking vegetables if the juice is discarded. *Note:* Riboflavin is destroyed by ultraviolet or sunlight; for example, a glass of milk exposed to light for four hours would lose up to 40 percent of its riboflavin.

Important: Do not add baking soda to vegetables when cooking; the sodium bicarbonate creates an alkaline solution in which great amounts of riboflavin can be lost.

Toxicity and Supplements

Riboflavin is considered one of the safest vitamins. One expert puts the minimum toxic dose at 1,000 mg, 588 times the U.S. recommended daily allowance. Excessive riboflavin is generally flushed out of the body through the kidneys within several hours.

FOODS RICH IN RIBOFLAVIN

The most riboflavin per weight regardless of calories

Liver of all types	Duck
Brewer's yeast	Goose
Milk	Smoked eel
Almonds	Yogurt
Cheese	Fortified cereals
Fish roe	Eggs
Wheat germ	Pork

RIBOFLAVIN SUPER-FOODS
THE MOST RIBOFLAVIN, THE FEWEST CALORIES

Here are 50 foods that rate exceptionally high in riboflavin content per calorie. Of the approximately 2500 foods in this book, these are tops in riboflavin nutrient density; they have the highest riboflavin-calorie ratios, giving you the most riboflavin for the fewest calories.*

	Food Rating	Riboflavin-calorie ratio (mg of Riboflavin per 100 calories)	Common Measure	Mg Riboflavin	Calories
1.	Beef, liver, braised	2.6	3 oz	3.5	137
2.	Lamb, liver, broiled	2	1.6 oz	2.3	117
3.	Mushrooms, raw	1.9	1 c	.1	5
4.	Calf, liver, fried	1.6	3 oz	3.5	222
5.	Pork, liver, braised	1.5	3 oz	1.9	141
6.	Brewer's yeast	1.5	1 tbsp	.3	23
7.	Chicken, livers, simmered	1.1	1 c	2.4	219
8.	Beet greens, fresh, cooked	1.1	½ c	.2	20
9.	Spinach, fresh, cooked	1	½ c	.2	21
10.	Broccoli, fresh, cooked	.7	½ c	.2	23
11.	Beef heart, braised	.7	3 oz	1.3	148
12.	Sausage, liver cheese	.7	1 oz	.6	86
13.	Pâté, chicken liver, canned	.7	1 oz	.4	57
14.	Chicken giblets, simmered	.6	1 c	1.4	228
15.	Roe, herring	.6	1 tbsp	.1	18
16.	Milk, dry, nonfat	.5	1 oz	.5	100
17.	Caviar	.5	1 tbsp	.2	46
18.	Roe, shad, cooked	.5	½ oz	.1	22
19.	Milk, skim	.5	1 c	.4	90
20.	Venison, stewed	.4	3 oz	.5	153
21.	Milk, lowfat, 1% fat	.4	1 c	.4	102
22.	Yogurt, skim milk	.4	4 oz	.3	63
23.	Braunschweiger (liver cheese)	.4	1 oz	.4	102
24.	Mung bean sprouts, cooked	.4	½ c	.1	31
25.	Buttermilk	.4	1 c	.4	99
26.	Oysters, smoked	.3	3 oz	.2	91
27.	Milk, lowfat, 2% fat	.3	1 c	.4	121
28.	Cheese, feta	.3	1 oz	.2	75
29.	Cheese, gjetost	.3	1 oz	.4	132
30.	Milk, whole, 3.3% fat	.3	1 c	.4	150
31.	Liverwurst	.3	1 oz	.3	93
32.	Oysters, raw	.3	3 oz	.2	56
33.	Cod, dried	.3	1 oz	.1	36
34.	Eggs	.2	1 large	.2	79
35.	Mackerel, boneless, broiled	.2	3 oz	.3	213
36.	Wheat germ	.2	½ c	.4	216
37.	Sardines, canned, tomato sauce	.2	.8 oz	.1	47
38.	Ham, extra lean, canned	.2	3 oz	.3	116
39.	Pork, lean, roasted	.2	3 oz	.4	207
40.	Turkey, dark meat, roasted	.2	3½ oz	.3	187
41.	Cheese, roquefort type	.2	1 oz	.2	105
42.	Cottage cheese, dry	.2	4 oz	.2	96
43.	Whiting, broiled/baked	.2	3 oz	.2	97
44.	Clams, raw	.2	3 oz	.2	65
45.	Bread, bran	.2	1 slice	.2	110

Food Rating	Riboflavin-calorie ratio (mg of Riboflavin per 100 calories)	Common Measure	Mg Riboflavin	Calories
Cereals: five with highest riboflavin-calorie ratio				
46. Total	1.7	1 oz	1.7	100
47. Product 19	1.6	1 oz	1.7	108
48. 100% Bran	1	1 oz	.8	76
49. Life	.6	1 oz	.6	104
50. All-Bran	.6	1 oz	.4	71

Source: Author's computer analysis from USDA data

*Excludes baby foods. Includes only foods for which one serving supplies a minimum of approximately 10 percent of the RDA.

RECOMMENDED DAILY DIETARY ALLOWANCES OF RIBOFLAVIN

Age	Milligrams
Birth–6 months	.4
6 months–1 year	.6
1–3	.8
4–6	1
7–10	1.4
Males	
11–14	1.6
15–22	1.7
23–50	1.6
51 and over	1.4
Females	
11–22	1.3
23 and over	1.2
Pregnant	add .3
Nursing	add .5

Source: National Academy of Sciences, Revised 1980

Niacin
So Much for So Little

Niacin, sometimes called B₃, is the term for a group of the B complex vitamins, including nicotinic acid and nicotinamide. Niacin is an essential, water-soluble nutrient. It is required by all living cells and is critical for the release of energy from carbohydrate, fat, and protein, and is necessary for DNA formation.

Who Is Deficient?

Virtually nobody needs to worry about getting enough niacin. The average American of all ages takes in well over the recommended dietary allowance (RDA) of "preformed niacin" in food, according to government figures. The U.S. Department of Agriculture's food-consumption surveys find that 67 percent of the population get more than 100 percent of the RDA. Only 9 percent eat less than 70 percent of the recommended niacin levels. Body chemistry adds even more by converting the amino acid tryptophan (found in protein foods) into niacin within the cells.

Your body is more likely to be awash in niacin than any other vitamin or mineral.

One warning: heavy drinkers may be deficient in niacin; pellagra, the classic niacin-deficiency disease, has been reported among alcoholics.

Pellagra: The Vanished Scourge

Pellagra—or *pelle agra* (rough skin)—was thought to be a disease endemic to Spain and Italy until 1907, when an epidemic of pellagra hit the southern part of the United States. In 1918 pellagra killed over ten thousand Americans, notably in small southern towns where niacin-poor corn, molasses, and pork fat were staples. Pellagra is the only deficiency disease ever to have been a major health problem in the United States. It disappeared after niacin emerged as a cure for it in the

1930s. Today, with the fortification of flour and cereals with the B vitamins, including niacin, pellagra and niacin deficiencies of any type are rare.

Since the B vitamins work together, current thinking is that pellagra does not result solely from a lack of niacin, but from multiple deficiencies of niacin, riboflavin, B_6, and the amino acid tryptophan.

SIGNS OF PELLAGRA
Early symptoms
Weakness
Apathy
Loss of appetite
Indigestion
Irritability
Headaches
Sleeplessness
Loss of memory
Signs of emotional instability

Classic advanced symptoms
Dermatitis
Diarrhea
Depression
(the 3-Ds, as they are called)
Additionally, psychosis with delirium, hallucinations, confusion, and stupor.

Niacin Antagonists and Helpers

Animal and/or human studies reveal that the following factors may affect how niacin is absorbed or utilized by the body; the extent of the effect depends on many unknowns, and the interaction may be important only if the antagonist or booster is of sufficient magnitude.

FACTORS THAT MAY BLOCK NIACIN, INCREASING NEED
Fructose (a simple form of sugar in fruits and primarily in processed foods using high-fructose corn sweeteners)
Alcohol

FACTORS THAT MAY BOOST UTILIZATION OF NIACIN
Thiamin
Vitamin B_6
Riboflavin

DRUGS THAT MAY DEPLETE NIACIN
Isoniazid

The Tryptophan Connection

Scientists trying to solve the pellagra-niacin puzzle discovered in 1945 that milk, low in niacin, nevertheless helped cure pellagra and that niacin-impoverished diets did not always cause pellagra. The reason: milk, as part of its protein, contains an amino acid called tryptophan, which is converted to niacin inside the body. Thus, much of the niacin your body eventually utilizes is not derived from foods high in niacin, but from protein foods high in tryptophan. The general rule is that 60 mg of tryptophan is converted in the cells to 1 mg of niacin.

That's why experts say that if you get enough protein, you do not have to worry about niacin. Animal protein contains 1.4 percent tryptophan; vegetable protein contains 1 percent. So, an adult who eats the recommended 60 grams of protein daily could potentially rack up 600 mg of tryptophan, or 10 mg of niacin. That, added to the widespread intake of preformed niacin in other foods, usually adds up to a generous supply.

Important: The food-content charts in the back of this book contain figures only for preformed niacin as determined by U.S. Department of Agriculture policy.

One reason niacin is a no-problem nutrient is that it is found widely in both plant and animal foods.

Foods That Have Niacin but Don't Release It

The niacin in rice and corn is locked up fairly tightly unless released by the presence of alkali, which helps make the vitamin available for use by the body. Alkali is used, for example, in preparing corn tortillas.

The niacin in wheat bran is a type generally unavailable for use by the body.

Only 30 percent of the natural niacin in cereal is bioavailable.

Cooking: Little to Worry About

Niacin is so resistant to heat, light, acid, alkali, and oxidation that very little is lost through processing or preparing food. Since it is water soluble, however, a great deal of the vitamin may leach out in water, so it is advisable, as with other nutrients, to use as little water as possible. Up to 50 percent of the niacin may be lost when vegetables are cooked in excess water.

Toxicity and Supplements

The most common side effect of niacin is the "niacin flush," caused by dilated blood vessels at doses as low as 75 mg of nicotinic acid daily; the flushing is not considered dangerous and disappears usually within half an hour. (Niacinamide, the form found in many vitamin supplements, does not cause flushing.) Other possible side effects from relatively low doses of nicotinic acid: headaches, nausea, cramps, and diarrhea.

Prolonged use of megadoses of nicotinic acid has been associated with jaundice, irregular heartbeat, promotion of gout, skin rashes, elevated plasma glucose, irritation of peptic ulcers, and other biochemical signs of liver damage.

Such side effects have not been reported from nicotinamide, even at doses of 3 to 9 grams daily.

Niacin: A Cholesterol Reducer

Megadoses of nicotinic acid (in the range of 3 to 6 grams daily) have been dramatically successful in lowering blood cholesterol and triglycerides in certain patients with heart disease. (Nicotinamide does not work.) But, because of fairly serious side effects, nobody should take megadoses except on the recommendation of a physician.

FOODS RICH IN NIACIN

The most niacin by weight regardless of calories

Beef and calf liver	Turkey
Tunafish	Mackerel
Codfish	Sardines
Chicken	Lamb
Rockfish	Peanuts
Swordfish	Enriched cereals
Salmon	Brewer's yeast
Rabbit	

NIACIN SUPER-FOODS
THE MOST NIACIN, THE FEWEST CALORIES

Here are 50 foods that rate exceptionally high in niacin content per calorie. Of the approximately 2500 foods listed in this book, these are tops in niacin nutrient density; they have the highest niacin-calorie ratios, giving you the most niacin for the fewest calories.*

	Food Rating	Niacin-calorie ratio (mg of Niacin per 100 calories)	Common Measure	Mg Niacin	Calories
1.	Tuna, canned in water	10.5	3 oz	14	135
2.	Tuna, raw	10.0	3 oz	11	113
3.	Bran, unprocessed	9.8	¼ c	3	31
4.	Lamb, liver, broiled	9.5	1.6 oz	11	117
5.	Chicken, light meat, roasted	9.2	3 oz	12	128
6.	Soup, escarole, canned	8.5	1 c	2	27
7.	Sturgeon, steamed	8.4	3 oz	8	99
8.	Cod, salted, dried	8.4	1 oz	3	36
9.	Tuna, fresh, broiled	8.1	3 oz	12	155
10.	Turkey loaf luncheon meat	7.6	2 sl	4	47
11.	Veal, cutlet, lean, cooked	7.4	3 oz	10	140
12.	Beef, liver, braised	6.6	3 oz	9	137
13.	Calf, liver, fried	6.3	3 oz	14	222
14.	Chicken, breast, meat & skin, fried	6.2	3.5 oz	13	218
15.	Salmon, steamed/poached	6.1	3 oz	8	126
16.	Tuna, canned in oil	6.0	3 oz	10	167
17.	Pork, liver, braised	5	3 oz	7	141
18.	Salmon, pink, canned	5.2	3 oz	7	130
19.	Swordfish steak, broiled	5.2	3 oz	8	148
20.	Rabbit, cooked	5.2	3 oz	9	182
21.	Veal, boneless, lean, roasted	5.1	3 oz	6	123
22.	Mackerel, canned	4.9	3 oz	9	182
23.	Halibut, fried	4.4	3 oz	7	153
24.	Turkey, breast, roasted	4.3	3½ oz	7	157
25.	Cod, smoked	4.1	3 oz	4	87
26.	Beef kidneys, simmered	4.1	3 oz	5	122
27.	Chicken, leg, broiled	4	1 medium	3	76
28.	Calf heart, braised	3.9	1 c	1	302
29.	Trout, broiled	3.8	3 oz	8	217
30.	Oysters, raw	3.8	3 oz	2	56
31.	Oysters, smoked	3.8	3 oz	3	106
32.	Bacon, Canadian, cooked	3.7	1 sl	2	43
33.	Ham, ext lean	3.7	1 sl	1	37
34.	Sardines, canned in oil	3.6	3 oz	6	172
35.	Trout, boneless, smoked	3.3	3 oz	5	153
36.	Lamb, chop, loin, lean, broiled	3.3	1 chop	4	116

	Food Rating	Niacin-calorie ratio (mg of Niacin per 100 calories)	Common Measure	Mg Niacin	Calories
37.	Turkey, light meat and skin	3.2	3½ oz	6	197
38.	Chicken meat, dark, roasted	3	3 oz	5	150
39.	Haddock, fillet, boneless, broiled	2.8	3 oz	3	102
40.	Chicken livers, simmered	2.8	1 c	6	220
41.	Shrimp, boiled	2.7	3 oz	3	102
42.	Venison, boneless, stewed	2.7	3 oz	4	153
43.	Peanuts	2.6	1 oz	4	165
44.	Ground beef, ext lean, broiled	2.2	3 oz	5	225
45.	Beef, top loin, lean, broiled	2.2	3 oz	4	176

Cereal: five with the highest niacin-calorie ratio

	Food Rating	Niacin-calorie ratio	Common Measure	Mg Niacin	Calories
46.	Total	10.0	1 oz	20	100
47.	Product 19	18.5	1 oz	20	108
48.	100% Bran	11.8	1 oz	9	76
49.	Wheat puffed, fortified	9.7	½ oz	5	52
50.	Rice, puffed, fortified	9	½ oz	5	57

Source: Author's computer analysis from USDA data

*Excludes baby foods. Includes only foods for which one serving supplies a minimum of approximately 10 percent of the RDA.

RECOMMENDED DAILY DIETARY ALLOWANCES
OF NIACIN

Age	Niacin Equivalents Milligrams*
Birth–6 months	6
6 months–1 year	8
1–3	9
4–6	11
7–10	16
Males	
11–18	18
19–22	19
23–50	18
51 and over	16
Females	
11–14	15
15–22	14
23 and over	13
Pregnant	add 2
Nursing	add 5

Source: National Academy of Sciences, Revised 1980

*One niacin equivalent is equal to 1 mg of preformed niacin or 60 mg of dietary tryptophan.

Vitamin B$_6$
Exciting New Discoveries

Vitamin B$_6$ is the common name for six water-soluble chemical compounds, including pyridoxine. B$_6$ has a vital role in many biochemical reactions in all organs and cells of the body; it helps to regulate blood glucose levels and is needed to synthesize hemoglobin and to convert fatty acids and amino acids. The influence of vitamin B$_6$ is so diverse that its deficiencies can show up in a variety of generalized symptoms.

Who Needs to Worry?

Vitamin B$_6$ is so severely deficient in the American diet that government officials brand it a "problem nutrient." The U.S. Department of Agriculture's latest ten-year food consumption survey found that only 22 percent of Americans past age one met the top recommended dietary allowances of B$_6$. About half of the population fell below 70 percent of the RDA. The consumption of vitamin B$_6$ foods declined almost steadily with age, becoming extremely low among the elderly.

Another study revealed that older people take in surprisingly little B$_6$. Of men and women over age 60 fully 50 percent of the females and 20 percent of the males ate foods with less than 50 percent of the recommended dietary allowance of vitamin B$_6$.

Important: Women of all ages are apt to consume diets marginal in B$_6$. According to USDA figures, a mere 8 percent took in 100 percent of the RDA's, and less than three-fourths managed to eat even 70 percent of the suggested dietary allowances. Teenage girls, too, are frequent targets of B$_6$-deficient diets. One recent survey of adolescent girls showed that 66 percent consumed less than the RDA. Biochemical tests revealed marginal or deficient B$_6$ status in one-third of the girls.

Breast Milk and the Pill: New Facts

At one time, it was thought that oral contraceptives seriously diminished vitamin B$_6$ status, and it was even suggested that B$_6$ be combined with the pill to prevent deficiencies. Because of better knowledge about how the drug reacts with B$_6$, much of the earlier concern has disappeared. Any such interference with the availability of B$_6$ for women on the pill is considered slight.

It has been suggested that women who breast-feed may endanger their infants by passing along milk with low levels of B$_6$, but, Dr. Robert Reynolds, at the USDA's Human Nutrition Research Center in Beltsville, Maryland and a leading authority on B$_6$, says that although lactating women eat much less B$_6$ than the RDA calls for, a study found no clinical signs of vitamin B$_6$ deficiency in either the women or their breast-fed infants. The milk was apparently not deficient in B$_6$.

Heavy drinkers of alcohol are very susceptible to B$_6$ deficiencies, and even high doses of B$_6$ do not correct the deficiency; alcohol has a potent capacity to destroy much B$_6$. There is even evidence that chronic drinking may impair the ability to utilize B$_6$. Alcoholics often have the classic symptoms of B$_6$ deficiency.

Do We Really Need That Much B$_6$?

Despite low intakes of B$_6$ throughout the population, there is no evidence of corresponding widespread overt symptoms of B$_6$ deficiency. Therefore, some experts argue that we may not need as much B$_6$ as once believed, and that the recommended dietary allowances for B$_6$ are actually set too high and should be lowered. The National Academy of Sciences committee, charged with making such changes, in 1985 did agree to lower the RDA for B$_6$ but their recommendations for this revision and others were not accepted.

WHAT ARE YOUR CHANCES OF GETTING TOO LITTLE B$_6$?

Age	% getting less than 100% RDA	% getting less than 70% RDA
Under 1	20	5
1–2	47	12
3–5	61	25
6–8	65	27

Age	% getting less than 100% RDA	% getting less than 70% RDA
Males		
9–11	65	26
12–14	61	25
15–18	63	28
19–22	74	46
23–24	77	42
35–50	80	44
51–64	80	43
65–74	86	54
75 and over	88	58
Females		
9–11	75	35
12–14	82	47
15–18	90	67
19–22	94	72
23–24	93	73
35–50	94	73
51–64	91	66
65–74	92	67
75 and over	92	69

Source: US Department of Agriculture

SYMPTOMS OF VITAMIN B$_6$ DEFICIENCY
Infants
Convulsive seizures
Weight loss
Abdominal distress
Vomiting
Hyperirritability

Adults
The three classic signs are:
Glossitis (inflammation of the tongue)
Fissures and cracks at the corners of the mouth
Patches of itchy, scaling skin.
Additionally, severe deficiencies may lead to anemia, depression, confusion, brain wave abnormalities, and convulsions.

Widespread Health Consequences

Vitamin B$_6$ although discovered about half a century ago, has stirred up very little interest until recently. In the 1970s with new discoveries about possible health roles for B$_6$, research on the vitamin picked up, and recently research into the vitamin has yielded some fascinating new information. Investigations of B$_6$ is now one of the hottest subjects around. Here are some of the exciting new findings on how B$_6$ may affect your health.

Because B$_6$ reacts so readily with all kinds of compounds in the body, it can have profound effects on a variety of health conditions that on the surface seem unrelated. However, there may be an underlying common mechanism which has not yet been discovered that explains the vitamin's influence on such seemingly different diseases and disorders.

• *Asthma.* Just by chance while screening seemingly normal adults for B$_6$ deficiencies, USDA scientists noticed that 15 had similar blood profiles, characterized chiefly by extraordinarily low levels of pyridoxal phosphate, the body's active form of B$_6$. It turned out that all 15 had asthma. When half of the individuals were given 50 milligrams of B$_6$ twice a day, their blood levels of B$_6$ did not go up significantly. In fact, they remained shockingly low. However, all of them reported a dramatic decrease in the frequency and severity of their asthmatic attacks while taking the vitamin supplement. Other studies have shown that asthmatic children also have fewer symptoms and attacks when given extra B$_6$.

Scientists don't know why asthmatics have such low levels of B$_6$. Speculation is that they may not metabolize it normally or may have a need for greater intakes. Research continues.

• *Cancers of certain types.* B$_6$ deficiencies have been related to skin problems, such as acne. Recent evidence links a deficiency with the potentially fatal skin cancer called melanoma. Preliminary studies found that one form of vitamin B$_6$ in a cream applied to the skin cancers of patients caused a dramatic regression. The amounts of B$_6$ in the blood of the patients also increased about nine times. Whether a lack of B$_6$ had anything to do with progression of the disease is unknown. Animal studies have revealed that mice, given B$_6$ and then injected with melanoma cells, have twice the resistance to developing cancer as mice not pretreated with B$_6$. The research is exciting, but preliminary.

There's also evidence that B$_6$ deficiencies may be related to breast and bladder cancer.

• *Carpal tunnel syndrome.* Many physicians now test anyone with this syndrome for vitamin B$_6$ deficiencies. The disorder results when a certain nerve in the wrist becomes compressed, causing tingling, numbness, weakness, pain and loss of function in the fingers and hand.

Surgery is often required to correct the problem. Numerous studies have found that people with the disorder are deficient in B_6 and often improve dramatically when given doses of B_6—50 to 150 milligrams a day. The B_6 apparently helps speed up the conduction of nerve signals through the hands.

• *Cardiovascular disease.* A flurry of research a few years ago heralded B_6 as a virtual magic bullet against heart disease. The theory was that vitamin B_6 deficiency helped precipitate arterial blood clots and thus was involved in clogged arteries and coronary heart disease. But since no confirming evidence of a mechanism of action was forthcoming, the theory fell into disfavor. Now the interest is back, and quite a few researchers, including some at Harvard, are finding suggestions that B_6 is somehow involved in heart disease.

For example, it is known that after heart attacks, patients often exhibit very low blood levels of B_6. One study also found that the levels of B_6 after a heart attack may predict how well the patient progresses. The higher the blood B_6 levels immediately following the heart attack, the more likely the patient is to recover faster, have less damage and survive. Additional long-term studies are underway to explain this phenomenon.

• *Diabetes.* Recent studies show that some forms of diabetes may be aggravated by B_6 deficiency and that adequate or supplemental doses of B_6 may help normalize glucose metabolism and reduce the need for insulin.

There is also a condition known as gestational diabetes in which pregnant women develop all the symptoms of diabetes, yet return to normal after delivery. Such women can be spotted during glucose tolerance tests by extremely low levels of B_6. By tracking B_6 status during a glucose tolerance test, scientists can determine which women have this disorder. Apparently, a change in hormonal status during pregnancy influences B_6 concentration in the blood.

• *Premenstrual syndrome (PMS).* A few years ago it was widely reported that B_6 helped relieve the symptoms of PMS, and gynecologists have prescribed it widely in high doses as a PMS treatment. In a few cases women, taking it on the advice of physicians, have been harmed by the high doses, for heavy doses of B_6 are not benign. Now, follow-up evidence indicates that B_6 has much less therapeutic effect on PMS symptoms than previously believed.

• *Sickle-cell anemia.* Recent research shows that those with sickle-cell anemia, an inherited disorder that strikes primarily blacks, are apt to have very low blood levels of vitamin B_6. In one study when patients were given 50 mg of B_6 twice a day over a two month period, the blood concentrations of B_6 went up, and in several cases, the number and duration of painful crises that often require hospitalization decreased.

However, the doses of B$_6$ did not bring the levels in the blood up to normal, suggesting that such persons may have unusually high requirements for B$_6$, perhaps because they metabolize B$_6$ differently.

Laboratory studies have shown that B$_6$ can inhibit the cells' sickling (resulting in odd-shaped blood cells roughly resembling a sickle), that causes the damage in the disease. Since evidence showing B$_6$ deficiencies in sickle-cell disease is new, much more research is now underway to determine the meaning of the finding.

• *Aging and senility.* Over the years there have been several reports that as people age, their vitamin B$_6$ blood levels decline. New USDA studies do confirm that men's B$_6$ blood levels go down as they age. It is not known whether this happens because they fail to metabolize B$_6$ as well or because they eat less food high in B$_6$. Fascinating new studies also reveal accelerated aging in the brains of rats severely deprived of B$_6$ and copper and sometimes chromium. The abnormal brain cells are similar in appearance to those found in elderly humans; there is some speculation, but no hard evidence that such combined deficiencies of B$_6$, copper, and chromium might be related to memory loss and dementia associated with aging.

HEALTH PROBLEMS THAT MAY BE LINKED TO VITAMIN B$_6$ DEFICIENCY

Research on animals and/or humans proves or suggests a connection between B$_6$ deficiency or unusual need for vitamin B$_6$ and:

Asthma

Carpal tunnel syndrome (a nerve disorder producing numbness, tingling, pain, weakness in hands and fingers).

Cancer, possibly melanoma, breast and bladder cancer

Diabetes (although there is no proof that B$_6$ prevents diabetes)

Coronary heart disease and atherosclerosis

Premenstrual syndrome (PMS)

Sickle-cell anemia

Aging and dementia

How Much Is Absorbed?

The amount of B$_6$ you get varies with the type of food. For example, the body seems better able to utilize B$_6$ in beef than in soy beans. The B$_6$ in fortified cereal may be poorly absorbed. One study found that only 18 to 44 percent of the B$_6$ in rice cereal was biologically available. The same study showed that the body utilized 100 percent of the B$_6$ in nonfat dry milk. Generally, however, it appears that about 70 percent of the B$_6$ in foods is actually utilized by the body.

The Vegetable Question

Recent research by Dr. James E. Leklem, an expert on B_6 at Oregon State University's Department of Foods and Nutrition, finds that a form of the vitamin in vegetables, called pyridoxine glycoside, which is measured as B_6, is simply not utilized by the body. After being absorbed from the digestive tract, much of the glycoside goes right through the blood stream and into the urine totally unchanged. This means that much of the B_6 in vegetables may be nutritionally wasted. Especially high in glycoside are the cruciferous vegetables—broccoli, cauliflower, brussels sprouts, and cabbage. Also high in glycoside are legumes and rice. More studies are underway to determine what this means—whether vegetarians are more apt to be deficient in B_6 for this reason. Meanwhile, it seems best not to depend heavily on these vegetables for your B_6 supply.

Vitamin B_6 Antagonists and Helpers

Animal and/or human studies reveal that the following factors may affect how vitamin B_6 is absorbed or utilized by the body.

FACTORS THAT MAY BLOCK B_6, INCREASING NEED
A high-protein diet
Alcoholism (vitamin B_6 deficiency is a severe problem in 20 to 30 percent of alcoholics)
Smoking (in one study pregnant smokers had double the risk of vitamin B_6 deficiency)
Dietary Fiber (small inhibitory effect)
Button mushrooms, (containing hydrazines)
Magnesium, zinc, or riboflavin deficiency (all three nutrients are required for conversion of B_6)
DRUGS THAT MAY DEPLETE VITAMIN B_6
Isoniazid (tuberculosis treatment and prevention)
Hydralazine (high blood pressure or blood vessel dilator)
L-dopa (Parkinson's)
Phenelzine (antidepressant)
Penicillamine (rheumatoid arthritis, lead poisoning)
Procarbazine (anti-cancer drug)

Cooking and Processing

B$_6$ is moderately susceptible to destruction. You save more B$_6$ by grilling or broiling meat than by roasting; losses can range from 20 to 55 percent. Both canning and cooking vegetables can destroy 20 to 30 percent of the B$_6$. You can lose some B$_6$ in milk by exposing it to sunlight or high heat.

Toxicity and Supplements

B$_6$ is quite safe in the diet and even nontoxic in moderate doses of supplements; no side effects have been apparent at 100 mg daily. But B$_6$ is not the innocuous vitamin once thought. Although B$_6$ is water-soluble and excesses are flushed out of the body to a great extent, high doses (500 to 6,000 mg per day) have produced neurological disturbances resulting in numbness of the feet, hands, and mouth and instability in walking. Damage has been confirmed by biopsies showing degeneration of certain nerve cells. According to one major report, victims generally recovered after they stopped taking megadoses of B$_6$, but some experienced minor abnormalities for two or three years. Interestingly, some victims were taking megadoses for relief of premenstrual water retention, sometimes upon the advice of a gynecologist.

WARNING: VITAMIN B$_6$ AND PARKINSON'S

Vitamin B$_6$ is an antagonist to the drug levodopa, commonly used to treat Parkinson's disease. The vitamin converts the drug into a form that cannot cross the blood/brain barrier, rendering the drug virtually ineffective. Experts advise those taking levodopa to restrict supplementary vitamin B$_6$ to less than 5 mg per day.

Other reported adverse effects from large doses of B$_6$ (upwards of 200 mg a day) are: nervousness, insomnia, frequent urination (the vitamin is apparently a diuretic for some people) irritability and wetting the bed for children. There is also some evidence that very high doses of the vitamin (500 mg a day) can slightly impair brain functioning.

FOODS RICH IN VITAMIN B$_6$

The most vitamin B$_6$ by weight regardless of calories

Whole-grain cereals	Peanut butter
Sunflower seeds	Sweet potatoes
Prunes	Currants
Liver	Soybeans
Filberts	Raisins
Walnuts	Chicken liver
Potatoes	Salmon
Bananas	Tuna
Turkey and chicken (white meat)	Mackerel
Dried apricots	Lobster
Pork and ham	Swordfish
Peanuts	

VITAMIN B$_6$ SUPER-FOODS
THE MOST VITAMIN B$_6$, THE FEWEST CALORIES

Here are 50 foods that rate exceptionally high in vitamin B$_6$ content per calorie. Of the approximately 2500 foods in this book, these are tops in vitamin B$_6$ nutrient density; that is, they have the highest vitamin B$_6$-calorie ratios, giving you the most vitamin B$_6$ for the fewest calories.*

	Food Rating	B$_6$-calorie ratio (mg of Vitamin B$_6$ per 100 calories)	Common Measure	Mg B$_6$	Calories
1.	Spinach, fresh, cooked	1.1	½ c	.2	21
2.	Soup, escarole, canned	.8	1 c	.2	27
3.	Tuna, raw	.7	1 oz	.8	113
4.	Bamboo shoots, canned	.7	1 c	.2	25
5.	Broccoli, fresh, cooked	.7	½ c	.2	23
6.	Vegetable juice cocktail, canned	.7	½ c	.2	22
7.	Sauerkraut, canned	.7	½ c	.2	22
8.	Brussels sprouts, frozen, cooked	.7	½ c	.2	33
9.	Bananas	.6	1 fruit	.7	105
10.	Tomato sauce, canned	.6	½ c	.2	37
11.	Beef liver, braised	.6	3 oz	.8	137
12.	Tuna, fresh, broiled	.5	3 oz	.8	155
13.	Carrots, fresh, cooked	.5	½ c	.2	35

	Food Rating	B$_6$-calorie ratio (mg of Vitamin B$_6$ per 100 calories)	Common Measure	Mg B$_6$	Calories
14.	Zucchini, Italian style, canned	.5	½ c	.2	33
15.	Carrot juice, canned	.5	½ c	.3	49
16.	Ham, lean	.5	1 oz	.2	34
17.	Watermelon, raw	.4	¹⁄₁₆ fruit	.7	152
18.	Chicken, light meat, roasted	.4	3 oz	.5	128
19.	Potato skin, boiled/baked	.4	1 skin	.4	115
20.	Salmon, smoked	.4	3 oz	.6	150
21.	Chicken, liver, simmered	.4	1 c	.8	219
22.	Turkey, light meat, roasted	.3	3½ oz	.5	157
23.	Pheasant, raw, w skin	.3	½	2.6	723
24.	Elderberries, raw	.3	1 c	.4	105
25.	Potato w skin, baked	.3	1 med	.7	220
26.	Squash, winter, baked	.3	½ c	.2	57
27.	Tomato, spaghetti sauce, canned	.3	1 c	.9	272
28.	Peas, green, fresh, cooked	.3	½ c	.2	67
29.	Yam, Hawaii, steamed	.3	½ c	.2	79
30.	Potatoes, instant mashed	.3	½ c	.4	137
31.	Calf liver, fried	.3	3 oz	.8	222
32.	Mackerel, broiled	.3	3 oz	.6	213
33.	Crab, steamed	.3	2 med	.3	89
34.	Peas, green, fresh cooked	.3	½ c	2	67
35.	Tuna, canned in water	.3	3 oz	.4	135
36.	Swordfish steak, broiled	.3	3 oz	.5	148
37.	Wheat germ	.3	¼ c	.3	108
38.	White potato, wo peel, boiled	.3	½ c	.3	67
39.	Plantain, cooked	.2	½ c	.2	89
40.	Mango, raw	.2	1 fruit	.3	135
41.	Avocado, raw	.2	1 fruit	.9	339
42.	Prunes, stewed	.2	½ c	.3	113
43.	Chicken, dark meat, roasted	.2	3 oz	.5	150
44.	Pork chop, loin, lean, broiled	.2	1 chop	.3	166
45.	Bulgur, canned	.2	⅔ c	.3	151

Cereals: five with the highest vitamin B$_6$-calorie ratio

46.	Total	2	1 oz	2	100
47.	Product 19	1.9	1 oz	2	108
48.	100% Bran	1.2	1 oz	.9	76
49.	All-Bran	.7	1 oz	.5	71
50.	Bran Buds	.7	1 oz	.5	73

Source: Author's computer analysis from USDA data

*Excludes baby foods. Includes only foods for which one serving supplies a minimum of approximately 10 percent of the RDA.

RECOMMENDED DAILY DIETARY ALLOWANCES
OF VITAMIN B$_6$

Age	Milligrams
Infants (birth to six months)	.3
6 months to 1 year	.6
1–3	.9
4–6	1.3
7–10	1.6
Males	
11–14	1.8
15–18	2
19 and over	2.2
Females	
11–14	1.8
15 and older	2
Pregnant	add .6
Nursing	add .5

Source: National Academy of Sciences, Revised 1980

Vitamin B$_{12}$

Deficiencies Serious, but Rare

Vitamin B$_{12}$ is the name given to an essential water-soluble substance that is critical for normal growth, healthy nerve tissue, and normal blood formation. B$_{12}$ is essential for cell replication and the synthesis of DNA, which carries the body's genetic codes.

Who Needs to Worry?

Dietary deficiencies of B$_{12}$ are extremely rare. Vitamin B$_{12}$ is one of the most widely consumed nutrients by all Americans, and the liver can store enough vitamin B$_{12}$ to last for three years or more. The body stores so much B$_{12}$ and uses it so sparingly (one-millionth of a gram per day) that a deficiency in people who consume any animal products is unusual, and studies show that even strict vegetarians rarely show signs of B$_{12}$ deficiency. Symptoms of a deficiency take many years to develop. However, if allowed to progress undetected and untreated, a B$_{12}$ deficiency can cause irreversible nerve damage.

According to a recent U.S. Department of Agriculture survey, 66 percent of Americans get *more* than 100 percent of the recommended dietary allowance (RDA) for B$_{12}$, and only 15 percent get less than 70 percent of the RDA. However, there may be problems as we age. The gradual decrease in some stomach functions with aging may destroy some of the ability to absorb vitamin B$_{12}$. Certain diseases in the elderly may also impair the ability to absorb B$_{12}$. Even so, they may only develop deficiency symptoms slowly because they have built up large stores of B$_{12}$.

Also, strict vegetarians and individuals with gastrointestinal disorders that produce an inability to absorb vitamin B$_{12}$ are in danger of vitamin B$_{12}$ deficiency.

B_{12}: The Animal Vitamin

Important: Vitamin B_{12} is unique in that it comes almost exclusively from animal foods: meat, fish, eggs, and milk. Plants cannot synthesize B_{12} and do not contain the vitamin unless they are contaminated with B_{12}-producing microorganisms. Certain types of seaweed may contain substances similar to B_{12} produced by microorganisms, as does tempeh, a fermented soybean food inoculated with a B_{12} brewing mold. But most of the "B_{12}" in such sources is not usable as B_{12} by humans. Some cereals are fortified with B_{12}. In the American diet, all significant amounts of B_{12} come from eating meat and dairy products.

At Highest Risk

Diet related. Strict vegetarians (called vegans) who eat no meat, fish, eggs, or dairy products. Although vegans may adapt to lower intakes, experts consider strict vegetarians virtually the only group susceptible to B_{12} deficiency from dietary inadequacies. Vegan infants and children in particular are in serious danger; they may develop B_{12} deficiency symptoms within two to three years, since they have no prior stores on which to draw. Alarming studies show that vegan babies and children deprived of any animal protein (except mother's breast milk) fail to grow properly and show signs of malnutrition, including B_{12} deficiency.

An adult who switches to strict vegetarianism will not be harmed immediately, because B_{12} deficiencies develop very slowly over many years. According to authority Dr. Victor Herbert, at the Bronx, New York, Veterans Administration Medical Center, it can take from ten to thirty years for signs of B_{12} depletion to show up in normal people who stop eating animal protein. Vegetarians, including infants and children, who eat eggs and/or milk products are generally not at risk for vitamin B_{12} deficiency.

Nondiet related. Generally, illness from B_{12} deficiency results not from low dietary intakes but from the inability to absorb the vitamin. Potential victims:

• People with Crohn's disease, chronic pancreatic insufficiency, and those who have had stomach or intestinal surgery, which frequently leads to malabsorption and B_{12} deficiency.

• Those with a genetic inability to metabolize or absorb B_{12}.

• Those who become depleted in stomach "instrinsic factor," needed to absorb B_{12}. These are usually older people.

• Some experts believe that even strict vegetarians who exhibit B_{12} deficiency symptoms may have some defect in utilizing the vitamin.

SYMPTOMS OF VITAMIN B$_{12}$ DEFICIENCY
Sore tongue
Weakness
Loss of weight
Back pains
Tingling or numbness in extremities
Apathy
Mental and nervous disorders such as memory loss and confusion

The Worst Danger: Pernicious Anemia

A vitamin B$_{12}$ deficiency leads to two distinct types of symptoms: a form of anemia, called pernicious anemia, and damage to the nervous system and brain.

Pernicious anemia is the classic vitamin B$_{12}$ deficiency disease. However, the cause is not inadequate ingestion but inadequate absorption. Although an essentially identical anemia can be caused by a B$_{12}$-depleted diet, classic pernicious anemia almost always results from the failure of the stomach to secrete a substance known as "intrinsic factor," which binds to the B$_{12}$ so that it can be absorbed. In rare cases the disease has appeared in infants, adolescents, and young adults. Much more frequently, however, the "intrinsic factor" disappears with decreasing gastric function in some people as they age, making them vulnerable to vitamin B$_{12}$ deficiency and pernicious anemia. Pernicious anemia may take years to appear; the most common age of diagnosis is around sixty. Although the defect is not always a genetic one, pernicious anemia does tend to "run in families."

Pernicious anemia not only involves blood-cell disturbances characterized as megaloblastic anemia, but, worse, can damage the nervous system, and will progress unless alleviated by vitamin B$_{12}$. Without adequate vitamin B$_{12}$ over a period of time, myelin, the protein sheath around nerve fibers and the spinal cord, deteriorates, leading to neurological symptoms. Whether the symptoms can be reversed depends on the extent of neurological damage.

HEALTH PROBLEMS THAT MAY BE LINKED TO VITAMIN B$_{12}$ DEFICIENCY
Research on animals and/or humans proves or suggests a connection between B$_{12}$ deficiencies and:
Pernicious anemia
Infertility (female and male)
Nervous system disorders
Walking difficulties

How Much B_{12} Do You Absorb?

Ordinarily, far less than half of the B_{12} in the diet is absorbed. As with most other vitamins and minerals, the more your body needs, the greater the percentage it absorbs; B_{12} absorption is increased during pregnancy, for example. If you take in more B_{12} than you need, your body stores some and washes the rest away in the urine. One study showed that oral intakes of 100 micrograms of B_{12} a day (33 times the RDA) resulted in absorption of only 1 percent.

Important: People with pernicious anemia who lack the intrinsic factor needed to absorb B_{12} get no value from the vitamin in food.

B_{12} Antagonists and Helpers

Animal and/or human studies reveal that the following factors may affect how vitamin B_{12} is absorbed or utilized by the body; the extent of the effect depends on many unknowns, and the interaction may be important only if the antagonist or booster is of sufficient magnitude.

FACTORS THAT MAY BLOCK VITAMIN B_{12}, INCREASING NEED
Vitamin C megadoses
Food fiber (both cellulose and pectin) in large amounts

DRUGS THAT MAY DEPLETE VITAMIN B_{12}
Cholestyramine (cholesterol reducer)
Colestipol (cholesterol reducer)
Cimetidine (antiulcer agent)
Ranitidine (antiulcer agent)
Colchicine (gout)

WARNING: DANGER FROM TOO MUCH VITAMIN C

Megadoses of vitamin C or other strong antioxidant substances can destroy B_{12} from food when mixed together. Studies show that only 500 mg per day can cut down on availability of vitamin B_{12} from foods. Taking 1 gram of vitamin C with each meal could induce vitamin B_{12} deficiency disease.

The Folacin-B$_{12}$ Connection

Vitamin B$_{12}$ and folacin are closely connected; deficiencies in either or both together can produce a type of anemia called megaloblastic, in which red blood cells fail to mature properly in bone marrow, and instead become abnormally large and misshapen. A folacin deficiency can happen rapidly, showing up in the blood within two weeks and in tissue stores within four months. On the other hand, a vitamin B$_{12}$ deficiency can be decades in the making.

It is important not to confuse the cause of megaloblastic anemia. High dietary levels of folacin (common in vegetarians) may alleviate the megaloblastic-anemia symptoms, such as fatigue and shortness of breath, even though the anemia results primarily from a vitamin B$_{12}$ deficiency. If, however, the vitamin B$_{12}$ deficiency goes undetected, progressive and irreversible neurological damage may develop. Thus, a vitamin B$_{12}$ deficiency can be hidden by adequate levels of folacin. It is important to determine whether a deficiency of folacin or of B$_{12}$ is responsible for the anemia.

Cooking: Few Losses

It's difficult to destroy B$_{12}$ during cooking, because the vitamin is very resistant to heat. Broiling meat or frying it on a griddle causes very little B$_{12}$ loss except on the surface of the meat, right on the griddle. However, boiling meat at high heat (for example, at 170 degrees centrigrade for forty-five minutes) can destroy up to 30 percent of the vitamin.

Toxicity and Supplements

B$_{12}$ is very safe, even in high doses, when taken orally. There is no evidence of harm because so little B$_{12}$ is absorbed, and excesses are flushed out of the body.

Although vitamin B$_{12}$ has been called the "pep pill," and it has been widely used by Americans to fight fatigue and increase energy, there is no magic in vitamin B$_{12}$ tablets for normal people. If you don't have a vitamin B$_{12}$ deficiency, more vitamin B$_{12}$ does nothing for you, say experts. In cases where the deficiency is caused by malabsorption problems, periodic injections of B$_{12}$ will almost always correct the deficiency. The only known therapeutic value of B$_{12}$ is in alleviating B$_{12}$ deficiency.

FOODS RICH IN VITAMIN B$_{12}$

The most vitamin B$_{12}$ by weight regardless of calories

Organ meats, especially kidneys and liver of all types
Liverwurst
Liver pâté

Milk, especially nonfat dry milk
Seafood, especially shellfish
Meat
Most cheeses

VITAMIN B12 SUPER-FOODS
THE MOST VITAMIN B$_{12}$, THE FEWEST CALORIES

Here are 50 foods that rate exceptionally high in vitamin B$_{12}$ content per calorie. Of the approximately 2500 foods in this book, these are tops in vitamin B$_{12}$ nutrient density; that is, they have the highest vitamin B$_{12}$-calorie ratios, giving you the most vitamin B$_{12}$ for the fewest calories.*

	Food Rating	B$_{12}$-calorie ratio (mcg of Vitamin B$_{12}$ per 100 calories)	Common Measure	Micro-grams B$_{12}$	Calories
1.	Clams, raw	78.9	5 clams	51	65
2.	Clams, canned	71.1	½ c	54	76
3.	Abalone, cooked	68.7	3 oz	83	120
4.	Beef liver, braised	43	3 oz	60	137
5.	Turkey, liver, simmered	28.1	1 c	66	237
6.	Oysters, raw	27.3	3 oz	15	56
7.	Oysters, smoked	27.3	3 oz	25	91
8.	Clams, breaded, fried	26.6	3 oz	42	158
9.	Chicken, liver, simmered	12.4	1 c	27	220
10.	Oysters, broiled/baked	10.5	3 oz	14	133
11.	Crab, steamed	10.1	2 med	9	89
12.	Squid, fried	9.5	3 oz	15	159
13.	Clam chowder, New England, canned	8.4	1 c	8	95
14.	Sausage, liver cheese	8.1	1 oz	7	86
15.	Roe, sturgeon (caviar)	6.9	1 tbsp	3	46
16.	Clam chowder, canned, Manhattan, chunky	5.9	1 c	8	133
17.	Roe, shad	5.9	½ oz	1	22
18.	Braunschweiger (liver sausage)	5.6	1 oz	6	102
19.	Salmon, canned	4.6	3 oz	6	130
20.	Mackerel, canned	4.2	3 oz	8	182
21.	Liverwurst, fresh	4.1	1 oz	4	93

Food Rating		B$_{12}$-calorie ratio (mcg of Vitamin B$_{12}$ per 100 calories)	Common Measure	Micrograms B$_{12}$	Calories
22.	Pâté, chicken liver, canned	4	1 oz	2	57
23.	Anchovy, canned	4	1 oz	2	49
24.	Salmon, smoked	4	3 oz	6	150
25.	Sardines, in oil, canned	3.9	3 oz	7	172
26.	Venison, stewed	3.5	3 oz	5	153
27.	Rabbit, wild, cooked	3.3	3 oz	6	182
28.	Squirrel, cooked	3.3	3 oz	6	182
29.	Herring, pickled	3.1	1 oz	2	62
30.	Eel, smoked	2.4	3 oz	7	280
31.	Tuna, raw	2.3	3 oz	2	113
32.	Beef, pressed, luncheon meat	2.1	1 oz	1	34
33.	Crab, soft shell, fried	2.1	1 crab	5	213
34.	Pâté de fois gras, canned (goose liver pâté)	2	1 oz	3	132
35.	Smelts, broiled/baked	2	3 oz	3	144
36.	Salmon, fresh, steamed/poached	1.9	3 oz	2	126
37.	Turkey, loaf	1.8	2 slices	1	47
38.	Tuna, fresh, broiled	1.7	3 oz	3	155
39.	Turkey soup, chunky, canned	1.6	1 c	2	134
40.	Sausage, Thuringer	1.3	1 oz	1	99
41.	Salami, beef	1.3	1 oz	1	74
42.	Flank steak	1.3	3 oz	2.6	207
43.	Beef steak, lean, broiled	1.2	3 oz	2	189
44.	Milk, skim	1.1	1 c	1	100
45.	Milk, dry, nonfat	1.1	¼ c	1	109

Cereals, fortified: five with highest B$_{12}$-calorie ratio

46.	Total	6.0	1 oz	6	100
47.	Product 19	5.6	1 oz	6	108
48.	100% Bran	3.5	1 oz	3	76
49.	Quisp	2.1	1 oz	2	118
50.	Maypo, cooked	1.7	½ c	1.5	85

Source: Author's computer analysis from USDA data

*Excludes baby foods. Includes only foods for which one serving supplies a minimum of approximately 10 percent of the RDA.

RECOMMENDED DAILY DIETARY ALLOWANCES OF VITAMIN B$_{12}$

Age	Micrograms
Birth–6 months	.5
6 months–1 year	1.5
1–3	2
4–6	2.5
7 and over	3
Pregnant	add 1
Nursing	add 1

Source: National Academy of Sciences, Revised 1980

Folacin
(also folic acid or folate)
Signs of Vegetable Malnutrition

Folacin is the name given a group of essential water-soluble vitamin compounds of very similar chemical structure, of which the most basic is folic acid. The name comes from the Latin for folium, *meaning foliage or leaf, because folic acid was first isolated from green leafy vegetables. Folacin is necessary for many metabolic processes, including the synthesis of DNA and RNA—cellular building blocks and carriers of the genetic code; thus, folic acid is vital in cell growth and division.*

Who Is Deficient?

Scattered studies have shown that perhaps one or two in ten Americans have marginal intakes of folacin. But the U.S. Department of Agriculture's first comprehensive nationwide scrutiny of the folacin intakes of women found alarming and surprising apparent deficiencies. The average American woman, aged nineteen to fifty, takes in only 210 micrograms of folacin a day—half the recommended level. The survey, conducted in 1985, uncovered profoundly deficient intakes among all women regardless of race, income, or geographic location. Although the survey did not include men, there is no reason to believe they have higher intakes. (However, some experts believe the RDA for folacin is too high, and should be reduced by half.) Youngsters aged one to five, according to the survey, on average did meet the RDAs.

Other reports spot certain segments of the population as frequent victims of folacin deficiency, namely the poor, the elderly, pregnant women, premature infants, alcoholics, or those with malabsorption diseases. The government's Ten State Nutrition Survey found "low levels" of folacin in the red blood cells of about 15 percent of white Americans and over 30 percent of black and Hispanic Americans. People admitted to hospitals are worse off. Surveys show 50 percent of the hospitalized in poor communities and 20 to 30 percent of those in other communities display signs of folacin deficiency.

Common victims of folic acid deficiency are chronic alcoholics.

Some experts say that about 90 percent of all alcoholics have folate deficiencies. As many as 60 percent of all alcoholics admitted to municipal hospitals, according to one study, have megaloblastic anemia caused by lack of folacin.

Pregnancy: A Special Problem

Pregnant women are also often vulnerable. Folacin is the only vitamin for which requirements double during pregnancy. Folacin blood concentrations drop drastically during pregnancy, and studies show that up to 25 percent of pregnant women may have blood cell changes signifying folacin deficiency, which can impair the growth and development of the fetus. In countries like the United States, from 2½ to 5 percent of pregnant women have megaloblastic anemia due to folic acid deficiency.

SIGNS OF FOLIC ACID DEFICIENCY
    Megaloblastic anemia
    Weakness
    Pallor
    Headaches
    Forgetfulness
    Sleeplessness
    Irritability

Anemia: The Worst Symptom

The most serious sign of folic acid deficiency is a type of anemia called megaloblastic anemia, which can be fatal if not treated. It is characterized by very large, misshapen, immature red blood cells. Symptoms are like those of anemia generally: tiredness, weakness, headaches, irregular heartbeat, breathing difficulty, etcetera. Additionally, there are symptoms peculiar to folate deficiency, including sore tongue (glossitis), intestinal problems such as diarrhea, loss of weight and appetite, and personality changes such as irritability and forgetfulness.

In the elderly an undetected folacin or vitamin B_{12} deficiency can be tragically mistaken for senile dementia (including Alzheimer's disease) or may aggravate the symptoms of existing dementia. Some studies have linked the severity of dementia in the aged with cell changes from folacin deficiency. And supplemental folacin therapy has reportedly caused improvements in patients with dementia, although most experts are skeptical of the results. Aging may also impair the ability to absorb folacin from foods.

Severe deficiency symptoms take about two to five months to show up, and disappear after about two weeks of treatment with folic acid.

The Vitamin B_{12} Connection

Even if you get enough folacin, it can be sabotaged by a lack of vitamin B_{12}. These two vitamins work closely together in the body, and B_{12} is essential to release folacin from bodily storage and get it into cells. Without sufficient B_{12}, folacin is of little use. Example: Strict vegetarians have high intakes of folacin (a vegetable vitamin) but low intakes of B_{12} (a meat vitamin). One fear is that in such cases high doses of folacin can mask symptoms of pernicious anemia (associated with insufficient B_{12}), allowing it to progress undetected to the point of irreversible nervous system damage. Consequently, the Food and Drug Administration limits the amount of folic acid that can be added to foods or nonprescription vitamin supplements. The government allows enough to protect against a folacin deficiency, but not enough to hide the symptoms of pernicious anemia.

HEALTH PROBLEMS THAT MAY BE LINKED TO FOLACIN DEFICIENCY

Research on animals and/or humans proves or suggests a connection between folacin deficiencies and:

Megaloblastic anemia
Depression
Dementia
Neuropsychological disorders, especially in the elderly
    (confusion, intellectual impairment, stupor)
Cervical dysplasia in women on the pill
Toxemia of pregnancy
Infections
Fetal damage, including neural-tube defects (spina bifida)
Cancer

How Much Folic Acid Do You Absorb?

On average, about half of the folic acid in the diet is absorbed, but it varies depending on many factors, including the food source of the folic acid. For example, studies have found widely varying absorption from different foods: brewer's yeast, 10 percent; romaine lettuce, 25 percent; wheat germ, 30 percent; egg yolk, 39 percent; cabbage, 47 percent; beef liver, 50 percent; spinach, 63 percent; dried lima beans, 70 percent; bananas, 82 percent; frozen lima beans, 96 percent.

Recommendation: Since you can never know how much folacin is being absorbed from a single food, get the vitamin from varied sources. In general, absorption is excellent from fresh, uncooked green leafy vegetables.

Folacin Antagonists and Helpers

Animal and/or human studies reveal that the following factors may affect how folacin is absorbed or utilized by the body; the extent of the effect depends on many unknowns, and the interaction may be important only if the antagonist or booster is of sufficient magnitude.

FACTORS THAT MAY BOOST UTILIZATION OF FOLACIN
Riboflavin
Vitamin C
B_{12}

FACTORS THAT MAY BLOCK FOLACIN, INCREASING NEED
Alcohol
Iron deficiency
Vitamin C deficiency
Diseases
  Infections
  Cancer
  Childhood and adult celiac disease
  Enzyme deficiencies
  Liver disease
  Uremia

DRUGS THAT MAY DEPLETE FOLACIN
Oral contraceptives
Phenytoin (anticonvulsant). **Warning:** Although anticonvulsants can lead to low levels of folacin, large supplemental doses of folic acid can increase seizures.
Sulfasalazine (anti-inflammatory drug)
Aspirin, high doses
Cholestyramine (blood-cholesterol depressant)
Cholestipol (blood-cholesterol depressant)
Triamterene (diuretic)
Antacids
Cancer chemotherapy drugs
Antibiotics

Folacin is the vegetable vitamin. Eating more vegetables and legumes is the perfect way to load up on folacin.

Cooking Cautions

Folic acid is extremely fragile, easily destroyed by heat, leaching, and light. One study by researchers at the University of British Columbia revealed the following losses in vegetables after 10 minutes of vigorous boiling in water: Cauliflower lost 84 percent; broccoli, 69 percent; spinach, 65 percent; cabbage, 57 percent; brussels sprouts, 28 percent; and asparagus, 22 percent. Another study found identical retention of folic acid from vegetables cooked in water or by microwave; however, the researchers noted that very little water was used in conventional cooking and none in the microwave cooking. Their conclusion: the amount of hot water used is the critical element rather than the method of cooking. Use as little hot water as possible. Ideally, cook vegetables in a wok as the Chinese do; just give them a brief stir-fry.

Just letting vegetables sit around at room temperature for two or three days destroys more than half of their folacin. Foods stored in a refrigerator for a couple of weeks lose little or no folacin.

Toxicity and Supplements

Folic acid is not acutely toxic; it is considered one of the safest of all vitamins for normal healthy people. One expert puts a minimum toxic dose at 400 milligrams, a thousand times more than the RDA.

However, megadoses can be dangerous to pregnant women by interacting to create dangerous zinc deficiencies. High doses of folic acid (1 milligram or more per day) can mask the symptoms of B_{12} deficiency and pernicious anemia. Also, patients with epilepsy controlled by anticonvulsants can start having convulsions again if they take megadoses of folic acid.

SIGNS OF FOLIC ACID POISONING
Muscle restlessness
Muscle jerking
Seizures

FOODS RICH IN FOLACIN

The most folacin regardless of calories

Sunflower seeds	Collards
Soybeans	Cashews
Spinach	Parsnips
Turnip greens	Avocados
Liver	Almonds
Asparagus	Dry beans
Brussels sprouts	Corn
Cereals	Beets
Filberts	Wheat germ

FOLACIN SUPER-FOODS
THE MOST FOLACIN, THE FEWEST CALORIES

Here are 50 foods that rate exceptionally high in folacin content per calorie. Of the approximately 2500 foods in this book, these are tops in folacin nutrient density; they have the highest folacin-calorie ratios, giving you the most folacin for the fewest calories.*

	Food Rating	Folacin-calorie ratio (mcg of Folacin per 100 calories)	Common Measure	Micro-grams Folacin	Calories
1.	Spinach, raw	884	½ c	54	6
2.	Spinach, fresh, cooked	634	½ c	131	21
3.	Turnip greens, fresh, cooked	592	½ c	85	15
4.	Chicken livers, simmered	490	1 c	1078	219
5.	Mustard greens, fresh cooked	489	½ c	51	11
6.	Asparagus, frozen, cooked	476	4 spears	81	17
7.	Asparagus, canned	479	½ c	115	24
8.	Spinach, canned	425	½ c	104	25
9.	Turkey, liver, simmered	394	1 c	932	237
10.	Okra, frozen, cooked	393	½ c	134	34
11.	Asparagus, fresh, cooked	392	½ c	88	22
12.	Spinach, frozen, cooked	384	½ c	102	27
13.	Brussels sprouts, frozen, cooked	241	½ c	79	33
14.	Chicken, giblets, cooked	239	1 c	545	228
15.	Broccoli, fresh, cooked	236	½ c	53	23
16.	Collards, frozen, cooked	211	½ c	65	31
17.	Beets, fresh, cooked	172	½ c	45	26

Food Rating	Folacin-calorie ratio (mcg of Folacin per 100 calories)	Common Measure	Micro-grams Folacin	Calories
18. Pâté, chicken liver, canned	160	1 oz	92	57
19. Beef liver, braised	137	3 oz	185	137
20. White beans, dry, cooked, no fat added	116	½ c	120	103
21. Red kidney beans, cooked, no fat added	110	½ c	114	103
22. Calf liver, cooked	109	3 oz	251	222
23. Bulgur, canned	105	⅔ c	158	151
24. Artichoke, cooked	101	1 medium	53	53
25. Pork liver, braised	99	3 oz	139	141
26. Cowpeas, green, cooked	96	½ c	86	89
27. Wheat germ	92	1 oz	100	107
28. Pigeonpeas, cooked	90	½ c	77	85
29. Parsnips, raw	89	½ c	45	50
30. Soybeans, green, cooked	79	½ c	100	127
31. Oranges, California, Valencias, raw	79	1 fruit	47	59
32. Peas, green, fresh, cooked	75	½ c	50	67
33. Parsnips, cooked	72	½ c	45	63
34. Corn, white, canned	62	½ c	52	83
35. Lima beans, dry, cooked	61	½ c	78	129
36. Bran, unprocessed	52	¼ c	16	31
37. Refried beans, canned	51	½ c	106	208
38. Soybean kernels, roasted	50	1 oz	64	129
39. Cantaloupe	49	½ fruit	45	94
40. Chickpeas, dry, cooked	48	½ c	70	146
41. Avocado, Florida	48	1 fruit	162	339
42. Muffin, English, whole wheat	47	1 muffin	61	130
43. Baked beans/tomato sauce, canned	43	½ c	67	156
44. Sunflower seeds	41	1 oz	65	162
45. Corn, fresh, white or yellow, cooked	43	½ c	38	89
Cereals: five with highest folacin-calorie ratio				
46. Product 19	370	1 oz	400	108
47. Corn Bran	186	1 oz	183	98
48. Cap'n Crunch	153	1 oz	182	119
49. Oats, instant	144	1 pkt	150	104
50. All-Bran	142	1 oz	100	71

Source: Author's computer analysis from USDA data

*Excludes baby food. Includes only foods for which one serving supplies a minimum of approximately 10 percent of the RDA.

RECOMMENDED DAILY DIETARY ALLOWANCES
OF FOLACIN*

Age	Micrograms
Birth–6 months	30
6 months–1 year	45
1–3	100
4–6	200
7–10	300
11 and over	400
Pregnant	add 400
Nursing	add 100

Source: National Academy of Sciences, Revised 1980

*An expert committee of the National Academy of Sciences in 1985 found these RDAs too high and recommended that they be reduced by about 50 percent.

Calcium
A Crippling Epidemic

Calcium is the most abundant mineral in the body, found in nearly all tissues. With phosphorus it combines to form calcium phosphate, the dense, hard material of the teeth and bones. Calcium is essential to keep the heartbeat regular, as well as nerves and muscles functioning normally, and helps blood to clot properly.

Who Is Deficient?

Widespread dietary deficiencies of calcium plus growing evidence of its health importance make calcium one of the hottest topics in nutritional research. Calcium has been dubbed "the nutrient of the 1980s"—a source of both concern and enormous potential benefit.

In the last few decades, the consumption of calcium has slipped to alarming levels. Deficiencies are so prevalent that government scientists label calcium a "problem nutrient." The U.S. Department of Agriculture's latest ten-year survey of the eating habits of over thirty-five thousand Americans found that 68 percent of the population does not meet the recommended dietary allowances (RDAs) for calcium.

The nutrient is particularly lacking in those who most need it and who may pay the highest price in later years: adolescent girls and middle-aged women. About eight out of ten women do not consume enough calcium. The average American woman eats from 500 to 600 mg of calcium per day—one-half that recommended by a National Institutes of Health committee. The average American male consumes about 750 mg daily.

SYMPTOMS OF SEVERE CALCIUM DEFICIENCY
    Irregular heartbeat
    Muscle spasms
    Convulsions
    Dementia
    Stunted growth
    Rickets
    Osteomalacia (adult rickets)

AMERICANS DEFICIENT IN CALCIUM INTAKE

68 percent

FEMALES DEFICIENT IN CALCIUM INTAKE

Age	Percent
15–18	87
35–50	84

Severe signs of calcium deficiencies are rare. More widespread and alarming are the symptoms of mild calcium deficiencies. Here is the latest medical evidence about the connection between dietary calcium and disease.

Calcium Protects Aging Bones

Calcium consumption is thought to be closely tied to osteoporosis, which afflicts about 20 million older Americans, mainly women over age sixty. Osteoporosis (which literally means *porous bones*) imperceptibly causes once-dense bones to become lighter, fragile, and honeycombed. The result is a skeleton so weak that vertebrae can collapse, producing what is called "dowager's hump." Minor falls can cause serious fractures, commonly in the hip; about 1.3 million fractures occur yearly in people aged forty-five and older with osteoporosis. By age ninety, osteoporosis produces hip fractures in about 32 percent of women and 17 percent of men.

Women in Most Danger

Women are more prone to osteoporosis than men because they have less bone mass to begin with and lose it faster with age. After age thirty-five nearly everyone starts losing bone. But in women, for five to ten years after menopause, bone loss accelerates dramatically as estrogen supplies diminish. (Synthetic-estrogen replacement helps prevent osteoporosis.) Some women can lose as much as 40 to 45 percent of their bone tissue over time.

The body's *absorption* of dietary calcium also decreases with age in both men and women. Thus, everybody's need for calcium actually increases with age. Certain women, partially for genetic reasons, are more vulnerable to osteoporosis and bone fractures. Among men, osteoporosis is a greater threat to those who are white (black men are less susceptible) and who smoke, drink more alcohol than average, and take calcium-robbing medications.

WOMEN AT HIGHEST RISK OF OSTEOPOROSIS
White and Oriental
Blond or red-haired, of northern European ancestry
Postmenopausal
Underweight
Small bone structure
Heavy alcohol users
Smokers
Heavy caffeine users
Those on a high-protein diet
Those with a family history (mothers, sisters, aunts, grandmothers with osteoporosis)

It's Never Too Early for More Calcium

Studies show that calcium produces denser bones, and the denser your bones when you are young, the more protected you are against osteoporosis in later life. After bone loss begins, typically after age thirty-five, greater intakes of calcium may arrest bone loss, some experts believe, but will not reverse it. That is why the most critical periods for high intakes of calcium are during adolescence and early adulthood. For example, one study found that females who drank more calcium-laden milk as children had denser bones, more resistant to osteoporosis in older age.

If you have not been so prudent, increasing your calcium in later life may help retard bone loss, although there is no proof that calcium is a remedy for osteoporosis. Some authorities believe loading up on calcium much after age thirty-five does little good. Nevertheless, a National Institutes of Health panel of experts in 1984 recommended drastic increases in calcium intake for older women. They noted that lab animals deprived of calcium develop osteoporosis and that surveys of the aged show lower rates of bone fractures in those who eat more calcium-rich dairy products.

DISEASES THAT MAY BE LINKED TO CALCIUM DEFICIENCY
Research on animals and/or humans proves or suggests a connection between calcium deficiencies and:
Osteoporosis
High blood pressure
Colon cancer

Arthritis
Leg cramps
Periodontal bone loss

Culprit in Gum Disease

There's evidence that bone loss due to persistent long-term calcium deficiency begins in the jaws. This leads some experts to speculate that periodontal bone and tooth loss is linked to calcium deficiency. One study showed that 1 gram of calcium supplementation per day for eighteen months reversed periodontal bone loss in 40 percent of those tested. In the other 60 percent the bone loss did not progress.

The Calcium–High Blood Pressure Connection

Impressive and growing evidence shows that high blood pressure among a large group of Americans is linked to calcium deficiency. Some researchers insist that perhaps 45 percent of those with hypertension (high blood pressure) are "calcium sensitive," and that calcium may be as or more important than sodium in regulating blood pressure. Pioneering this scientific research are Dr. David A. McCarron, an internist at the Oregon Health Sciences University, and Dr. John Laragh, a Cornell University cardiologist.

Some of the findings: Hypertensive people eat fewer calcium-rich foods. Women with osteoporosis are more than twice as likely to have both diastolic and systolic high blood pressure as women of the same age without osteoporosis. A major study of about eight thousand men aged forty-five to sixty-four by the National Heart, Lung and Blood Institute revealed that non-milk drinkers were twice as likely to have high blood pressure as those who drank a quart of milk a day.

Several studies show that calcium supplements can lower high blood pressure, especially in those with low calcium blood levels and a high sodium intake. According to Dr. Laragh, among a group of hypertensive patients who were "calcium sensitive" (had low blood levels of ionized calcium), 60 percent (sixteen out of twenty-six) showed a drop in blood pressure with 2 grams of calcium-carbonate pills per day. The average drop was from 160/94 mm Hg to 128/81 mm Hg. Dr. Laragh estimates that from one-third to one-half of all hypertension patients (ten to twenty million) can benefit from increased calcium. Although calcium supplements were used in the study, Dr. Laragh notes that some people with mild hypertension (with diastolic blood pressure readings of

90–104 mm Hg) related to calcium deficiency can lower blood pressure through a high-calcium diet.

However, there is evidence that heavy doses of calcium can also raise blood pressure in some hypertensives (apparently those not "calcium sensitive"). Thus, if you have high blood pressure, don't self-medicate with calcium without medical supervision; you could do yourself more harm than good.

One study at the University of Texas Health Science Center found that about 20 percent of mild hypertensives, given 800 mg of calcium a day, had a dramatic *increase* in blood pressure. An equal percentage registered large drops in blood pressure with the same dose.

It is unclear how a deficiency of calcium affects blood pressure, and some authorities still dispute the connection. But others speculate that some hypertensives have a genetic metabolic defect making them respond abnormally to calcium. Current thought holds that high blood pressure is related not to calcium alone but to the intricate combined effects of several minerals, including sodium, phosphorus, and potassium. Those who seem to benefit most from calcium are the so-called salt reactors, who experience higher blood pressure from excessive salt. Some researchers believe that the higher calcium intake counteracts the blood-pressure–raising effects of sodium.

Calcium and Colon Cancer

Two or three glasses of milk a day may help prevent colorectal cancer because of milk's high calcium and vitamin D content, according to a major study of about two thousand middle-aged men. Those who drank no milk were three times more likely to come down with colorectal cancer than those who drank a couple of glasses a day. Other studies have shown that calcium alone apparently renders bile acids less toxic in the colon; bile acids are implicated in the cause and progression of colon cancer.

Recent research by Dr. Martin Lipkin and colleagues at New York's Memorial Sloan-Kettering Cancer Center found that calcium supplements "quieted"—or reduced the growth rate of—cancer-prone cells lining the colon of patients at high risk because of a family history of colon cancer. Their theory is that the calcium blocked the effect of bile acid.

How Much Do You Absorb?

Your body does not absorb all the calcium you take in. An average adult absorbs from 20 to 30 percent of the calcium in the diet. The amount of calcium absorbed depends on need and other factors, including calcium antagonists in foods and drugs. For example, a pregnant woman generally absorbs more calcium from the same amount of milk than she did before she was pregnant—50 percent versus 20 or 30 percent. Growing children absorb 50 to 60 percent of the calcium they ingest. The elderly have an impaired ability to absorb calcium. One study showed that calcium absorption past the age of sixty fell dramatically—by one-third between the ages of seventy and eighty, compared with ages twenty to sixty. After age eighty, calcium malabsorption was severe.

Calcium Antagonists and Helpers

Animal and/or human studies reveal that the following factors may affect how calcium is absorbed or utilized by the body; the extent of the effect depends on many unknowns, and the interaction may be important only if the antagonist or booster is of sufficient magnitude.

FACTORS THAT MAY BOOST UTILIZATION OF CALCIUM
Vitamin D
Protein
Exercise
Lactose (milk sugar)
Vitamin C
Sunshine

Vitamin D is considered the most essential in utilizing calcium. Without vitamin D, much calcium would simply be flushed out of the body. Most vitamin D comes from exposure to the sun; ultraviolet rays trigger the body's production of vitamin D. Additionally, you get some vitamin D in foods, such as fortified milk (about 98 percent of all milk sold is fortified with vitamin D), liver, and tuna, but this type of vitamin D must be "activated" or converted to a hormone called calcitriol before the body can use it. One study shows that as people age, their ability to activate vitamin D diminishes. Thus, some people may need more vitamin D if they eat few vitamin D foods and are not in the sun. The hormone calcitriol may emerge as a drug for increasing calcium absorption and fighting osteoporosis.

Current recommendations for vitamin D are 400 international units for those under age sixty-five and 600 to 800 IUs after age sixty-five.

Some people may need vitamin D supplements, but take them with caution.

Vitamin D is toxic in high doses and can lead to dangerously high levels of calcium in the blood, causing damage to the arteries and kidneys. In fact, chronic overdoses of vitamin D can alter calcium metabolism so as actually to trigger bone *loss*. Since people differ greatly in their reactions to vitamin D, it is difficult to say how much is toxic. According to one study, as little as 2,000 IUs of vitamin D daily has produced loss of calcium in bones. The NIH expert committee warned against more than 600 to 800 IUs of vitamin D per day except on a physician's recommendation.

FOODS HIGH IN VITAMIN D

	IU
Milk, fortified with vitamin D: 1 c	100
Eel, smoked: 3½ oz	6400
Salmon, canned: 3½ oz	500
Sardines, canned: 3½ oz	300
Shrimp, canned: 3½ oz	105
Chicken liver, simmered: 3½ oz	67
Pork liver, cooked: 3½ oz	51
Smoked link sausage, pork and beef: 1 link (about 2⅓ oz)	32
Egg, chicken: 1 medium egg	23
40% Bran Flakes: ¾ c	100
Product 19: ¾ c	200

FACTORS THAT MAY BLOCK CALCIUM, INCREASING NEED

• *Alcohol.* Bone loss and osteoporosis can be quite dramatic even in young alcoholic males. Alcohol per se may inhibit calcium absorption; also, alcohol interferes with the utilization of vitamin D needed for calcium absorption. One study showed that male social drinkers had nearly two and a half times the risk of osteoporosis as nondrinking males.

• *Smoking.* Smokers have a higher risk of osteoporosis than nonsmokers. A Mayo Clinic study found that male cigarette smokers had a 2.3 times greater risk of the disease. A California study estimated that women smokers lost about twice as much bone mass as nonsmokers.

• *Sodium.* Perhaps helping to explain a link between high blood pressure and calcium, a Dutch study found that doubling the sodium intake from 3,000 mg to 6,000 mg daily resulted in a 20 percent greater excretion of calcium by the kidneys.

• *High-fat foods.* Eating excessively fatty foods may increase calcium demands, because too much fat combines with calcium, converting it to insoluble fatty globs the body cannot absorb.

YOU MAY NEED EVEN MORE CALCIUM IF:

You are a heavy smoker or drinker; eat a diet high in caffeine, protein, fat, sodium, phosphorus, food fiber, or phytates (agents found in whole-grain foods); are under great stress; are sedentary; have certain diseases; are taking certain drugs.

• *Stress.* Some studies show that excessive worry or strain may deplete calcium, even though intake is normal.

• *Lack of exercise.* Physical activity, especially "weight bearing" exercise, such as walking, jogging, biking, aerobics, and jumping rope, are thought to somehow promote calcium utilization. Bedridden or immobilized people suffer drastic and rapid calcium bone loss. Conversely, athletes have denser bones than nonathletes. Exercise may even trigger new bone growth. The playing arms of tennis players have denser bones than do their nonplaying arms.

• *Caffeine.* One recent study showed that caffeine increases the body's need for calcium. Researchers at Washington State University noted that an older man or woman would have to consume an extra one-third cup of milk or one-half ounce of cheddar cheese to make up for the calcium loss caused by two cups of coffee.

• *Food fiber.* There is considerable evidence showing that when you eat more food fiber—both from grains and fruits and vegetables—your calcium levels drop. The solution is not to cut out high fiber but to compensate by eating more calcium. A rough estimate by one researcher is to increase your intake of calcium by 150 mg for every 25 grams of extra fiber. Some research shows that the body may adapt in time to a high-fiber diet, overcoming the calcium deficit.

• *Phytates or phytic acid* (agents found in whole-grain foods). Phytates are reported to bind numerous minerals, including calcium, lowering absorption.

• *Certain diseases.* The following conditions suppress the absorption of calcium: primary biliary cirrhosis; severe Crohn's disease (inflammatory bowel disease); chronic kidney failure; diabetes; hypoparathyroidism.

Calcium Enemy Number One

Although many green leafy vegetables are high in calcium, some are not considered good calcium sources. The reason: they are also high in oxalic acid, or oxalates. The oxalates retard the body's absorption of the calcium. Thus, when you eat spinach, the calcium value to the body may range from 50 percent to zilch, according to different studies. Exactly how much of the calcium is destroyed by oxalates is unknown, but it probably depends on how much of each you eat. If the calcium content is high—for example, as in milk—a little oxalate from chocolate will probably make little difference in calcium bioavailability.

Although much more research is needed on this hazard, the best current advice is: Do not depend on foods high in both oxalates and calcium as good calcium sources.

POOR SOURCES OF CALCIUM
(Foods high in both calcium and oxalic acid)

Food	Oxalic acid mg per 100 grams
Beets, boiled	109
Green beans, raw	43.7
Green beans, cooked	29.7
Rhubarb, stewed	447
Spinach, boiled	571

DRUGS THAT MAY DEPLETE CALCIUM
Antacids that contain aluminum
Cholestyramine (lowers blood cholesterol)
Furosemide (diuretic)
Anticonvulsant medications
Thyroid medication (high doses)
Corticosteroids (taken over long periods)
Tetracycline (antibiotic)
Isoniazid (a tuberculosis treatment and prevention drug)

Food Sources of Calcium

By far the best sources of calcium are dairy products. However, even if you are lactose intolerant (lacking the capability to easily digest lactose or "milk sugar" in many dairy products), you can get high amounts of calcium from other foods. Yogurt without added milk solids is okay for most lactose intolerant persons. You can buy lactase and add it to milk. Some dairy products, such as low-lactose milk and cheese, are available in many parts of the country. And numerous other foods, such as canned sardines, mackerel, and salmon *with bones,* have high amounts of calcium.

Important: Fish without bones has little or no calcium.

The Cow without the Calories

Many high-calcium foods are dairy products, which connote high fat and high calories. But many low-fat dairy products have as much, sometimes more, calcium than high-fat whole milk and cheeses. Remember, the calcium is contained in the milk, not in the fat. Taking out the fat does not affect the calcium content at all. Sometimes food processors *add* nonfat milk solids to low-fat dairy products to thicken them. That explains why yogurt, for example, often has even more calcium than the milk from which it was made. Skim milk is an excellent low-calorie, high-calcium drink.

Important: Don't depend on cream cheese and Neufchâtel or cottage cheese for your calcium. They are not good sources. Other cheeses are excellent calcium sources, although they are usually high in fat. Few people realize that the calcium content of cheeses varies considerably. For example, American processed cheese has only half as much calcium per ounce as Parmesan.

HOW CHEESES RANK: THE TOP TWENTY

	Milligrams of calcium per ounce
Parmesan	355
Romano	301
Gruyère	287
Swiss	272
Processed Swiss	219
Provolone	214
Monterey	211
Mozzarella, part skim	207
Edam	207
Cheese food, Swiss	205
Cheddar	204
Muenster	203
Tilsit	198
Gouda	198
Colby	194
Brick	191

	Milligrams of calcium per ounce
Caraway	191
Roquefort	188
Port du Salut	184
American processed	174

Source: Author's computer analysis of USDA data

Cooking to Preserve Calcium

Calcium is not lost from the pasteurization, homogenization, heating, or drying of milk. Modest amounts of calcium can leach into the water when cooking vegetables. Since calcium and other minerals are concentrated near the skin, you save calcium by cooking vegetables unpeeled.

Food: Better and Safer

It is better to get calcium through foods because for one reason it is better absorbed. There is some evidence that milk prevents bone loss better than do pure calcium-carbonate pills. Further, it is almost impossible for healthy people to get too much calcium from the diet because the small intestine prevents excess calcium from being absorbed. Occasionally that safeguard breaks down and high blood calcium levels lead to calcification of the kidneys and other organs. This is more likely to happen in the presence of too much vitamin D.

Toxicity and Supplements

Some experts worry that Americans are overdosing on calcium supplements. Dr. Walter Mertz, head of the Department of Agriculture's Human Nutrition Research Center, warns that rats stuffed with calcium end up with calcified and encrusted internal organs. If you do take calcium, keep it within the bounds of the RDAs, or the NIH expert committee's recommendations, which set 1,500 mg daily as the maximum safe dose—unless a physician advises higher amounts.

Estimate how much calcium you get from your diet, and then add only the amount of supplement necessary to bring the level to the appropriate RDA for calcium. Calcium carbonate is usually considered the cheapest and most concentrated supplement. For best absorption, take the supplement at intervals, not all at once. Washing the pills down with a little milk may increase absorption. Avoid dolomite and bone-meal calcium supplements, which may be contaminated with poisonous metals such as lead.

POSSIBLE ADVERSE EFFECTS OF EXCESSIVE CALCIUM SUPPLEMENTS

Kidney stones in some susceptible persons

Constipation (notably from calcium-carbonate tablets)

Acidic stomach

High blood pressure complications

Nausea

Milk-alkali syndrome—a serious, unusual condition characterized by early warning signs of nausea, headache, and weakness (caused by a heavy diet of milk or cream with high doses of calcium carbonate—8 grams or so per day)

FOODS RICH IN CALCIUM

The most calcium regardless of calories

Milk	Canned mackerel, salmon, and
Cheese	sardines with bones
Yogurt	Filberts
Smelts	Kale
Almonds	Collards
Caviar	Tofu

CALCIUM SUPER-FOODS
THE MOST CALCIUM, THE FEWEST CALORIES

Here are 50 foods that rate exceptionally high in calcium content per calorie. Of the approximately 2500 foods in this book, these are tops in calcium nutrient density; they have the highest calcium-calorie ratios, giving you the most calcium for the fewest calories.*

	Food Rating	Calcium-calorie ratio (mg of Calcium per 100 calories)	Common Measure	Mg Calcium	Calories
1.	Bok choi, cooked	775	½ c	79	10
2.	Turnip greens, fresh, cooked	685	½ c	99	14
3.	Collards, frozen, cooked	583	½ c	179	31
4.	Collards, fresh, cooked	557	½ c	74	13
5.	Kale, frozen, cooked	428	½ c	90	19
6.	Dandelion greens, fresh, cooked	424	½ c	73	17
7.	Broccoli, fresh, cooked	393	½ c	89	23
8.	Yogurt, plain, skim milk	357	4 oz	225	63
9.	Milk, skim	353	1 c	316	90
10.	Milk, dry, nonfat	347	¼ c	377	109
11.	Parmesan cheese	302	1 oz	336	111
12.	Milk, 1% fat	300	1 c	300	102
13.	Yogurt, plain, lowfat	289	4 oz	207	72
14.	Buttermilk	288	1 c	285	99
15.	Romano cheese	275	1 oz	302	110
16.	Mozzarella cheese, part skim	261	1 oz	207	80
17.	Okra, frozen, cooked	260	½ c	88	34
18.	Milk, lowfat, 2% fat, fortified	258	1 c	352	137
19.	Swiss cheese	256	1 oz	213	83
20.	Gruyere cheese	245	1 oz	286	117
21.	Swiss cheese, processed	231	1 oz	220	95
22.	Sardines, with bones, canned in tomato sauce	228	.8 oz	108	47
23.	Sardines, with bones, canned in oil	215	3 oz	371	172
24.	Provolone cheese	215	1 oz	214	100
25.	Tilsit cheese	206	1 oz	198	96
26.	Edam cheese	205	1 oz	205	100
27.	Yogurt, coffee, vanilla, low-fat	200	4 oz	194	97
28.	Monterey cheese	199	1 oz	212	106
29.	Ricotta, part skim	197	½ c	337	171
30.	Yogurt, plain, whole milk	197	4 oz	137	70
31.	Gouda cheese	196	1 oz	198	100
32.	Muenster cheese	195	1 oz	203	104
33.	Milk, whole, 3.3% fat	194	1 c	291	150
34.	Cheese spread, American	193	1 oz	157	82
35.	Feta cheese	187	1 oz	140	75
36.	Brick	181	1 oz	162	90
37.	Roquefort cheese	179	1 oz	188	105
38.	Cheddar cheese	179	1 oz	205	114
39.	Caraway cheese	179	1 oz	191	107
40.	Bean curd (tofu)	178	½ c	118	66
41.	Cheese food, American	175	1 oz	163	93

	Food Rating	Calcium-calorie ratio *(mg of Calcium per 100 calories)*	Common Measure	Mg Calcium	Calories
42.	Colby cheese	174	1 oz	165	95
43.	Cod, salted, dried	173	1 oz	63	36
44.	Cheese, processed American	164	1 oz	174	105
45.	Yogurt, fruit, low-fat	161	4 oz	172	115
46.	Oats, instant, fortified, plain	156	1 pkt	164	105
47.	Limburger cheese	152	1 oz	141	93
48.	Blue cheese	149	1 oz	150	100
49.	Salmon, with bones, canned	147	3 oz can	191	130
50.	Mackerel, with bones, canned	144	3 oz	263	182

Source: Author's computer analysis from USDA data

*Excludes baby foods. Includes only foods for which one serving supplies a minimum of approximately 10 percent of RDA. Also excludes foods high in oxalates.

RECOMMENDED DAILY DIETARY ALLOWANCES OF CALCIUM

Age	Milligrams
0–6 months	360
6 months–1 year	540
1–10	800
11–18	1200
19–39	800*
40 and over	800*
Pregnant or nursing	add 400

Source: National Academy of Sciences, Revised 1980

*A National Institutes of Health committee on osteoporosis in 1984 branded this too low. They recommend:

Women until menopause	1000
Postmenopausal women not taking estrogen	1500
Postmenopausal women taking estrogen	1000

Sodium
Wretched Excesses

Sodium is a silver white mineral, an essential nutrient in our diet. More than 90 percent of the sodium we eat comes from sodium chloride, salt (NaCl). Salt is 40 percent sodium and 60 percent chlorine. The detrimental health element in salt is believed to be sodium, not chlorine.

Who Is at Risk?

Practically everybody overdoses on sodium. The amount of sodium Americans consume is truly astounding. According to several surveys, the average American eats from 2,500 to 6,000 mg of sodium per day—ten to twenty-five times the amount needed for good health. The worst offenders: men between the ages of eighteen and forty-four and girls from six to fourteen years old. A 1985 food-consumption survey by the Department of Agriculture found that the average child eats an astonishing 2,000 mg of sodium a day, not even counting that added by the salt shaker. Even some infants are consuming up to 2,500 mg of sodium daily—over a teaspoon of salt! The normal human requirement is but one-tenth of a teaspoon.

Our needs for sodium are so minuscule that healthy adults can get by on little more than the minimum requirement for infants. From 200 to 250 mg (equal to one-tenth of a teaspoon of salt) per day are fully enough to support all bodily functions. For centuries our vegetarian forefathers survived well on such minimal sodium intakes. "What's so frightening is how little sodium our body needs," said former Food and Drug Administration commissioner Arthur Hull Hayes, Jr., an expert in hypertension. "In fact, the only sodium we need is the amount we lose every day. And that is really a rather small amount."

"Common sense tells even the uninitiated that it is wise to limit salt intake. Indeed, if salt were a new food additive, it is doubtful that it would be classified as safe and certainly not at the level most of us consume," observed Dr. Mark Hegsted, former head of Human Nutrition at the U.S. Department of Agriculture and now a professor at Harvard.

HOW MUCH SODIUM WE EAT:

4,000 to 6,000 mg daily

HOW MUCH SODIUM WE NEED TO SURVIVE:

200 to 250 mg daily

Salt Cravings: Inborn and Acquired

A craving for salt is a powerful animal instinct, of thirty million years' duration, says Dr. Derek Denton, an Australian physician and worldwide expert on salt. Sensing sodium depletion, the brain sends urgent signals that stop only when the appetite for salt is satisfied. All species of animals, including humans, will go to extreme measures to meet the biological demands for sodium in order to survive. However, this biological craving appears only when the body is severely deprived of sodium, and was apparently developed as an evolutionary protection in days when our ancestors were vegetarians and got little salt in their diet. But rare today is the person who suffers sodium deficiency leading to biological cravings.

Salt (sodium chloride) is 40 percent sodium. One teaspoon of salt contains about 2,000 mg of sodium.

Learning to Love Salt

The modern taste for excessive salt is learned—conditioned by habit-forming supplies of sodium in the diet, according to many experts. After studying a group of Canadian youngsters as infants and again at age four, Dr. David L. Yeung, at the University of Toronto, concluded that a taste for salt depends on how much salt children were fed as infants, and how much salt their parents eat.

Dr. Yeung also found that the salt intake rose abruptly when the infants started on cow's milk and table foods. The salt intake of infants in the study jumped dramatically at a rate of 80 mg increase per month when they began drinking cow's milk. As soon as they began eating table foods—from months eight through ten, the salt intake rose a striking 120 mg per month. At one year of age the babies were eating an average 920 mg daily, and after fifteen months over 1,000 mg daily— two and a half to three times more than Canada's recommended daily intake of sodium.

Dr. Yeung followed the infants in the study until age four, and found that those who were eating excessive salt at that age were often the same ones who had been fed high amounts of salt as infants.

Another study, at the Monell Chemical Senses Center in Philadelphia, found that if you cut back on salt, you may for the next twenty-four hours or so desire more salty foods. But if you hang in there, the desire goes away, and you begin to prefer food with less salt. After salt restriction, your taste buds in fact become more salt sensitive, and foods taste more salty to you than previously—so you prefer salty foods less.

Is Anybody Deficient?

It's virtually impossible to have a chronic deficiency of sodium because it is so widespread in food, and requirements are so slight. Even heavy exercisers are usually in no danger of salt depletion. One study by Dr. David Costill, an exercise physiologist at Ball State University, found that even when athletes underwent strenuous exercise and sweated off two quarts of water at a time, they had enough sodium in their diets to weather it by replacing only lost fluid with plain water. Dr. Costill notes that you lose about 1,000 mg of sodium for every quart of sweat. Further, he says, if you keep up strenuous exercise in hot weather, your body begins to adapt and secretes only one-third to one-half of the normal amount of sodium in sweat, as protection against possible sodium depletion.

However, other experts note that a few people who exercise and sweat profusely in hot weather may deplete their sodium stores and experience deficiency symptoms of weakness, nausea, diarrhea, severe muscle cramps, and mental confusion.

To avert that, if you are sweating heavily (more than three quarts of fluid), you need to replace salt. The National Academy of Sciences Food and Nutrition Board recommends that you replace the first three pounds of fluid lost with plain water. After that, use 2 to 7 grams (one-third to a little over a teaspoon) of salt for each additional quart of fluid lost.

Warning: Don't take salt tablets unless recommended by a physician. These tablets are so concentrated that they can even further throw off your body's sodium balance, leading to severe dehydration.

Health Consequences: Heart Disease and Stroke

Some experts blame too much salt for promoting an epidemic of heart disease and stroke by causing or aggravating high blood pressure (hypertension.) About sixty million Americans have "essential hypertension" with silent symptoms and cause unknown. High blood pressure somehow accelerates atherosclerosis (hardening of the arteries). As a rule of thumb, the higher the blood pressure, the greater the danger of cardiovascular disease. Some experts claim that even chronic mild or moderate elevated blood pressure raises the risk of catastrophic illness and death. If you have "definite" high blood pressure (diastolic, or lower number, above 90), you are:

• Eight times more likely than average to have a stroke (high blood pressure is the number-one cause of strokes)

• Three times more likely than average to have a heart attack

• Five times more likely than average to suffer congestive heart failure

At especially high risk of high blood pressure are blacks (twice the risk of whites), the overweight, and those whose parents have high blood pressure. Vegetarians generally have less high blood pressure.

The Sodium–High Blood Pressure Puzzle

More than half a century ago, scientists began to suspect a connection between too much sodium and high blood pressure. The suspicion has now become a full-scale investigation. Although the extent and nature of the connection is still controversial, the growing consensus is that excessive sodium is a strong factor in promoting high blood pressure in certain people. The British medical journal *Lancet* calls high blood pressure a type of "salt poisoning."

Here is the main evidence:

• Studies of populations throughout the world show a direct correlation between high-salt diets and the number of people with high blood pressure. The greater the amount of salt consumed, the greater the chance of high blood pressure. In one study, by the late Lewis K. Dahl, of the Brookhaven National Laboratory in Upton, New York, ten percent who ate a high-salt diet had high blood pressure, and 7 percent who ate moderate amounts of salt had the disease, compared with only 1 percent who ate little salt.

• *The Japanese.* There is much good to be said about the classic Japanese low-fat diet, but when it comes to salt consumption, the Japanese are the worst. Their rate of high blood pressure and stroke is also astronomical. The Japanese, with a diet high in soy sauce, miso, and salted fish, commonly consume 25 grams of salt a day (10,000 mg of sodium). In parts of the north, Japanese often eat 50 grams of salt daily—about 10 teaspoons. From 40 to 60 percent of the adult population is reported to have high blood pressure and a stroke rate 170 percent higher than ours.

• *Primitive peoples.* Cultures that exist on low-sodium diets as our prehistoric ancestors did have virtually no high blood pressure—the Maori tribesmen, the Kalahari bushmen of Africa, the Aita of the Solomon Islands, and the Indians of the Amazon Basin. Among some the diet contains a mere 500 mg of sodium a day. Studies also show that their blood pressure does not increase with age as it does in industrialized countries. But—a crucial point—when these people who have not grown up eating salt move to more civilized settings where they eat more salt, processed food, and fat, they develop essentially the same high rates of blood pressure as everybody else.

• *Animals on sodium.* In numerous studies with rats, pigs, chickens, and monkeys, a high-sodium diet has induced high blood pressure within months or years. There's also evidence that feeding genetically susceptible animals high amounts of sodium as infants predisposes them to high blood pressure in later life. The same animals did not develop high blood pressure when not given salt early in life. The younger the animal, the more susceptible to sodium, indicating that high blood pressure may be a long-term problem with its origins in high salt consumption during infancy.

• *Genetic factors.* Interestingly, experimenters found that the reaction to sodium was determined by genetic differences. Some animals are "sodium sensitive" (prone to high blood pressure from salt) and some "sodium resistant" (don't develop high blood pressure even with sodium overloads). Also, when kidneys from salt-sensitive rats were transplanted to salt-resistant rats, the rats with the new kidneys developed high blood pressure when fed sodium, indicating genetic susceptibility.

• *Human experiments.* There is strong evidence that cutting down on salt lowers blood pressure. A landmark study by Dr. Graham MacGregor at London's Charing Cross Hospital found that a moderately restricted salt intake lowered blood pressure by an average of 6 percent in patients—about the same as a diuretic or a beta blocker would do. A Mayo Clinic study showed that patients on low-salt diets were much more likely to achieve normal blood pressure than those who ate more salt. Studies have also demonstrated that a low-salt diet can lower blood pressure in people with normal readings, indicating that a low-salt diet may *prevent* as well as treat high blood pressure.

WHEN IS BLOOD PRESSURE TOO HIGH?

	Diastolic (lower reading)
Normal	under 85
High-Normal	85–89
Mild high blood pressure	90–104
Moderate high blood pressure	105–114
Severe high blood pressure	115 and over

HEALTH PROBLEMS THAT MAY BE LINKED TO SODIUM EXCESSES

Research on animals and/or humans proves or suggests a connection between excessive sodium and:

High blood pressure, leading to stroke, heart, and kidney disease
Obesity
Water retention

At Highest Risk: The "Salt Sensitive"

Some humans, like animals, are apparently "sodium reactors" —genetically prone to high blood pressure. Experts estimate that at least 15 to 20 percent of the population has some genetic abnormality reducing their ability to excrete excessive salt, which triggers high blood pressure. It is generally agreed that most of these may benefit enormously from reduced sodium intakes. Unfortunately, there is no widely available test to identify such people. The only proof: when cutting down on sodium lowers blood pressure. Treating high blood pressure with diet is also preferable to the risk of side effects from drugs.

How much sodium or salt should people with high blood pressure eat? The important thing seems to be that they eat less than they do now. Says one expert, "As little as possible." One major study showed significant drops in blood pressure when persons cut their sodium intake in half—from 4,400 mg to 1,900 mg daily. Another two-year study showed that blood pressure dropped—to normal in some cases—when sodium intake went down from 4,400 to 3,600 mg—an 18 percent reduction. Some experts consider 1,100 mg—the National Academy of

Sciences' low range—best for people with or at risk of high blood pressure.

The American Medical Association says the general policy among physicians is to recommend that people with high blood pressure consume a maximum of 2,000 mg of sodium a day (1 teaspoon of salt). That includes both salt from the table and in processed foods which are the primary source of sodium.

WARNING: Pregnant women should not restrict sodium intake. The well-known desire for salty foods during pregnancy (pickles, for example) apparently serves a compelling biological need. Physicians used to prescribe diuretics and a low-sodium diet during pregnancy—but recent information shows that practice to be potentially dangerous. Most experts now advise pregnant women to eat as much salt as their taste dictates.

No Problem for Some?

But what about the millions of other Americans who do not have high blood pressure or a family history denoting a genetic predisposition? Should they too cut back on sodium? Dr. James C. Hunt, chancellor of the University of Tennessee Center for the Health Sciences, and a prominent hypertension researcher, argues that there is no biological reason for 90 percent of the sodium we consume, so there can be no harm in such reductions and possibly great benefit. Also, some experts doubt that hypertension is entirely genetically controlled; they contend that excessive salt in early life may cause later onset of high blood pressure even in people not genetically predisposed.

On the other hand, Dr. James W. Woods, professor of medicine and cardiology at the University of North Carolina, says: "We do know that hypertension tends to aggregate in families, and with that history, people are well advised to moderate their intake of salt. But unless one has hypertension or a family history of it, I don't think one can make a compelling case for major diet modification." Dr. Norman Kaplan, a high blood pressure specialist at the University of Texas Health Science Center in Dallas, says that both those with and those without high blood pressure should eat less salt, but he adds that a person with normal blood pressure, no family history of high blood pressure, and older than forty-five or fifty is quite unlikely to develop high blood pressure and "can probably go ahead and eat what he damn well pleases."

Sodium Antagonists

DIETARY FACTORS THAT MAY HELP COUNTERACT THE DETRI-
MENTAL EFFECTS OF SODIUM
Potassium
Calcium
A low-fat diet
Weight loss
Dietary fiber
Protein restriction

Potassium May Counteract Sodium Excesses

If you eat too much sodium, you should also be sure you eat a lot of potassium. There's a chance the potassium can help neutralize the damaging effects on blood pressure. In 1928 a scientist noted that increased sodium raised blood pressure, but that increased potassium lowered it. Since then, numerous studies show that potassium has a protective effect against high amounts of sodium in the diet, ameliorating high blood pressure. The beneficial effect is most pronounced when the diet is exceptionally high in sodium.

In some cases there was little or no potassium effect when the sodium intake was low or moderate. Some experts say that our caveman ancestors were protected from high blood pressure by generous intakes of potassium from fruits and vegetables, as well as low intakes of sodium.

Thus, it is no surprise that high potassium consumption seems also to protect modern vegetarians from high blood pressure. In one study, meat eaters and vegetarians ate about the same amounts of sodium, but the vegetarians who ate more potassium had lower blood pressure. The conclusion was that the high consumption of potassium in the fruits and vegetables helped to counteract the blood-pressure–raising effects of sodium.

More Calcium, Too

Other reports show that increasing calcium intake can help blunt the effects of sodium, helping to keep blood pressure lower.

High amounts of sodium also increase your need for calcium. One study shows that doubling the amount of sodium—from 3,000 to 6,000 mg daily—caused a 20 percent increase in loss of calcium from the body.

Sodium Interacts with Drugs

More sodium means more drugs. If you are on high blood pressure medication, especially diuretics, a high-sodium diet can necessitate larger doses of drugs to bring blood pressure down, increasing chances of side effects.

WHERE SODIUM IS FOUND IN THE DIET

	Percent
Naturally in foods	about 10
Processed foods	about 75
Salt added in home cooking or at the table	15

Source: Center for Science in the Public Interest

Hidden Sodium: You Can't Always Tell by the Taste

You can readily spot the high salt in foods like pickles, olives, nitrite-cured meats, sauerkraut, potato chips, and pretzels. The problem is that many processed foods don't actually taste salty; the excess sodium is concealed. Often the sodium taste is masked by stronger flavors and spices. Only salt lying on the surface, as on potato chips and peanuts, tweaks our taste buds and is readily noticeable.

Some foods you would least suspect contain the most sodium. Would you believe, for example, that ounce per ounce Kellogg's corn-flakes has twice as much sodium as Planter's cocktail peanuts? Or that two slices of Pepperidge Farm white bread has more sodium than an ounce of Lay's potato chips? Or that one-half cup of prepared Jell-O instant chocolate-flavor pudding has more sodium than three slices of Oscar Mayer bacon? (Source: *Consumer Reports* magazine.)

Salt Is Not the Only Sodium

OTHER COMMON SOURCES OF SODIUM IN PROCESSED FOODS TO BEWARE OF BESIDES SALT (sodium chloride)
- sodium nitrite (a curing agent in meats)
- sodium phosphate (an emulsifier found especially in processed cheeses)
- sodium bicarbonate, or baking soda (found in baked goods)

- monosodium glutamate (MSG—a flavor enhancer)
- sodium bisulfite (a preservative and antioxidant)
- sodium propionate (a preservative)
- sodium saccharin (an artificial sweetener)

How to Read Sodium Labels

Products with nutritional labeling (about one-half of all foods) are now required to note the amount of sodium along with other nutrients. Manufacturers may even offer sodium information even if they do not carry other nutritional information. Here are the meanings of terms that can be used on labeling, according to the Food and Drug Administration.

Sodium free—less than 5 mg per serving
Very low sodium—less than 135 mg per serving
Low sodium—140 mg or less per serving
Reduced sodium—75 percent reduction in sodium from that usually found in a product
Unsalted, no salt added, without added salt—foods processed without salt which ordinarily have it; for example "no salt added" pretzels or potato chips

---

Recommendation: If a product contains less than 135 mg of sodium per serving, consider it *safe*. If it contains more than that, check the grocery shelves for a "no-salt added" version.

Source: Center for Science in the Public Interest

Ways to Cut Back on Sodium

- Use fresh or frozen vegetables, which are lower in sodium.
- Drain the juice in canned vegetables, substituting water for heating (gets rid of 30 percent of the sodium).
- Rinse canned tuna with tap water for a minute. It will remove 80 percent of the sodium, according to an experiment at Duke University Medical Center.
- Gradually cut back on the use of the salt shaker. One study showed that using a salt shaker with smaller holes cut back dramatically on the amount of salt used.
- Taste food *before* you salt it. According to one study, only one out of four people does. Salting is a habit.

- Substitute herbs and other seasonings for salt.
- Reduce the amount of salt called for in recipes.
- In restaurants, ask for dishes to be cooked without salt.

Sodium Chloride Toxicity

In sudden high doses, salt has caused severe poisoning, cerebral hemorrhages, kidney damage, permanent brain damage, and even death. Babies have died in hospital nurseries when salt was accidentally substituted for sugar in formulas. One seventeen-year-old girl who downed four glasses of salt water (150 grams of salt, or 60 grams of sodium) within an hour and a half developed severe toxic symptoms. Experts say that 3 grams of sodium chloride per kilogram (2.2 lbs) of body weight could be a lethal dose. Injections of high doses of sodium chloride into pregnant animals have produced offspring with birth defects—mainly clubfoot and other abnormalities of the feet and toes.

ESTIMATED SAFE AND ADEQUATE DAILY INTAKE OF SODIUM

Age	Milligrams Sodium
Infants	
birth–6 months	115–350
6 months–1 year	250–750
Children	
1–3	325–975
4–6	450–1350
7–10	600–1800
11 and over	900–2700
Adults	1100–3300

Source: National Academy of Sciences Food and Nutrition Board, Revised 1980

THE 50 SALTIEST FOODS
(by common measure)

	Sodium mg
1. Salt, table: 1 tsp	2000
2. Cod, dried, salted: 1 oz	1960
3. Sauerkraut juice: 1 c	1904
4. Pickles, dill: 1 lrg (about 4 in long)	1827
5. Manhattan clam chowder, canned: 1 c	1808
6. Chicken broth, from cube: 1 c	1536
7. Ham, boneless, roasted: 3 oz	1177
8. Black bean soup, canned: 1 c	1197
9. Beef broth, from cube: 1 c	1152
10. Soy sauce: 1 tbsp	1029
11. Cream of potato soup, canned: 1 c	1000
12. Beef, dried: 1 oz	984
13. Oyster stew, canned: 1 c	980
14. Peppers, red or green, canned: ½ c	958
15. Chicken gumbo soup, canned: 1 c	954
16. Tuna, canned: 3 oz	930
17. Salmon, smoked: 1 oz	890
18. Hot chili peppers, canned: 1 pepper	856
19. Olives, green: 10	827
20. Ham, luncheon: 2 slices	810
21. Sauerkraut, canned: ½ c	780
22. Herring, smoked, kippered: 3 oz	765
23. Pretzels: 1 c	756
24. Canadian style bacon: 2 slices	719
25. Sardines, canned oil: 3 oz	700
26. Kielbasa: 1 oz	687
27. Corn grits, instant w imitn ham bits: 1 pkt	657
28. Salami, pork: 1 oz	642
29. Frankfurters, turkey: 1	641
30. Turkey luncheon meat, loaf: 2 slices	608
31. Pepperoni: 5 slices	560
32. Roquefort cheese: 1 oz	513
33. Luncheon meat, beef, thin sliced: 1 oz	470
34. Frankfurter, beef: 1	462
35. Cheese spread, processed, American: 1 oz	461
36. Parmesan cheese: 1 oz	449
37. Peppered loaf luncheon meat: 1 slice	435
38. Luncheon meat, olive loaf: 1 oz	423
39. Sausage, thuringer: 1 oz	412

		Sodium mg
40.	Cottage cheese: 4 oz	459
41.	Cheese, blue: 1 oz	395
42.	Wheaties: 1 oz	355
43.	Total cereal: 1 oz	352
44.	Cornflakes: 1 oz	352
45.	Caviar: 1 tbsp	352
46.	Golden Grahams cereal: ¾ c	346
47.	Rice Krispies: 1 c	340
48.	Romano cheese: 1 oz	340
49.	Bacon, cooked: 3 slices	303
50.	Smoked link pork sausage: 1 link	240

Source: Author's computer analysis of USDA data

Iron
The Dangers of Being Female

Iron, the fourth most abundant element in the earth's crust, is a trace mineral essential for life. Its main job is to transport oxygen around the body—via hemoglobin in red blood cells and myoglobin in the muscles. Iron is also essential for the proper functioning of many biochemical reactions, especially in relation to the enzyme system. Iron deficiency—with and without anemia—is a serious worldwide problem.

Who Needs to Worry?

Iron is in such short supply in the average American diet that it has consistently been labeled a "problem nutrient" by government nutritionists. According to the federal government's National Health and Nutrition Examination Survey (1980) of about twenty-eight thousand Americans of all ages, only 43 percent of the entire population takes in as much iron as authorities recommend. Most at risk of deficiencies: females of all ages and youngsters between ages one and two. Shockingly, only 4 percent of children aged one to two take in the recommended dietary allowance of iron. The average youngster that age eats only 55 percent of the recommended iron—an all-time low for any nutrient at any age.

YOUR CHANCES OF EATING AN IRON-DEFICIENT DIET

	Percent
Child, age 1–2	96
Adult male	10
Female, age 12–50	95

The Alarming Female Condition

A look at females between the ages of twelve and fifty is equally disconcerting. Virtually every American female from puberty to menopause is lacking iron in the diet. Only 5 to 7 percent meet the RDA for iron and about three-fourths of these take in under 70 percent of the suggested iron. The average female of that age is getting only 60 percent of her optimum needs. Women of reproductive age need much more iron than men because iron is lost during menstruation and pregnancy. Women on average lose over ½ mg of iron per day during menstruation. Pregnancy puts critical strains on iron requirements that an alarming proportion of women do not meet.

Further, individual women differ dramatically in their iron requirements— depending on the amount of iron lost from menstruation. Ten percent of women, for example, consistently lose more than 1.4 mg of iron per day, three times more than the average. Twenty percent of all women have no iron stores whatever, and 8.5 percent are anemic, according to one study.

Adequate iron is especially difficult to achieve for women who are on low-calorie diets. In fact, it is estimated that women eating the typical American diet have to consume approximately 3,000 calories a day to get enough iron. Women after menopause, who cease to lose iron monthly, do not have severe iron-deficient diets.

Who is *not* deficient in iron? Usually, males older than nineteen. Roughly 80 to 90 percent of men eat the daily recommended doses of iron. The average adult male takes in about 150 percent the amount of iron his body needs. However, elderly men, paying little attention to nutrition, may also take in too little iron.

WHO NEEDS MORE IRON: INTAKES BY AGE

Age	% getting less than 100% of RDA	Average intake (% of RDA)
Children (male and female)		
Under 1 (not being breastfed)	40	156
1–2	96	55
3–5	82	80
6–8	36	115
Males		
9–11	55	103
12–14	88	82
15–18	67	92

Ages	% getting less than 100% of RDA	Average intake (% of RDA)
19–22	15	155
23–34	11	158
35–50	11	156
51–64	13	154
65–74	17	142
75 and over	21	140
Females		
9–11	67	92
12–14	94	65
15–18	93	62
19–22	95	59
23–34	95	60
35–50	95	61
51–64	41	113
65–74	46	108
75 and over	50	106

Source: U.S. Department of Agriculture, Food Consumption Survey

Tired, Iron-Poor Blood

What happens if you don't get enough iron? Anemia, from lack of iron in the diet, is the most common nutritional-deficiency disease in the country. Most vulnerable: teenaged girls, young women, infants, and elderly men. Anemia, characterized by low hemoglobin—that substance in red blood cells that carries oxygen around the body—literally causes tissues to become oxygen starved. The body's efficiency slows down, causing muscle weakness, fatigue, listlessness, a tendency to tire easily, and slow recovery from exertion and exercise. One study of women found that their "work performance" quadrupled when they put more iron in their diets. Another showed more-normal heartbeats and quicker recovery from exercise when their anemia was corrected with increased iron.

Although anemia is the "end stage" of severe iron deficiency, mild iron deficiency can produce harm quite unrelated to anemia or oxygen-starved tissues. Scientists now know that iron plays a critical part in enzymatic reaction to keep metabolism functioning smoothly. Growing research reveals that lack of iron can produce subtle harm to intellectual capabilities, notably in children.

SYMPTOMS OF IRON DEFICIENCY
(Both related and unrelated to anemia)

Increased risk of Infection
Immune disorders
Maternal and fetal death and illness
Poor job performance
Decreased gastric-juice secretion
Reduced enzyme activity and malfunction
Decreased growth rate
Muscle weakness
Decreased exercise tolerance
Fatigue
Dizziness
Shortness of breath
Rapid heartbeat
Tingling in fingers and toes

In children
Irritability
Hyperactivity
Learning problems
Shortened attention span
Poor motivation
Poor intellectual performance

Iron Deficiency Affects the Brain

Mounting evidence shows that even iron-deficient infants without anemia have signs of impaired mental development and abnormal behavior, possibly due to changes in the brain's chemical messengers (neurotransmitters) induced by iron deficiency. Studies link iron shortages in children to shortened attention span, lack of intellectual motivation, diminished intellectual performance, hyperactivity, reduced attentive-

---

Caution: Other factors cause anemia besides iron deficiency, so do not medicate yourself with iron to cure suspected anemia. For example, pernicious anemia is *not* caused by an iron-deficient diet, nor is it cured by increased iron. Pernicious anemia is an absorption disorder that produces a vitamin B_{12} deficiency. The disease is treated with vitamin B_{12}.

ness, and lower IQ. Iron-deficient children often show restlessness and irritability that disappear after treatment with iron. Electroencephalograms (EEGs) reveal different brain-wave patterns in iron-deficient youngsters. Many experts now accept the view that some learning disabilities can be associated with iron deficiency.

HEALTH PROBLEMS THAT MAY BE LINKED TO IRON DEFICIENCY
Research on animals and/or humans proves or suggests a connection between iron deficiencies and:

Anemia

Plummer-Vinson syndrome (obstruction of the esophagus)

Cancers of certain types

Infections

Behavior problems in infants and children

The Other Side of the Coin: Too Much Iron

For a segment of the population, iron excess, not deficiency, is a major problem. They have an inherited defect in regulating iron absorption. This can cause "iron overload," or hemochromatosis, a life-threatening condition. Such persons must be extremely cautious in keeping their iron intakes low. Recent studies suggest that iron-storage disease is much more common than previously suspected, and often goes undiagnosed. Some experts worry that chronic consumption of high amounts of iron supplements even by normal people could cause long-term storage of iron in the liver, leading to serious problems in later life.

How to Get More Iron in Your Diet

Important fact: There are two types of iron in the diet—heme and nonheme. Heme iron is more potent; it is found only in animal tissues. Animal tissue iron is about 40 percent heme iron, and 60 percent nonheme iron. *All* of the iron in vegetables, beans and grains is nonheme iron.

This distinction is critical, because it affects dramatically how well your body actually absorbs the iron you eat. Some people eat enough iron but are still quite deficient, because the iron never gets absorbed. It is destroyed in that rough-and-tumble intestinal battlefield where the individual components of the diet fight it out, obliterating and neutralizing one another. Thus, it is a matter not only of getting enough iron, but of making sure it survives that hazardous intestinal journey fairly intact.

Of the two, heme iron is by far the stronger contender for survival. Heme iron, from meat, is readily absorbed and is relatively immune to the onslaught by other dietary components. Furthermore, if heme iron accompanies nonheme iron, the nonheme iron is much more likely to be absorbed also. That means that if you eat only a little iron-containing meat, fish, or poultry with vegetables (as the Chinese commonly do), you absorb more of the nonheme vegetable iron. A mere 3½ ounces of meat, for example, can increase nonheme-iron absorption in a meal by as much as ten times. Some experts suspect that amino acids in meat convey the benefit. Nobody knows for sure.

Why Animal Iron Is a Better Source

Heme iron in meat, poultry and fish is more potent, although only an estimated average of 25 to 35 percent of it is absorbed. One study among Swedish soldiers eating a mixed diet found that although heme iron supplied only 6 percent of the iron in their diet, it accounted for one-third of the amount absorbed.

Nonheme iron alone is extremely fragile and is susceptible to being wiped out by all kinds of intestinal substances such as food fibers, phosphates, proteins, acids, and tannins. This is too bad because most of the iron we eat is nonheme iron. However, there are simple ways of bolstering its bioavailability.

Three things essentially determine how much total iron you absorb: (1) the amount of iron in the food; (2) the composition of the meal, namely interactions determining the absorption of nonheme iron; (3) whether you are iron deficient—the more iron your body needs, the more you absorb, as much as 2 to 3 mg more of nonheme iron per day than expected.

Breast Milk: Best Iron for Infants

The iron in breast milk (like zinc) is readily absorbed by infants— about 50 percent of the iron is absorbed, more than from any other food. The iron in cow's milk, for an unknown reason, is not as well assimilated. Breast milk alone usually provides adequate iron at least for the first six months. After that, the iron intake of many infants falls alarmingly. One analysis found that of infants (under age one), 70 percent did not receive 100 percent of the recommended dietary allowance for iron and 47 percent did not receive even two-thirds of the recommended amount.

The Old Vitamin C Trick

Soak some iron wire in a little sherry or vinegar, or embed some iron nails in slices of apple. Then remove the bits of iron and drink the elixir or eat the apple. That's the way our ancestors used to cure iron-deficiency anemia. And modern science says they were absolutely right. They had discovered centuries earlier the amazing ability of vitamin C or citric acid to potentiate the absorption of iron in the body. It's a trick that can boost by hundreds of percent the amount of iron that gets in your system. In fact, researcher Elaine R. Monsen, of the University of Washington's Divison of Human Nutrition, Dietetics and Foods, calls vitamin C "the most useful and readily found therapy for iron deficiency."

All you have to do is add vitamin C (in foods or synthetic vitamins) to a meal, and the amount of total iron absorbed from food soars. And the amount of iron absorbed goes up in direct proportion to the amount of vitamin C consumed. Adding orange juice to breakfast boosted the iron absorbed by 200 percent. Eating a papaya (66 mg of vitamin C) with a meal increased iron absorption by 500 percent.

In another study, subjects ate two vegetarian meals with the same amount of nonheme iron—5.8 mg. One meal consisted of navy beans, rice, cornbread, and an apple, the other of cauliflower, red kidney beans, white bread, cottage cheese, and pineapple. The difference is that the first meal had only 7 mg of vitamin C, the second meal, 74 mg of C. Even though both meals had the same amount of iron, diners absorbed 2.2 percent of the iron from the first meal, compared with 16.9 percent of the iron from the second meal—768 percent more! All because of the vitamin C.

Tea, the Giant Iron Killer

One caveat: The absorption of iron plunged when tea was added to a meal. For example, when tea instead of coffee was consumed with breakfast, in one study, the percentage of iron absorbed sank from 16 percent to 3 percent. Studies in Israel, where tea is commonly given to infants, found that tea-drinking babies were ten times more likely to have anemia—33 percent were anemic, compared with only 3.5 percent of non-tea-drinking babies.

The reason: tea, and to a lesser extent, red wine, contains tannins that form an insoluble complex with nonheme iron, rendering it less absorbable. Tea has no harmful effect on meat-type heme iron. How much tea it takes to interfere depends on many variables. Dr. Eugene Morris of the Vitamin/Mineral Nutrition Laboratory at USDA says the tannins in "two mugs of moderately strong tea *could* interfere with iron availability." However, vitamin C can significantly reverse the iron-blocking effects of tea and similar inhibitors in direct proportion to the amount of C consumed.

Important: Vitamin C and the mysterious factor in meat, fish, and poultry greatly promote the absorption of nonheme iron *only if consumed at the same time, in the same meal with the iron-containing foods.* It is essential to have the vitamin C and the iron in the small intestine at *the same time* for the beneficial reaction to occur. For example, if you consume vitamin C, even in high doses, four hours before a meal, it has little impact on the iron absorption.

IRON BOOSTERS
What to Drink with a Meal to Influence
Iron Absorption

Orange juice	Excellent
Wine, white	Good
Coffee, red wine	Poor
Tea	Worst

Getting Iron the Old-Fashioned Way

Cooking food, especially acidic food, in iron pots and pans adds lots of nonheme iron to your diet. Dr. Walter Mertz, director of the USDA's Human Nutrition Research Center, equates the passing of the usage of iron pots and pans with the beginning of epidemic anemia among women of child-bearing age.

One classic study compared foods cooked in glass dishes with those cooked in iron skillets. When cooked in the iron skillet, apple butter had 112 times more iron; spaghetti sauce, 29 times more; gravy, 14 times more; potatoes, 8 times more; beef hash, 3 times more. Even scrambling eggs in an iron skillet doubled the amount of iron.

Recommendation: If you want a little more iron in your diet, cook nonacidic foods in iron—they pick up some of the iron; if you want a lot more iron, cook acidic foods in iron. If you are worried about iron overload, do not use iron utensils.

Iron Antagonists and Helpers

Animal and/or human studies reveal that the following factors may affect how iron is absorbed or utilized by the body; the extent of the effect depends on many unknowns, and the interaction may be important only if the antagonist or booster is of sufficient magnitude.

FACTORS THAT MAY BOOST IRON UTILIZATION
Vitamin C either from foods or supplements
Meat
Fish
Poultry
Fruit (containing high vitamin C)
Sauerkraut (contains lactic acid)
Citric acid (in citrus fruits and wine)
Oral contraceptives

FACTORS THAT MAY BLOCK IRON, INCREASING NEED
Tannins (in tea and red wine)
Phytates or phytic acid
Phosphates
Soy-protein products
Dietary fiber
Manganese
Wheat bran

DRUGS THAT MAY DEPLETE IRON
Aspirin (long use or overuse may cause iron-deficiency anemia)
Indomethacin (anti-inflammatory agent)
Cholestyramine (blood-cholesterol depressor)
Antacids (when taken with meals)
EDTA (food additive and chemical commonly used in chelation
therapy)

Does Fiber Rob You of Iron?

Numerous studies show that fiber in the diet can "bind up" iron in the body, preventing its utilization. However, it is unclear how serious a problem this is. There is evidence that this binding is strongly blocked by the presence of even low amounts of vitamin C. Also, nobody knows whether the problem is fiber itself, the binding process, phytates (substances that occur along with fiber in whole-grain foods) or other unknown factors, or a combination of all of them.

Wheat bran appears to block the absorption of iron. The kind of fiber in vegetables and fruits may not have an effect. And in one study, bran muffins without the phytate still depressed the amount of iron absorbed.

Soy Products: A Question

Soybean products are fairly high in iron, but the iron is in a form not readily utilized by the body. However, a study at the University of Kansas now finds that tofu (bean curd) is an exception. For some unknown reason, during the making of tofu the iron is somehow liberated. The iron in tofu is three times more available for bodily use than the iron in whole, dehulled soybeans or other soy products.

Toxicity and Supplements

There is little danger in getting a toxic dose of iron from food. Daily intakes of 25 to 75 mg are unlikely to cause problems in healthy persons. However, iron supplements are another matter: About two thousand cases of iron poisoning happen yearly in the United States, mainly to youngsters who accidentally eat iron-supplement pills. The deadly dose for a two-year-old is about 3 grams; for an adult, 200–250 mg per kilogram (2.2 lbs) of weight. The minimum toxic dose for iron is estimated at 100 mg, about five and a half times the RDA of 18 mg.

When diet is not enough. Because of the grave deficiencies of iron and the difficulty for women in getting sufficient iron in the average diet without overindulging in calories, iron supplements are often recommended, especially for premenopausal females. Iron supplements are also regularly prescribed for infants, very young children, women with heavy menstrual periods, pregnant and nursing women, frequent blood donors of both sexes, and those with iron-deficiency anemia. During pregnancy relatively small doses of 30 to 60 mg a day are recommended by experts. General advice is to take the pills between meals.

COMMON SIDE EFFECTS OF IRON SUPPLEMENTS
    Upset stomach
    Constipation
    Diarrhea
    Abdominal pain
    Dark brown or black stool

FOODS RICH IN IRON

The most iron by weight regardless of calories

Liver, all types
Brewer's yeast
Beef steak
Pumpkin, sunflower, and
　squash seeds
Beef kidneys
Sorghum molasses
Fish roe
Oysters
Soybeans
Liver sausage
Wheat germ

Pine nuts
Dried lima beans
Clams
Potatoes with skin
Cashew nuts
Sardines
Dried apricots, peaches, raisins,
　and prunes
Dried kidney beans
Cod
Turkey
Chicken

IRON SUPER-FOODS
THE MOST IRON, THE FEWEST CALORIES

Here are 50 foods that rate exceptionally high in iron content per calorie. Of the approximately 2500 foods in this book, these are tops in iron nutrient density; they have the highest iron-calorie ratios, giving you the most iron for the fewest calories.*

	Food Rating	Iron-calorie ratio (mg of Iron per 100 calories)	Common Measure	Mg Iron	Calories
1.	Spinach, fresh, cooked	15.5	½ c	3	21
2.	Pork, liver, braised	11	3 oz	15	141
3.	Sauerkraut juice, canned	11	1 c	3	24
4.	Turnip greens, canned	10.8	½ c	2	17
5.	Oysters, raw	8.3	3 oz	5	56
6.	Oysters, smoked	8.3	3 oz	8	91
7.	Clams, raw	8	3 oz	5	65
8.	Oysters, canned	7.8	3 oz	6	81
9.	Sauerkraut, canned	7.7	½ c	2	22
10.	Clams, canned	7.2	½ c	5	76
11.	Lamb, liver, broiled	6.9	1.6 oz	8	117
12.	Brewer's yeast	6.1	1 tbsp	1	23
13.	Calf, liver, fried	5.4	3 oz	12	222
14.	Chicken, livers, simmered	5.4	1 c	12	219
15.	Beef, kidneys, cooked	5.2	3 oz	6	122
16.	Sorghum molasses	4.9	2 tbsp	5	105
17.	Clams, meat, steamed	4.8	3 oz	4	93

Food Rating	Iron-calorie ratio (mg of Iron per 100 calories)	Common Measure	Mg Iron	Calories
18. Pâté, chicken liver, canned	4.6	1 oz	3	57
19. Beef, heart	4.6	3 oz	6	148
20. Turkey, liver, simmered	4.6	1 c	11	237
21. Caviar, sturgeon	4.5	1 tbsp	2	46
22. Beef liver, braised	4.2	3 oz	6	137
23. Pumpkin, canned	4.1	½ c	2	41
24. Oysters, broiled/baked	4.1	3 oz	5	133
25. Cherries, sour, red, canned, water	3.7	½ c	2	43
26. Chicken, giblets, simmered	3.7	1 c	9	228
27. Potato skin, baked	3.6	from 1 potato	4	115
28. Sausage, liver cheese	3.6	1 oz	3	87
29. Pork, kidneys, cooked	3.5	3 oz	5	128
30. Clams, breaded, fried	3.5	3 oz	6	158
31. Oysters, fried	3.4	3 oz	5	165
32. Venison, boneless, cooked	3.3	3 oz	5	153
33. Bulgur, canned	3.3	⅔ c	5	151
34. Snails (escargots), wo shell, cooked	3.2	1 oz	1	37
35. Artichoke, cooked	3.1	1 med	2	53
36. Potatoes, instant, mashed	3.1	½ c	4	136
37. Mussels, canned	3	¾ c	6	218
38. Pumpkin and squash seeds	2.9	1 oz	4	148
39. Sardines, canned, mustard sauce	2.8	2 sardines	1	47
40. Cod, salted, dried	2.8	1 oz	1	36
41. Braunschweiger (liver sausage)	2.6	1 oz	3	102
42. Wheat germ	2.6	1 oz	3	108
43. White beans, dry, cooked	2.3	½ c	1	103
44. Lentils, dry, no fat added, cooked	2.3	½ c	2	101
45. Mussels, cooked	2.2	3 oz	3	138

Cereals: five with highest iron-calorie ratios

Food Rating	Iron-calorie ratio	Common Measure	Mg Iron	Calories
46. Total	18	1 oz	18	100
47. Product 19	16.7	1 oz	18	108
48. 40% Bran Flakes, Kellogg's	8.8	1 oz	8	93
49. Wheat, puffed, fortified	8.7	½ oz	4	52
50. Cream of wheat, cooked	8	1 c	10	129

Source: Author's computer analysis from USDA data

*Excludes baby foods. Includes only foods for which one serving supplies a minimum of approximately 10 percent of the RDA.

RECOMMENDED DAILY DIETARY ALLOWANCES OF IRON

Age	Milligrams
Birth–6 months	10
6 months–4 years	15
4–10	10
Males 11–18	18
Males over 18	10
Females 11–50	18
Females over 50 (postmenopausal)	10
Pregnant	Iron Supplements 30–60
Nursing	Iron Supplements 30–60

Source: National Academy of Sciences, Revised 1980

Potassium
Low Intakes, New Concerns

Potassium is a silver-white metallic element, the third most abundant element in the body, after calcium and phosphorus. Intake is essential for life. Potassium, like sodium, performs as an "electrolyte," carrying a tiny electrical charge that governs muscle functioning, including that of the heart. Potassium aids in the transmission of nerve impulses, release of insulin, proper functioning of digestive enzymes, and helps maintain a delicate fluid balance inside and outside the cells. A potassium imbalance can shut down the heart instantly.

Who Needs to Worry?

Many Americans undoubtedly take in too little dietary potassium, especially women who have comparatively low-calorie diets. The Food and Drug Administration's Selected Minerals in Food Survey (1976, '77, '78) found that the average consumption of potassium was 1,193 mg per 1,000 calories eaten. That means that an adult would have to eat about 1,600 calories per day to get the bare minimum potassium that experts consider adequate—1,875 mg—and at least 2,100 calories daily to take in a middling range of 2,500 mg of potassium, considered desirable by most experts. The average American woman, according to a 1985 U.S. Department of Agriculture survey, consumes 1,660 calories a day. Another study showed that people on a 3,900-calorie-per-day diet took in potassium in the high ranges of about 4,600 mg per day.

SYMPTOMS OF POTASSIUM DEFICIENCY
Muscle cramps and spasms
Lethargy
Muscular weakness
Irritability
Abnormal heartbeat that can result in sudden death

The Delicate Life-Death Balance

Both too much and too little potassium creates dangerous electrolyte imbalances, seriously upsetting the body's metabolic processes. For example, there is a delicate balance between sodium and potassium. Potassium is located almost entirely in the interior of living cells; almost all sodium is located outside the cells in the extracellular spaces—in blood plasma and other fluids. So delicate is the electrical balance that the heart stops beating if potassium blood levels rise to three to four times normal. Slightly higher potassium levels shut down muscle contractions and nerve electrical impulses.

On the other hand, too little potassium causes similar symptoms—such as muscle inactivity, irregular heartbeat, and cardiac arrest. A sudden loss of only 6 percent of the body's potassium would cause instant death. The interaction between levels of potassium and sodium and possibly calcium is thought to have a significant impact on health, especially cardiovascular functions, including blood pressure. People taking certain diuretics for high blood pressure must take special care to get enough potassium to replace the amounts lost through the urine. (Unless they are taking potassium-sparing diuretics.)

Sudden deaths from fasting, starvation, low-calorie liquid protein diets, and severe diarrhea have come from heart failure linked to electrolyte disturbance and potassium depletion.

Not surprisingly, one of the first signs of potassium deficiency is lack of energy, especially in muscular activity. A study published in the *Journal of the American Medical Association* revealed that people with low potassium intakes had weaker grips than did those with normal amounts of potassium in the diet. The authors concluded that a chronic potassium deficit can apparently sap muscle strength and persist for months.

Potassium and Heart Disease

In prehistoric days our ancestors ate a diet very high in potassium and low in sodium. Today, we eat about one-third as much potassium as primitive man. And some experts think that is a mistake. "There is no reason to think that our requirements for potassium are any less," says Dr. Louis Tobian, Jr., chief of the hypertension section at the University of Minnesota. Dr. Tobian is convinced that a low potassium intake is linked to heart disease and stroke. He points out that blacks in the South and the people of Scotland eat about half the amounts of potassium as the rest of us and have among the highest rates of heart attack and stroke in the world.

In animal experiments, Dr. Tobian found that rats with salt-induced hypertension developed 50 percent less kidney disease when given potassium supplements equivalent to the potassium intake of prehistoric humans. In other research, he found that potassium protected rats from fatal strokes. In animals with high blood pressure, 40 percent of those fed a diet "normal" in potassium suffered small strokes, evidenced by bleeding in the brain; none of the rats on a high-potassium diet showed any evidence of brain hemorrhage. Dr. Tobian maintains that the extra potassium kept the artery walls elastic, able to withstand increased pressure and ward off stroke.

The All Important
Potassium–Sodium Ratio

It's not just how much potassium you eat. Equally important is how much potassium you consume in relation to the daily intake of sodium. It is called the potassium–sodium ratio. The Food and Nutrition Board of the National Academy of Sciences recommends eating six-tenths of a gram of sodium for every gram of potassium: .6 to 1. But that's hardly the norm for those eating the typical American diet. According to a recent one-year study by the U.S. Department of Agriculture, in the Washington, D.C., area, a group of twenty-eight adults ate far too little potassium in relationship to sodium. They ate 1.3 grams of sodium daily for every gram of potassium—about half the amount of potassium and twice the amount of sodium as recommended.

The author of the study, Dr. James C. Smith, chief of the USDA's Vitamin and Mineral Nutrition Laboratory in Beltsville, Maryland, pointed out that people who consume high levels of dietary potassium may excrete more sodium in the urine. But individuals who eat too much sodium in relationship to potassium may disturb the delicate balance in tissue fluids inside and outside body cells. He says a ratio too light on potassium and too heavy on sodium may lead to high blood pressure in individuals susceptible to the disease.

The Potassium–High
Blood Pressure Link

Much current research centers on the theory that increased potassium may reduce high blood pressure, especially in those with high salt intakes and a genetic susceptibility to hypertension. Vegetarians, who eat a diet rich in potassium, have less hypertension than meat eaters, even when both consume similar amounts of salt. Several studies show that potassium supplements can reduce the blood pressure of those who already have hypertension. For example, researchers at St. Mary's Hospital in London produced modest reductions in diastolic blood pressure in healthy men by giving them potassium pills—equal to the potassium in about three oranges, bananas, or vegetable servings per day.

However, a well-controlled study showed that this did not work in those who were on low-sodium diets. Thus, it appears that potassium can blunt the blood-pressure–raising effects of sodium in some people predisposed to hypertension. Animal studies show that potassium can reduce sodium-induced high blood pressure by up to 25 percent; in humans, the reduction of arterial pressure has been from 3 to 10 percent. It is uncertain how much potassium is needed for beneficial results, or by what mechanism potassium helps control blood pressure.

Since a higher-potassium, lower-salt diet is "natural" to the human species, some experts see no harm—and much potential benefit—in eating more potassium-rich foods such as fruits and vegetables, which are also beneficial in other ways. Increasing dietary potassium may help guard against heart disease, high blood pressure, and stroke in some people. However, the evidence is far from conclusive.

Important: Do not eat more potassium or take potassium supplements in attempts to counteract the effects of a high-sodium diet. This not only may not work in many people, but might actually be damaging to others. More potassium should not be used as an excuse to continue eating lots of salt.

Beware: Potassium "Salt Substitutes"

By avoiding salt, many people encounter another danger—overdosing on potassium in salt substitutes. Numerous cases have been reported in the medical literature of problems from unintentionally or intentionally consuming salt substitutes high in potassium. Near-fatalities have been reported, as well as heart failure. Don't use a salt substitute if you are taking potassium-sparing diuretics. If you do use salt substitutes, do not overdo it; using salt substitutes as liberally as salt can be dangerous.

People with healthy kidneys can usually handle widely fluctuating amounts of potassium, but the elderly and people with certain diseases cannot. At high risk of problems from salt substitutes: patients with chronic or acute kidney failure, acidosis, cardiovascular diseases treated with potassium-sparing diuretics, and the elderly. People with kidney disease or oliguria (low urine output) should not use salt substitutes.

Even low-sodium soups with high potassium content can be dangerous to people with renal failure who are on kidney dialysis.

POTASSIUM CONTENT OF SOME SALT SUBSTITUTES

	Potassium mEq per teaspoon
Morton's Salt Substitute	70
No Salt	68
Diamond Crystal	66
Adolph's Salt Substitute	65
Featherweight K Salt Substitute	49
Nu-Salt	55
Morton's Seasoned Salt Substitute	50
Adolph's Seasoned Salt Substitute	33
Morton's Lite Salt	40

Source: Danielle Riccardella, M.S., and Johanna Dwyer, D.Sc., *Journal of the American Dietetic Association*, April 1985

Potassium Antagonists and Helpers

Animal and/or human studies reveal that the following factors may affect how potassium is absorbed or utilized by the body; the extent of the effect depends on many unknowns, and the interaction may be important only if the antagonist or booster is of sufficient magnitude.

FACTORS THAT MAY BOOST UTILIZATION OF POTASSIUM
Vitamin C

FACTORS THAT MAY BLOCK POTASSIUM, INCREASING NEED
Alcoholism, chronic
Magnesium deficiency

DRUGS THAT MAY DEPLETE POTASSIUM
Thiazides (diuretics)
Furosemide (duiretic)
Ethacrynic acid (diuretic)
Senna (laxative)
Phenolphthalein (laxative)
Bisacodyl (laxative)

The Problem with Processed Foods

Processing, canning, or freezing foods reduces potassium and, most important, changes the natural balance between potassium and sodium. In fact, the ratio is severely reversed. Canning peas, for example, according to Department of Agriculture experts, slashes the amount of potassium in half while often raising the amount of sodium by 200 percent. Turning corn into cornflakes reduces the potassium by about 65 percent.

Because the potassium in food occurs in soluble form, considerable amounts may be lost in the water when cooking vegetables and fruits.

The best way to preserve potassium in vegetables: Don't peel them; this causes loss of potassium no matter how they are cooked. Bake, steam, or stir-fry.

Toxicity and Supplements

It is virtually impossible to get too much potassium from food. Generally, the body senses a dangerous increase and flushes away the excess. In tests, 200 mg of potassium per kilogram (2.2 lbs) of body weight did not cause toxic effects in healthy individuals. However, potassium overdoses could be toxic to those with diseases of the kidney, heart, or liver. Injections of potassium into a vein can stop the heart.

Potassium toxicity is usually seen only in patients taking potassium supplements or in cases of kidney failure. Toxic signs are similar to deficiency symptoms.

Warning: Although it makes sense to increase dietary amounts of potassium by eating more vegetables and fruits, et cetera, no one already suffering from hypertension, especially those with poor kidneys, should take potassium supplements or other sources of high potassium except on the advice of a physician. Because of the potential danger, a prescription is required for therapeutic doses. Supplements of potassium may be needed, especially for those on certain diuretics.

FOODS RICH IN POTASSIUM

The most potassium by weight regardless of calories

Brewer's yeast	Figs
Nonfat dry milk	Peanuts
Dried apricots and peaches	Potatoes
Wheat germ	Dry lima beans
Pumpkin and squash seeds	Avocados
Currants	Sardines
Raisins	Swordfish
Almonds	Pork
Prunes	Turkey

POTASSIUM SUPER-FOODS
THE MOST POTASSIUM, THE FEWEST CALORIES

Here are 50 foods that rate exceptionally high in potassium content per calorie. Of the approximately 2500 foods in this book, these are tops in potassium nutrient density; that is, they have highest potassium-calorie ratios, giving you the most potassium for the fewest calories.*

	Food Rating	Potassium-calorie ratio (mg of Potassium per 100 calories)	Common Measure	Mg Potassium	Calories
1.	Beet greens, fresh, cooked	3367	½ c	654	20
2.	Bok choi, fresh, cooked	3092	½ c	315	10
3.	Amaranth, cooked	3052	½ c	423	14
4.	Chard, swiss, fresh, cooked	2745	½ c	483	18
5.	Spinach, fresh, cooked	2026	½ c	419	21
6.	Mushrooms, raw	1480	1 mushroom	67	5
7.	Sauerkraut juice, canned	1400	1 c	339	24
8.	Molasses, blackstrap	1374	¼ c	2400	175
9.	Tomato juice, canned	1294	½ c	268	21
10.	Tomatoes, fresh	1040	1 tomato	254	24
11.	Beets, fresh, cooked	1006	½ c	265	25
12.	Okra, fresh, cooked	1006	½ c	257	26
13.	Tomato sauce, canned	983	½ c	452	37
14.	Tomatoes, canned	883	½ c	265	24
15.	Cantaloupe, raw	883	½ fruit	825	94
16.	Squash, acorn, cooked	780	½ c	446	57
17.	Carrot juice, canned	703	½ c	360	49

	Food Rating	Potassium-calorie ratio (mg of Potassium per 100 calories)	Common Measure	Mg Potassium	Calories
18.	Squash, winter, butternut, baked	703	½ c	290	41
19.	Potatoes, flesh, raw	687	½ c	407	59
20.	Papaya, raw	659	1 fruit	780	117
21.	Bran Buds	648	1 oz	474	73
22.	Brewer's yeast	645	1 c	152	23
23.	Marinara sauce, canned	623	1 c	1061	171
24.	Apricots, raw	617	3 fruit	313	51
25.	Artichokes, fresh, cooked	598	1 medium	316	53
26.	Apricots, dried	579	10 halves	482	83
27.	Yam, cooked	578	½ c	455	79
28.	Chicken broth, canned	548	1 c	427	78
29.	Kiwifruit	544	1 fruit	252	46
30.	Wheat bran, unprocessed	526	¼ c	162	31
31.	Parsnips, raw	503	½ c	251	50
32.	All-Bran cereal	496	1 oz	350	71
33.	Milk, nonfat, dry	495	¼ c	538	109
34.	Minestrone, chunky, canned	481	1 c	612	127
35.	100% Bran	464	1 oz	354	76
36.	Lima beans, green, fresh, cooked	463	½ c	484	104
37.	Yogurt, plain, skim milk	457	4 oz	288	63
38.	Parsnips, cooked	455	½ c	287	63
39.	Milk, skim	447	1 c	418	90
40.	Lima beans, dry, cooked	443	½ c	572	129
41.	Nectarine, raw	439	1 fruit	288	67
42.	Avocado, Florida	436	1 fruit	1484	339
43.	Potato, in skin, boiled	436	½ c	295	68
44.	Orange juice, fresh	432	4 fl oz	236	56
45.	Bananas	430	1 fruit	451	105
46.	Peaches, dried	417	10 halves	1295	311
47.	Soybeans, dried, cooked	415	1 c	972	234
48.	Plantain, cooked	401	½ c	358	89
49.	Prune juice, canned	387	1 fl oz	88	23
50.	Peas, blackeye, cooked	387	½ c	344	89

Source: Author's computer analysis from USDA data

*Excludes baby foods. Includes only foods for which one serving supplies a minimum of approximately 10 percent of the estimated adequate and safe amount.

ESTIMATED SAFE AND ADEQUATE DAILY DIETARY INTAKES OF POTASSIUM

Age	Milligrams
Birth–6 months	350–925
6 months–1 year	425–1275
1–3	550–1650
4–6	775–2325
7–10	1000–3000
Adolescents 11 and over	1525–4575
Adults	1875–5625

Source: National Academy of Sciences, Revised 1980

Zinc
A Powerful Protector

Zinc is a trace mineral essential to health. The human body contains about 2.2 grams of zinc—more than any other trace element except iron. Zinc is concentrated mainly in the skin, hair, nails, eyes, and prostate gland. The mineral is crucial for cell multiplication, tissue regeneration, sexual maturity, and proper growth. Zinc, a vital player in the enzymatic system throughout the body, helps regulate the immune system, insulin metabolism, normal taste, and vision, and speeds wound-healing.

Who Needs to Worry?

For many years nobody worried about zinc deficiency. Then, in the early 1960s, to their great surprise scientists discovered severe and profound abnormalities including dwarfism among adolescent males in Egypt and Iran eating zinc-poor diets of unleavened bread and beans. Since then, investigators have linked zinc to a long and ever-growing list of health problems. The potent and subtle damage to the body of even small scarcities of this mineral is increasingly the subject of intriguing and far-reaching speculations in medical journals.

In the United States, *severe* zinc deficiencies rarely exist. However, authorities believe that persistent *low-grade* or sub-clinical zinc deficiency is undoubtedly taking an unrecognized toll on the health of millions of Americans who have no detectable symptoms and are totally unaware that they lack zinc. As Dr. Harold H. Sandstead, at the Department of Preventive Medicine, University of Texas at Galveston, and a leading authority on zinc, puts it: "Mild, potentially damaging zinc deficiency is not a rare phenomenon in the United States."

At High Risk

Although zinc deficiency can appear in all ages and segments of the population, major concern centers on children, females—especially pregnant women—and the elderly. According to a recent USDA study, only 8 percent of the participants met the full recommended daily allowances of zinc. Women, because of lower calorie intakes, suffer the worst. The Department of Agriculture's 1985 nationwide survey revealed the average intake of zinc for women to be a scant 9.2 mg per day—60 percent of the recommended amount. American women eat only half the calories required to get enough zinc from an ordinary diet.

Children also may be at special risk. A study in Denver of apparently healthy children from well-to-do homes uncovered signs of marginal zinc deficiency, such as poor appetite, substandard growth, and impaired taste, which were corrected by increased zinc intake. Similarly, the diets of adolescent males and teenaged and college women are often deficient in zinc. Even breast-fed infants may not get enough zinc—many consume only half the recommended quotient because of zinc-deficient mothers.

Of growing concern, as a result of animal studies, are pregnant women—who may risk birth complications and deformed infants because of zinc deficiencies—and zinc-deficient elderly, who may be rendered more susceptible to infections, and a variety of so-called autoimmune diseases, including diabetes and arthritis. Because of poor nutrition and progressive inability to absorb zinc, the elderly are prime candidates for zinc malnutrition. Surveys show that older people often consume only one-half to two-thirds of the RDA for zinc. Aging may also seriously impair the ability to absorb zinc.

MAJOR SIGNS OF ZINC DEFICIENCY
Loss of appetite
Stunted growth in children
Skin changes
Small sex glands in boys
Delayed sexual maturation
Impotence
Loss of taste sensitivity
White spots on fingernails
Delayed wound-healing
Dull hair color

The First Sign: Loss of Taste and Smell

Taste and smell dysfunction is one of the earliest signs of mild or severe zinc deficiency, affecting an estimated four million Americans. One theory is that zinc deficiency may chemically change saliva, altering taste. Is this why the elderly frequently lose their sense of taste and smell? Maybe, partly. The evidence is unclear. Increased zinc may or may not restore lost taste and smell. Even so, it's a good idea for elderly people to eat more zinc-rich foods because of the great risk of mild, undetected deficiency.

Subtle Health Damage

Since zinc is a key element in turning numerous body functions on and off, it is not surprising that a lack of zinc could wreak such widespread, though often subtle, havoc among cells governing everything from mental processes to reproduction. Since zinc, relatively speaking, is a fairly new ground for scientific study, the clues to the real importance of zinc are just coming in. Here are some that may or may not prove out:

Anorexia Nervosa—Connected with Zinc Deficiency?

Because anorexia (severe loss of appetite) is one of the classic signs of acute zinc deficiency, some researchers speculate that anorexia nervosa in humans may be influenced by zinc deficiency. Indeed, according to experiments by Dr. Craig McClain, associate professor of medicine and director of the division of gastroenterology at the University of Kentucky School of Medicine at Lexington, rats deprived of zinc developed anorexia-bulimia–like symptoms, eating only one-third their usual diet. Zinc reversed their bizarre eating habits. Dr. McClain in another study found nine women with bulimia to be extremely low in zinc—but it is unclear whether the deficiency was the result or the cause of their eating disorder.

HEALTH PROBLEMS THAT MAY BE LINKED TO ZINC DEFICIENCY

Research on animals and/or humans proves or suggests a connection between zinc deficiencies and:

Low sperm counts (which generally return to normal after correction of mild deficiencies)

Night blindness (a zinc deficiency interacts with a vitamin A deficiency to exacerbate night blindness)

Cancer of some types (notably prostate and esophagus)

Anorexia nervosa and bulimia

Alcoholism

Diabetes

Rheumatoid arthritis

Gum disease

Osteoporosis

Immune-system malfunctioning

Lead poisoning

Dementia associated with aging

Low-birth-weight babies

Fetal and maternal complications

Birth malformations

Learning disabilities

Frightening, Long-Term Genetic Damage

A study of mice, done at the University of California at Davis, found astounding results of zinc deficiency that persisted for several generations. When pregnant mice were fed a diet moderately deficient in zinc, their offspring exhibited a malfunctioning immune system for the first six months of life. More alarming, the second and third generations also showed signs of poor immunity—even though they were fed a zinc-plentiful diet! Somehow the impaired immune system induced by zinc deficiency in the womb was transmitted from generation to generation in the form of a subtle birth defect or mutation.

Birth defects among infants of zinc-deficient women are becoming a major worry to scientists. Studies show that women with low blood-zinc levels at midterm have more complications during delivery and give birth to children with higher rates of malformations. Because zinc is so critical to fetal development of the brain, the birth defects may be subtle—in the form of behavior abnormalities and learning disabilities. This was pointed up dramatically in a study of monkeys. Those deprived of zinc through most of the third trimester gave birth to infants that were less active, less exploratory, and less playful, suggesting what are called "behavioral birth defects."

More striking, the young monkeys later in life showed distinct learning disabilities—which, inexplicably, they seemed to outgrow by age three. Studies of rats also show drastic detrimental effects to the brain in offspring of mothers who are zinc deficient. More research needs to be done to find out whether learning disabilities can develop in human children born to zinc-deficient mothers.

Researchers have found thought disturbances and subtle brain-wave changes in electroencephalograms (EEGs) in humans with mild zinc deficiencies. A British study found that elderly patients with dementia in one hospital had significantly lower blood levels of zinc. The researchers speculate that there may be a connection because zinc deficiency can interfere with the transmission of brain chemicals.

Zinc Fights Infections

There is little question that zinc is somehow vitally connected to the immune system and consequently to colds, infections, and an ever-growing list of what scientists call "autoimmune" diseases, in which antibodies perversely launch attacks on healthy tissue. Apparently the zinc–immunity connection is delicate: too little zinc may impair the immune system, but so can too much zinc consumed in supplements.

The key seems to be the degree of "deficiency." If you are deficient in zinc, your immune system just can't work up to par. Animal studies show that without zinc the body "forgets" to release antibodies against foreign invaders. This may be especially true for the elderly, because the immune system does slow down with age, a process that could be aggravated by a chronic deficiency in zinc. In humans, moderate zinc supplements increased the number of T-lymphocytes (infection-fighting cells) in zinc-deficient persons. A study reported in the *American Journal of Medicine,* May 1981, by Belgian researchers concluded that the "addition of zinc to the diet of old persons could be an effective and simple way to improve their immune function." For a month, elderly people who took 50 mg of zinc a day produced more antibodies and other infection-fighting cells.

There's some evidence that rheumatoid arthritis, an autoimmune disease, may be associated with zinc deficiency. Preliminary studies show that those with rheumatoid arthritis have lower zinc levels, and zinc may help reduce inflammation of the joints. But that is still very iffy. Similarly, another metabolic disease, diabetes, may be linked to zinc deficiency. A recent study in the *American Journal of Medicine,* found that 25 percent of a group not dependent on insulin injections had low blood-zinc levels and possibly problems absorbing zinc. The connection, though possible, is still vaguely understood.

Zinc: The Sex Nutrient

Oysters have long been reputed to be an aphrodisiac. That bit of folklore may have legitimacy, for oysters are packed full of zinc, and without enough zinc many men may be infertile or impotent. According to a foremost zinc researcher, Dr. Ananda S. Prasad at Wayne State University in Detroit, even mild zinc deficiency can induce dramatic decline of the male hormone testosterone and of sperm counts, rendering the male infertile. Zinc deficiencies in childhood are well recognized as blocking sexual maturation. There is also evidence that some impotent males became potent again when zinc deficiencies were corrected. Men who are infertile or impotent may need to take in more zinc, although the causes of reproductive dysfunction may be multiple—psychological as well as physical.

DISEASES THAT LEAD TO ZINC DEFICIENCY
Alcoholism
Cirrhosis of the liver
Diarrhea
Crohn's disease (inflammatory bowel disease)
Ulcerative colitis
Sickle cell anemia
Cystic fibrosis
Rheumatoid arthritis

Kidney disease

Acrodermatitis enteropathica (an inherited zinc deficiency, necessitating therapeutic doses of zinc)

How Much Zinc Do You Absorb?

Estimates of how much zinc you actually absorb from food range all over the place: one study found from 60 percent zinc absorption among children to a mere 2 percent among the elderly. The National Academy of Sciences puts the average figure for Americans at around 40 percent.

Zinc, perhaps more than any other nutrient, undergoes a hazardous journey through the intestinal tract before it finds its proper niche in the chemical soup of cells. How much of it finally gets there depends on how much of it has been diverted or excreted along the way.

Thanks to body wisdom, as with other nutrients, you absorb far more zinc if your diet is low in zinc. Generally, starting at about age twenty-five, the ability to absorb zinc steadily declines with age. A study of elderly men showed the average amount of zinc absorbed to be a scant 16 percent.

Zinc Interactions Make the Difference

The amount of use you get from zinc is unpredictable because it depends heavily on the rest of your diet. How you combine foods is just as important as how much zinc you eat. Some scientists are beginning to believe that harmful zinc deficiencies may be caused not so much by deficiencies in intake but by deficiencies in utilization. The early studies among children in the Middle East, for example, documenting the horrible effects of zinc deficiency, tied the problem not to a zinc-deficient diet but to a combination of foods that made the zinc unavailable to the body.

Let's face it: because of all the other things you have to think about, you cannot always be aware of which foods are the most beneficial to your zinc status, but here are some facts to consider that may make a difference.

Meat and Seafood: Better Sources

Generally, the less meat you eat, the greater the chances of zinc deficiency. Not only are meat and seafood high in zinc, but for some reason zinc from these sources is more readily absorbed and less vulnerable to attacks from other nutritional elements in the digestive tract. This problem is of great concern to vegetarians. Despite conflicting studies, the consensus is that you are better off to get zinc from meat, poultry, and especially seafood, instead of from plants, because it's more likely to reach its final destination in the body unscathed.

If you are a vegetarian, you have to be careful to get enough zinc. One study showed that vegetarians eating zinc in *excess* of the recommended amounts still ended up zinc deficient, apparently because the zinc was canceled out by other dietary elements, including some in the very zinc-carrying vegetables and grains eaten. However, this is somewhat mitigated by the observation that vegetarians may adapt by absorbing higher rates of zinc.

Mother's Milk: The Winner

For some mysterious reason, known only to nature, if you want your infant better zinc-nourished, you should breast feed. Breast-fed infants have higher levels of zinc in their blood—even though human and cow's milk contain similar levels of zinc. The baby is better able to absorb zinc from human milk than from cow's milk or infant formula. However, breast milk is no guarantee of safety; a nursing mother deficient in zinc will not supply needed amounts, and a deprived infant may also become critically deficient. Studies show that the majority of breast-fed infants receive only 50 to 70 percent of the recommended zinc intake.

Zinc Killers: Phytate and Fiber

Although numerous factors can ruin zinc's bioavailability, the two worst are food fiber and naturally occurring compounds called phytates, also known as phytic acid. Some authorities suggest that even drinking too much coffee, which is high in phytates, could induce zinc deficiency by causing chemical reactions in the digestive tract that wash away the zinc. Other studies show that eating oysters, which are high in zinc, and dried beans, which are high in fiber and phytates, at the same time robs the body of about 65 percent of the zinc from the oysters. If you combine enough tortillas or corn chips with oysters (an oyster burrito?) you might as well forget about any zinc benefit from the oysters: it is entirely wiped out.

Most scientists believe that phytic acid, rather than fiber in foods, is the primary agent blocking the body's utilization of zinc. These two agents occur together in many foods, such as grains, beans, and nuts.

Don't Give Up Whole-Grain Foods

Does that mean you should stop eating less-processed, high-fiber foods like whole-grain breads and cereals because of the possibility of fiber overkill? No. Definitely not. Experts like Dr. Walter Mertz, head of the U.S. Department of Agriculture's Human Nutrition Laboratories, do not see fiber in the diets of most people as a significant threat to zinc adequacy. Even though high-fiber foods can bind up zinc, reducing its utilization by the body, such foods are often such superior sources of zinc that it makes little difference.

Food processing steals zinc as well as other nutrients. White bread has about one-fourth as much zinc as unrefined wheat; degermed cornmeal, half the zinc of dry corn; and polished rice, less than one-third the zinc of unprocessed grain.

On the other hand, a lower percentage of the zinc in unprocessed grains is absorbed. One study showed that you absorb 38.2 percent of the zinc in white bread, but only 16.6 percent of the zinc in whole-wheat bread. But still whole-wheat bread turns out to be a better zinc source in the long run because of the higher amounts of zinc in whole grains. Despite the blocking effect, you end up with a *total of more zinc*: .15 mg from the white bread, and .22 mg from the whole-wheat bread.

Anyone on an extremely high-fiber diet, however, should take precautions to get enough zinc, and certain other minerals—namely calcium and iron—which can also be depleted by fiber.

Most important, some experts contend, is something called a phytate–zinc molar ratio. That's the proportion of phytate to zinc in a food. If you consistently eat foods with a high ratio—10 or more—you may be in danger of losing much of the zinc you eat and of compromising your zinc balance. As you can see from the chart below, the worst offenders are dried beans, rice, and some whole-grain products. This, of course, does not mean you should not eat these foods, but only that you should be aware of the interactions in case you are worried about zinc. Notice also that coffee, tea, and cocoa can rob you of zinc. Meat, poultry, and seafood do not contain phytate.

THE PHYTATE–ZINC RATIO OF SOME FOODS
(The higher the figure, the more apt the food is to block the utilization of zinc by phytate)

	Phytate-zinc molar* ratio
Dried lima beans, raw: ¼ c	79
Dried navy beans, boiled: ½ c	34
Rye bread: 1 slice	58
Bread, white: 1 slice	11
Bread, whole wheat: 1 slice	21
Carrots, raw: 1	2
Chickpeas, cooked: ½ c	14
Cocoa, dry powder: 1 tbsp	33
Coffee, brewed: 1 c	6–40
Coffee, instant: 1 c	4–6
Corn, whole kernel, canned: ½ c	8
Corn chips: 1 oz	41
Cornflakes: 1 oz	16
Farina, cooked: 1 c	7
Granola: 1 oz	29
Macaroni, cooked: ½ c	16
Meat	0
Oatmeal, cooked: ½ c	22
Peanut butter: 1 tbsp	42
Peas, canned: ½ c	3
Popcorn, popped: 1 c	15
Potatoes, cooked, peeled: ½ c	20
Poultry	0
Rice, white, dry: ¼ c	99
Rice cereal, dry: 1 oz	16
Seafood	0
Tea, brewed	.5–5
Tea, instant	7–11
Tomatoes, canned: ½ c	3
Wheat bran: 1 oz	54
Wheat cereal, flakes: 1 oz	62
Wheat flour, all purpose: 1 c	40
Whole wheat flour: 1 c	34
Wheat germ: 1 tbsp	28

Source: Barbara F. Harland, Donald Oberleas, *Journal of the American Dietetic Association*, October 1981, and the *Journal of American Oil Chemists*, September 1985

*Molar means 1 gram of molecular weight

Zinc Antagonists and Helpers

Animal and/or human studies reveal that the following factors may affect how zinc is absorbed or utilized by the body; the extent of the effect depends on many unknowns, and the interaction may be important only if the antagonist or booster is of sufficient magnitude.

FACTORS THAT MAY BOOST UTILIZATION OF ZINC
Red wine
Lactose
An unidentified agent in human milk

FACTORS IN ADDITION TO DIETARY FIBER AND PHYTATE THAT MAY BLOCK ZINC, INCREASING NEED
Protein (The more protein and phosphorus you eat, the more zinc you need. A USDA analysis of zinc intakes of elderly men and women found that men who ate 81 grams of protein a day and 1.25 grams of phosphorus needed 10.1 mg of zinc daily to maintain adequate zinc levels. Women needed only 6.5 mg of zinc daily because they ate less protein and phosphorus.)

Calcium. High calcium intakes enhance phytate's ability to bind tightly to zinc, decreasing zinc absorption.

Oxalic acid (A recent USDA study found that foods high in oxalic acid [oxalates] can dramatically block the absorption of zinc when combined with a high-fiber diet. When spinach, high in oxalic acid, was eaten along with high-fiber foods, very little zinc was absorbed. When cauliflower was substituted for the spinach, the zinc was absorbed.)

Folic acid supplements (200 mcg or more daily)

Supplements of riboflavin, B_6, and B_{12}

Iron (primarily nonheme, or vegetable, iron—not heme, or animal, iron)

DRUGS THAT MAY DEPLETE ZINC
Corticosteroids
Anti-cancer drugs
Diuretics
Laxatives
Iron supplements
Penicillamine

Important Advice to Pregnant Women

Beware of high supplements of folic acid. Dr. Harold Sandstead warns that certain kinds of folate in supplements can block the intestinal absorption of zinc, creating a possibly dangerous deficiency. Such deficiencies of zinc have been linked to birth defects and complications. Dr. Sandstead advises: Have your blood levels of zinc tested early in pregnancy. Eat zinc-rich foods, especially red meat and liver, at least once a week. Don't get much more than 800 micrograms of folate a day. Avoid zinc supplements if possible; they depress absorption of copper.

Toxicity and Supplements

Zinc is considered of low acute toxicity in humans. About 2 grams or more will cause acute gastrointestinal irritation and vomiting. Around 500 mg is considered the minimum toxic dose. Some people have taken ten times the RDA for zinc for months or years without noticeable toxic effects. However, recent reports reveal subtle damage from high doses of zinc, such as impaired immune systems and blood-cholesterol changes.

A study in the *Journal of the American Medical Association,* September 21, 1984, warned against megadoses of zinc supplements: "Excessive intake by healthy persons could have deleterious effects, both immunologic and cardiovascular," according to the author, Dr. Ranjit Kumar Chandra, at Newfoundland's Memorial University. Supplements ten to twenty times the recommended dietary allowance of zinc—150 to 300 mg—for six weeks produced the detrimental effects.

Another report notes severe anemia from copper deficiency related to zinc supplements of 150 mg a day for only fourteen months. Megadoses of zinc (160 mg daily) can also depress levels of protective HDL-type cholesterol. The National Academy of Sciences warns against zinc supplements of more than 15 mg daily without medical supervision.

SYMPTOMS OF ZINC OVERDOSE
Stomach upset
Nausea
Vomiting
Bleeding in the stomach (ultimately anemia)
Accidental zinc poisoning has led to kidney failure and death.

FOODS RICH IN ZINC

The most zinc in weight regardless of calories

Shellfish, especially oysters
Wheat germ
Whole-grain cereals
Pumpkin, watermelon, sunflower,
 and squash seeds
Peanuts
Pecans

Brazil nuts
Nonfat dry milk
Turkey, dark meat
Pork
Pine nuts
Cheese
Dry beans
Lentils

ZINC SUPER-FOODS
THE MOST ZINC, THE FEWEST CALORIES

Here are 50 foods that rate exceptionally high in zinc content per calorie. Of the approximately 2500 foods in this book, these are tops in zinc nutrient density; that is, they have the highest zinc-calorie ratios, giving you the most zinc for the fewest calories.*

	Food Rating	Zinc-calorie ratio (mg of Zinc per 100 calories)	Common Measure	Mg Zinc	Calories
1.	Oysters, wo shell, raw	113.2	3 oz	63	56
2.	Oysters, smoked	113.2	3 oz	103	91
3.	Oysters, breaded, fried	36.9	3 oz	61	165
4.	Oyster stew, w/milk, canned	7	1 c	10	134
5.	Squid, boiled	4.8	3 oz	4	82
6.	Wheat germ	4.4	1 oz	5	108
7.	Crab, meat, steamed	4.3	2 medium	4	89
8.	Pork, liver, cooked	4.1	3 oz	6	141
9.	Bran, unprocessed	3.9	¼ c	1	31
10.	Pot roast, lean, good, braised	3.9	3 oz	7	189
11.	Carp, baked/broiled	3.4	3 oz	5	161
12.	Luncheon meat, beef	3.3	1 oz	1	35
13.	Spinach, fresh, cooked	3.3	½ c	1	21
14.	Calf's liver, cooked	3.2	3 oz	7	222
15.	Lamb, shoulder, lean, boneless, cooked	3.2	3 oz	4	128
16.	Mussels, fresh, cooked	2.9	3 oz	4	138
17.	Tenderloin, lean, good, broiled	2.9	3 oz	5	167
18.	Beef brisket, lean, cooked	2.9	3 oz	6	205
19.	Chicken, liver, simmered	2.8	1 c	6	219

	Food Rating	Zinc-calorie ratio (mg of Zinc per 100 calories)	Common Measure	Mg Zinc	Calories
20.	Clams, canned	2.6	½ c	2	76
21.	Clams, raw	2.6	3 oz	2	65
22.	T-bone steak, lean, broiled	2.5	3 oz	5	182
23.	Venison, stewed	2.4	3 oz	4	153
24.	Turkey, dark meat, roasted	2.4	3½ oz	5	187
25.	Lobster, meat, steamed/ boiled	2.3	3 oz	2	81
26.	Luncheon meat, corned beef, jellied	2.3	1 oz	1	46
27.	Pumpkin and squash seeds, roasted	2.3	1 oz	3	148
28.	Squid, fried	2.2	3 oz	3.5	159
29.	Luncheon meat, peppered loaf	2.2	1 oz	1	42
30.	Luncheon meat, luxury loaf	2.2	1 oz	1	40
31.	Goat, boneless, boiled	2.1	3 oz	4	177
32.	Veal chop, lean, cooked	2.1	3 oz	4	177
33.	Pork, shoulder, lean cooked	1.9	3 oz	4	207
34.	Scallops, broiled/baked	1.9	3 oz	2	106
35.	Carp, fried	1.9	3 oz	4	226
36.	Luncheon meat, honey loaf	1.9	1 oz	1	36
37.	Cheese, processed, American, lowfat	1.8	1 slice	1	38
38.	Turkey liver, cooked	1.8	1 c	4	237
39.	Watermelon seeds, dried	1.8	1 oz	3	158
40.	Chunky pea and ham soup, canned	1.7	1 c	3	184
41.	Sausage, lebanon bologna	1.7	1 oz	1	64
42.	Yogurt, plain, skim milk	1.7	4 oz	1	63
43.	Sesame butter, tahini	1.7	1 oz	3	172
44.	Ham, extra lean (approx. 5% fat)	1.6	2 slices	1	74
45.	Sardines, in oil, canned	1.5	3 oz	2	172

Cereals: five with the highest zinc-calorie ratio

46.	All-Bran	5.3	1 oz	4	71
47.	Bran Buds	5.1	1 oz	4	73
48.	40% Bran Flakes, Kellogg's	4	1 oz	4	93
49.	Nutri-Grain (cereal)	3.7	1 oz	4	102
50.	Special K	3.4	1 oz	4	111

Source: Author's computer analysis from USDA data

*Excludes baby foods. Includes only foods for which one serving supplies a minimum of approximately 10 percent of the RDA.

RECOMMENDED DAILY DIETARY
ALLOWANCES OF ZINC

Age	Milligrams
Birth–6 months	3
6 months–1 year	5
1–10	10
11 and over	15
Pregnant	add 5
Nursing	add 10

Source: National Academy of Sciences, Revised 1980

Magnesium
A Mineral of Major Concern

Magnesium is an essential mineral, necessary to keep every major biological process functioning, including glucose metabolism, protein and nucleic-acid synthesis, muscle contractions, electrical balance of cells, and transmission of nerve impulses. About half of all magnesium is found in the bones and is one of the three "bone minerals," along with calcium and phosphorus. In fact, magnesium and calcium are biologically locked together in the performance of many vital processes. A deficiency of magnesium also affects the metabolism of calcium, potassium, and sodium.

Widespread, Serious Deficiencies

Magnesium is commanding increased attention as researchers discover ever-more disease and health connections with magnesium and, at the same time, widespread marginal deficiencies. Surveys consistently show that very few Americans get enough magnesium. According to the U.S. Department of Agriculture's food-consumption survey, only 25 percent of all Americans meet the recommended dietary allowance (RDA) for magnesium. An alarming 39 percent consume less than 70 percent of the RDA, indicating that magnesium is a "problem nutrient." One recent study even found that people getting over 100 percent of the RDA for magnesium still showed biological insufficiencies of the mineral. Because of current low-calorie, low-complex-carbohydrate diets, the amount of magnesium in the typical American diet has dropped drastically—from an average 475 mg per person in 1900 to 245 mg today.

Who Is at High Risk?

Most likely to suffer magnesium deficiencies are teenagers, women—notably pregnant women—the elderly, alcoholics, diabetics, users of diuretics and digitalis, and heavy exercisers. Alcohol is very destructive to magnesium. About 80 percent of alcoholics are quite deficient in magnesium. Recent research also shows that people who are hyper-reactive to stress (so-called Type A personalities) have extremely low levels of magnesium. A magnesium deficiency frequently also is associated with deficiencies in calcium and potassium.

Experts are not as worried about severe magnesium deficiencies as about marginal deficiencies. Increasing evidence links low levels of magnesium with numerous diseases and conditions. However, the interpretation of the evidence is quite controversial.

YOUR CHANCES OF DEFICIENT INTAKES OF MAGNESIUM

Age	Percent getting less than 100% RDA	Percent getting less than 70% RDA
0–1 year	11	3
1–2	26	7
3–5	52	16
6–8	55	16
Males		
9–11	70	27
12–14	81	43
15–18	81	44
19–22	74	43
23–34	69	32
35–50	70	30
51–64	69	29
65–74	77	38
75 and over	83	44
Females		
9–11	72	27
12–14	84	45
15–18	88	55
19–22	90	62
23–34	85	54
35–50	85	48
51–64	78	41
65–74	85	45
75 and over	84	47

Source: U.S. Department of Agriculture Food-Consumption Survey

SYMPTOMS OF SEVERE MAGNESIUM DEFICIENCY
(Generally seen only in people with certain diseases such as alcoholism, malnutrition, kidney disease, malabsorption disorders, and hyperparathyroidism)

> Loss of appetite
> Apathy
> Nausea
> Vomiting
> Diarrhea
> Muscle contractions
> Tremors
> Confusion
> Depression
> Loss of coordination
> Convulsions

The Heart-Disease Connection

A recent flurry of scientific research ties low levels of magnesium to cardiovascular problems, notably heart disease, hypertension, and stroke. Some of the evidence:

• People who live in areas with soft water have the lowest magnesium levels and the highest incidence of heart disease. Conversely, people who drink hard water have lower rates of heart disease, stroke, and hypertension. What makes water hard are the two minerals, magnesium and calcium. Water is sometimes naturally soft because it lacks magnesium and calcium, but many people artificially "soften" their hard water through devices that remove the magnesium and calcium.

• The magnesium connection may even help explain why people with Type A personalities are more susceptible to heart disease. Dr. Jean-Georges Henrotte and colleagues at the University of Paris find that type As, who are hyper-reactive to stress, produce more chemicals that flush magnesium out of red blood cells. This self-induced chronic magnesium deficiency, set off by stress, Dr. Henrotte says, could give rise to high blood pressure and coronary heart disease. Additionally, other researchers believe that magnesium deficiency can trigger blood-vessel spasms, shutting off oxygen to parts of the heart, and sudden death from heart failure.

A Key to High Blood Pressure

• Studies by Dr. Lawrence Resnick, a cardiologist at Cornell University Medical Center, show that people with high blood pressure consistently have lower levels of magnesium in their red blood cells, and that drops in blood pressure are accompanied by increases in cell levels of magnesium. A Swedish study showed that people taking diuretics to lower blood pressure had much better results when they also increased their intake of magnesium. Such patients are often magnesium depleted.

• A study by Drs. Burton M. and Bella Altura, the State University of New Health Science Center at Brooklyn found that rats fed diets severely deficient in magnesium developed high blood pressure. Further, the blood vessels were most constricted in animals lacking magnesium. The researchers theorize that magnesium regulates the sodium-calcium exchange pump that helps control blood pressure. Thus, too little magnesium, especially when coupled with high amounts of sodium, opens the "gateway" for too much calcium to flood the cells, producing contractions of blood vessels and high blood pressure. It appears that several minerals are involved in the complex puzzle of high blood pressure.

• Additionally, Dr. Burton Altura says that the influx of calcium can lead to coronary artery spasms, ischemia (lack of blood supply to vessels or heart muscle), the death of heart tissue, and fatal heart attacks. He notes that one thing many victims of fatal heart attacks have in common is "strikingly low magnesium levels."

• There is also evidence that consuming more magnesium helps depress blood cholesterol, lessening heart-disease risk.

• Physicians have a much more difficult time controlling the fibrillation (potentially fatal rhythmic disturbances of the heartbeat) in patients with low blood levels of magnesium.

It is important to note that although the relationship between cardiovascular disease and magnesium deficiency is the subject of intense study, not all experts agree that there is substantial evidence to confirm it.

HEALTH PROBLEMS THAT MAY BE LINKED TO MAGNESIUM DEFICIENCY

Research on animals and/or humans proves or suggests a connection between magnesium deficiencies and:

Ischemic heart disease
Cardiac dysrhythmia
High blood-cholesterol levels
Premenstrual syndrome (PMS)
High blood pressure
Type A behavior
Migraines
Lead poisoning
Kidney stones
Diabetic retinopathy (a complication of diabetes that can lead to blindness)
Depression

How Much Magnesium Do You Absorb?

From 30 to 50 percent of magnesium in the diet is absorbed.

Magnesium Antagonists and Helpers

Animal and/or human studies reveal that the following factors may affect how magnesium is absorbed or utilized by the body; the extent of the effect depends on many unknowns, and the interaction may be important only if the antagonist or booster is of sufficient magnitude.

FACTORS THAT MAY BOOST UTILIZATION OF MAGNESIUM
    Protein
    B_6

FACTORS THAT MAY BLOCK MAGNESIUM, INCREASING NEED
    Food fiber
    Oxalic acid in foods
    Calcium
    Phosphorus
    Alcohol
    Stress
    Strenuous exercise (According to an Israeli study, after a 120-kilometer march by extremely physically fit men, their magnesium levels fell sharply within three days and remained low for three months.)

DRUGS THAT MAY DEPLETE MAGNESIUM
    Thiazides (diuretics)
    Furosemide (diuretic)
    Ethacrynic acid (diuretic)

Washed Away by Processing

Magnesium, high in whole grains, is destroyed during processing. For example, whole-grain wheat contains 1,502 parts per million (ppm) of magnesium, white flour only 299 ppm. Vegetables lose magnesium into cooking water; one-half to three-fourths can leach out during vigorous boiling of vegetables like carrots, celery, and parsnips. Preferably, steam or bake vegetables to preserve magnesium.

Toxicity and Supplements

Magnesium is of low toxicity. About 6,000 mg is considered a minimum toxic dose. The primary sign of too much magnesium is diarrhea. Magnesium sulfate is sold as a laxative.

Magnesium is sometimes used therapeutically in relatively high doses. For example, since insufficient magnesium may lead to potentially deadly disruptions of the heartbeat, the mineral has been used successfully to treat cardiac dysrhythmias.

Because magnesium is so scarce in the diets of most Americans, a low-dose supplement in the range of 200 to 400 mg daily (not exceeding the RDA dose) may be good insurance. But megadoses of magnesium could be harmful especially to people with certain heart and kidney problems. High doses could also upset the fragile balance of other nutrients in normal people, and should be used only on the advice of a physician.

FOODS RICH IN MAGNESIUM

The most magnesium regardless of calories

Wheat bran	Whole-wheat flour
Tofu (soybean curd)	Fish
Wheat germ	Nuts
Dried beans	Peanut butter
Bulgur wheat	Cereals
Pumpkin, watermelon, sunflower, and squash seeds	Green vegetables
	Dried apricots

MAGNESIUM SUPER-FOODS
THE MOST MAGNESIUM, THE FEWEST CALORIES

Here are 50 foods that rate exceptionally high in magnesium content per calorie. Of the approximately 2500 foods in this book, these are tops in magnesium nutrient density; they have the highest magnesium-calorie ratios, giving you the most magnesium for the fewest calories.*

Food Rating	Magnesium-calorie ratio (mg of Magnesium per 100 calories)	Common Measure	Mg Magnesium	Calories
1. Chard, swiss, fresh, cooked	430	½ c	76	18
2. Spinach, fresh, cooked	378	½ c	79	21
3. Bran, unprocessed	282	¼ c	87	31
4. Amaranth, cooked	262	½ c	36	14
5. Beet greens, fresh, cooked	252	½ c	49	20
6. Snails (escargots), cooked	229	1 oz	85	37
7. Broccoli, fresh, cooked	207	½ c	47	23
8. Okra, fresh, cooked	178	½ c	46	25
9. Navy bean sprouts, raw	151	½ c	53	35
10. Bean curd (tofu)	142	½ c	94	66
11. Pumpkin and squash seeds	102	1 oz	152	148
12. Bulgur, canned	97	⅔ c	147	151
13. Watermelon seeds	92	1 oz	146	158
14. Artichoke, cooked	89	1 med	47	53
15. Clams, raw	85	3 oz	55	65
16. Clams, canned	85	½ c	65	76
17. Wheat germ	84	1 oz	91	108
18. Squash, acorn, cooked	77	½ c	43	57
19. Sunflower seeds	62	1 oz	100	162
20. White beans, dry, cooked	58	½ c	60	103
21. Clams, steamed	57	3 oz meat	53	93
22. Black, brown & boyo beans, dry, cooked	53	½ c	52	98
23. Beans, lima, green, fresh, cooked	52	½ c	63	104
24. Almonds	52	1 oz	86	167
25. Bread, whole wheat	49	1 slice	27	63
26. Pinto, calico, mexican beans, dry, cooked	46	½ c	47	102
27. Cowpeas, cooked	46	½ c	41	89
28. Cashew nuts	45	1 oz	74	163
29. Pine nuts	45	1 oz	66	146
30. Filberts or hazelnuts	45	1 oz	85	187
31. Shrimp, canned	43	3 oz	42	99
32. Soybeans, green, cooked	43	½ c	54	127
33. Muffins, English, whole wheat	42	1 muffin	54	130
34. Whole wheat, cracked	42	1 c	168	400
35. Red kidney beans, dry, cooked	41	½ c	43	103
36. Clams, smoked, canned in oil	41	3 oz	62	151
37. Bread, sprouted wheat	40	1 slice	25	63
38. Milk, skim	39	1 c	36	90

Food Rating	Magnesium-calorie ratio (mg of Magnesium per 100 calories)	Common Measure	Mg Magnesium	Calories
39. Scallops, broiled/baked	39	3 oz	42	106
40. Soybean kernels, roasted	38	1 oz	49	129
41. Split peas, green/ yellow, dry, cooked	37	½ c	43	116
42. Watermelon, raw	34	1/16 fruit	52	152
43. Brazil nuts	34	1 oz	64	186
44. Walnuts, black	33	1 oz	57	172
45. Pita, whole wheat	32	1	62	190
Cereals: five with highest magnesium-calorie ratio				
46. All-Bran	150	1 oz	106	71
47. Bran Buds	123	1 oz	90	73
48. Bran Chex	81	1 oz	73	91
49. 40% Bran Flakes, Ralston Purina	74	1 oz	68	92
50. Roman Meal, plain, cooked	74	1 c	109	147

Source: Author's computer analysis from USDA data

*Excludes baby foods. Includes only foods for which one serving supplies a minimum of approximately 10 percent of the RDA.

RECOMMENDED DAILY DIETARY ALLOWANCES OF MAGNESIUM

Age	Milligrams
Birth–6 months	50
6 month–1 year	70
1–3	150
4–6	200
7–10	250
Males	
11–14	350
15–18	400
19 and over	350
Females	
11 and over	300
Pregnant	add 150
Nursing	add 150

Source: National Academy of Sciences, Revised 1980

Copper

Authorities recently have become extremely worried about copper deficiencies. Copper is an essential trace mineral, and it's estimated that humans need about 2 to 3 mg per day. Numerous studies, however, show that Americans eat less than half that much, a mere 1 mg per day. According to experts at the U.S. Department of Agriculture, most Americans are dangerously deficient in copper. Surveys show that only 25 percent of the population consumes 2 mg of copper per day.

What are the possible consequences?

• *Heart disease.* Dr. Leslie M. Klevay, research leader at the USDA's Grand Forks Human Nutrition Research Center in North Dakota, contends that copper deficiency is "a major contributor to the development of coronary heart disease." In fact, he believes that it is the single most important dietary cause—outranking even fatty foods.

In government experiments, rats were fed diets (two to three times more deficient in copper) than the typical American diet. Researchers say that virtually everything was wrong with the test animals. They were anemic (since copper is needed for iron metabolism); they had high levels of blood cholesterol and triglycerides; they had glucose intolerance; and mainly they had abnormal arteries and hearts, clogged with fat and diseased by inflammation. Many of the animals died suddenly, often from ruptured hearts.

• *Central nervous system disorders.* Copper deficiency decreases the concentration of at least two neurotransmitters, dopamine and norepinephrine, and may have damaging effects on myelin, the protein sheath surrounding the spinal cord.

• *Anemia, similar to that produced by iron-deficiency.* A possible explanation is that copper is essential for iron metabolism.

• *Bone disorders,* in which bones fracture spontaneously.

Copper deficiency is promoted by other nutrients in the diet that block the absorption of copper:

• Diets high in fructose and other sugars that contain fructose, such as sucrose (ordinary table sugar), dramatically increase the severity of copper deficiency in rats.

• High levels of vitamin C impair copper absorption and aggravate copper deficits.

• High levels of zinc cause copper deficiencies. Daily supplements of 50 mg of zinc per day may interfere with copper absorption.

• Fiber and phytates in food block absorption of copper.

If you want better absorption of copper, be sure you get enough calcium. Studies show that 1 gram of calcium a day raises the level of copper stored in the liver and lowers blood cholesterol.

Supplements

Don't use copper supplements, because they can interfere with other minerals, and only 10 to 15 mg a day can be toxic.

It's best to get your copper from foods. However, it is difficult to get enough copper in the diet without eating lobster, liver, and oysters.

FOODS RICH IN COPPER

The most copper regardless of calories

Shellfish	Nuts and seeds
Liver	Meat
Fresh vegetables	

THE MOST COPPER FOR THE FEWEST CALORIES

	Milligrams per 1,000 calories
Oysters	212
Liver	32
Lobster	19
Yeast, dried	18
Crab meat	9
Vegetables, fresh	2.5
Fruit, fresh	2
Nuts and seeds	1.9
Fish	1.9
Flour, whole wheat	1.5

Source: Dr. Walter Mertz, U.S. Department of Agriculture

ESTIMATED SAFE AND ADEQUATE DAILY DIETARY INTAKES OF COPPER

Age	Milligrams
Birth–6 months	.5–.7
6 months–1 year	.7–1
1–3	1–1.5
4–6	1.5–2
7–10	2–2.5
11 and over	2–3

Source: National Academy of Sciences, Revised 1980

Chromium

Studies show that virtually nobody gets enough chromium, and the consequence may be increased risk of diabetes and heart disease. New evidence reveals a link between glucose intolerance and low levels of the essential trace mineral chromium. Although research on chromium is too scant to warrant firm conclusions, it appears that marginal deficiencies in chromium are widespread and worsen with age. One recent study by Dr. Richard Anderson and colleagues at the U.S. Department of Agriculture's Human Nutrition Center in Beltsville, Maryland, found that 100 percent of thirty-two adults tested consumed less than the 50 to 200 micrograms of chromium recommended as adequate by the National Academy of Sciences. Another study put the average at 33 micrograms per day for men and 25 micrograms for women.

Other studies show that chromium continuously decreases in human tissues throughout life. For example, children under age ten average ten times more chromium in liver tissue than adults over age thirty. Dwindling supplies of chromium in the body may partly account for the fact that the rate of glucose intolerance rises with age. Marginal deficiencies may induce no health troubles at first, but over a period of years chromium-induced glucose intolerance may worsen to the point of severity known as diabetes.

The Diabetes Connection

There is ample evidence that low chromium is linked to diabetes. One study showed diabetics to have low levels of chromium. Experts also know that in some people increasing chromium intakes can correct impaired glucose tolerance, characteristic of diabetes. In a recent study of seventy-six people, Dr. Anderson found that twenty had abnormally high glucose levels. When given 200 micrograms of chromium every day for three months, the glucose levels of the twenty fell dramatically. Conversely, in other studies, Dr. Anderson has found that chromium supplements also help "normalize" the glucose levels of those suspected of being hypoglycemic—having low blood sugar. In that case, increased chromium helped raise blood-sugar levels. Thus, too little chromium may also contribute to that condition known as hypoglycemia.

Increasing intakes of chromium, experts say, might help prevent both high blood sugar (diabetes) and low blood sugar (hypoglycemia) from developing. As for using chromium to treat diabetes, there is little evidence that that will work. It appears that the worse the glucose intolerance, the less the effects of increased chromium.

The richest source of chromium is brewer's yeast. Dr. Walter Mertz, a prominent authority on chromium, says a tablespoon of brewer's yeast per day might be advisable to help ward off diabetes in people who have a family history of the disease.

Low chromium is also implicated as a cause of heart disease. Here's some of the evidence:

• In animals, injections of chromium caused a regression of athero-sclerosis, by helping reduce cholesterol-plaque in arteries.

• Blood levels of chromium were lower in a group of patients with coronary artery disease than in those without heart disease.

• Taking in more chromium—about 200 micrograms a day—raised levels of "good" HDL-type cholesterol, thought to protect against heart disease.

It is difficult to get chromium from typical diets; you usually have to eat at least 3,000 calories per day to get adequate amounts. Dr. Anderson says he sees nothing wrong with a little supplementary chromium (high doses may be dangerous to diabetics). However, you can also get enough from food if you are selective.

Certain beers are remarkably high in chromium, much of it coming from contamination during processing. For example, a USDA analysis

---

FOODS RICH IN CHROMIUM

The most chromium regardless of calories

Brewer's yeast	Cheese
Whole grains	Mushrooms
Liver and other organ meats	Prunes
Oysters	Asparagus
Potatoes with skins	Rhubarb
Egg yolks	Beer and wine
Nuts	

found that an average 12 ounces of beer contained 2½ micrograms of chromium, about 5 percent of the recommended amount. One Carling's beer, produced in Baltimore, contained about 26 micrograms, half the daily adequate intake. Dr. Anderson believes this may help explain why moderate drinking of alcohol, beer in particular, has been tied in some studies to lower risk of heart disease.

ESTIMATED SAFE AND ADEQUATE DAILY DIETARY INTAKES OF CHROMIUM

Age	Milligrams
Birth–6 months	.01–.04
6 months–1 year	.02–.06
1–3	.02–.08
4–6	.03–.12
7–10	.05–.2
11 and over	.05–.2

Source: National Academy of Sciences, Revised 1980

Selenium

Is selenium one of the more recently discovered trace minerals that helps ward off cancer, heart disease, perhaps even aging? Many scientists have high hopes for the protective power of selenium, a micronutrient required by the body in very minute amounts. Journals are flooded with scientific papers on selenium, and although the results are promising, there is no consensus yet on exactly how important selenium is, how it protects, and how many people are potentially deficient.

Here is some of the evidence:

• *Cancer.* There is little question that low bodily levels of selenium are associated with increased risk of various types of cancers. Whether the low selenium is a cause or an effect of the cancer is uncertain. Animal studies consistently show that high levels of selenium inhibit cancer development. Tests on cancer patients show that they often have low levels of selenium. People who live in areas where the soil is low in selenium seem to have higher rates of cancer. One comprehensive survey in the United States found that both men and women who lived in counties where plants were high in selenium had lower rates of lung, colon, rectum, bladder, esophagus, and pancreas cancer. Women living in the counties had less breast, ovarian, and cervical cancers.

• *Heart disease.* Severe deficiencies of selenium in the diet have been linked to a potentially fatal children's heart disease called Keshan disease (enlarged heart), common in parts of China. Other studies link low levels of selenium to increased risk of stroke, heart attack, and angina.

Other evidence suggests that selenium may help keep the immune system functioning properly and, because it is an antioxidant, help protect cells from destruction by toxic agents in the body.

Also, selenium works closely with vitamin E. If you are low in selenium, the potential harm from vitamin E deficiency is accentuated.

Since selenium can be toxic in high doses, it is not advisable to take supplements beyond 200 micrograms a day.

Although the content of selenium in plants varies depending on the soil, analyses find that the selenium in whole-wheat flour, whole-wheat bread, and wheat bran is in a form easily utilized by the body. Thus grains are a valuable source of selenium. The availability of selenium from organ meats is also high and reliable since animals, unlike plants, tend to conserve and accumulate selenium. Seafood is high in selenium, but it may not be so readily absorbed by the body. Studies show that the selenium in canned tuna, for example, is about one-third as available to the body as the selenium in whole-wheat bread. Dairy products are a poor source of selenium.

FOODS RICH IN SELENIUM
Micrograms per 100 grams (3½ ounces)

Swordfish, raw	284
Lobster, canned	79
Sugar Crisp cereal	78
Sunflower seeds	77
Salmon, canned	75
Tuna, canned	72
Cracked-wheat bread	67
Shrimp, cooked or canned	64
Egg noodles, macaroni, spaghetti	64
Brazil nuts	63
Special K cereal	63
Salmon, raw	60
Oysters, raw	57
French bread	56
Beef liver, cooked	56
Haddock, cooked	48
Egg, whole	44
Whole wheat bread	44
Cheerios cereal	40
Rye bread	38
Ham	35

Source: U.S. Department of Agriculture

ESTIMATED SAFE AND ADEQUATE DAILY
DIETARY INTAKES OF SELENIUM

Age	Milligrams
Birth–6 months	.01–.04
6 months–1 year	.02–.06
1–3	.02–.08
4–6	.03–.12
7 and over	.05–.2

Source: National Academy of Sciences, Revised 1980

Vitamin E

Vitamin E, a fat-soluble antioxidant, also called tocopherol, is of increasingly high interest, possibly as some protection against the development of cancer. Information about vitamin E and where to find it in foods is included in this book for that reason, although there is no evidence of substantial vitamin E deficiencies. However, the fundamental role of vitamin E in the body is still not well understood. Vitamin E supplements are medically used to correct some problems, but many wild claims for therapeutic megadoses of vitamin E have not held up.

Here is some of the evidence about the health effects of vitamin E:

Vitamin E deficiencies can increase the tendency of blood to clot. High doses (300 to 800 IUs per day) can relieve a condition known as "intermittent claudication"—pains in the calves due to narrowing arteries. Vitamin E in normal people may also influence certain prostaglandins, chemical substances that help control numerous bodily processes. Certain neurological disorders have been associated with severe vitamin E deficiencies; the problems disappeared with correction of the deficiencies.

Additionally, vitamin E deficiencies interfere with the proper utlization of vitamin A and iron. Studies in animals find that low levels of vitamin E can help induce iron-deficiency anemia by somehow promoting abnormal iron metabolism. High levels of iron can also destroy vitamin E. Research with children shows that correcting vitamin E deficiencies boosts their blood levels of vitamin A. Apparently, adequate vitamin E helps protect vitamin A in the body. However, animal studies suggest that very large doses of vitamin E can actually reduce absorption of the vitamin.

It is doubtful that many people, with the possible exception of those on very low-calorie, low-fat diets, are deficient in vitamin E by current standards. In fact, the consumption of vitamin E is increasing because of a rise in the use of polyunsaturated oils—a rich source of E. At the same time, the more polyunsaturated fat you eat, the more vitamin E you need.

Although vitamin E, like vitamin A, is fat soluble, and thus is stored in tissue, vitamin E is relatively nontoxic in comparison with vitamin A. Experts generally consider doses of 200 to 600 mg daily of tocopherol to be safe.

Vitamin E primarily comes from plants, is most concentrated in vegetable oils, and rarely is found in meat, because animals do not manufacture the vitamin; they receive it only from other foods.

FOODS RICH IN VITAMIN E

Oils: 1 tablespoon	Milligrams
Coconut	.5
Corn	11.2
Olive	1.7
Palm	4.7
Peanut	3.3
Safflower	5.1
Sesame seed	3.9
Soybean	12.6
Sunflower seed	8.6
Wheat germ	34

Other foods	
Almonds, blanched: 1 oz	6
Cashews, roasted: 1 oz	3.1
Corn, whole: 1 oz	1.6
Lima beans, dry: 1 oz	2.2
Margarine, corn-oil stick: 1 tbsp	8
Margarine, corn, soybean-oil stick: 1 tbsp	9.5
Margarine, safflower, soybean, tub: 1 tbsp	6.8
Peanuts, roasted: 1 oz	3.1
Rice bran: 1 oz	4.2
Shortening, soybean: 1 tbsp	13.7
Soybeans, dry: 1 oz	5.8
Sunflower seeds: 1 oz	15
Wheat bran: 1 oz	2.5
Wheat germ: 1 oz	8

Source: U.S. Department of Agriculture

RECOMMENDED DAILY DIETARY ALLOWANCES
OF VITAMIN E

Age	Milligrams expressed as tocopherol equivalents
Birth–6 months	3
6 months–1 year	4
1–3	5
4–6	6
7–10	7
11–14	8
Males 11 and over	10
Females 11 and over	8
Pregnant	add 2
Nursing	add 3

Source: National Academy of Sciences, Revised 1980

How to Read the Charts

The following food composition charts are extracted from the U.S. Department of Agriculture's databases and are in common serving sizes as designated by government experts. The charts list twenty-one common nutritional elements chosen by the author, in consultation with government officials, as the nutrient information most commonly sought.

At the time this book went into production the USDA had updated thirteen of twenty-three categories in its ongoing revision of *Handbook 8*. Those revised sections, extracted in the following charts, are dairy and egg products; breakfast cereals; poultry products; fruits and fruit juices; soups, sauces, and gravies; fats and oils; spices and herbs; baby foods; vegetables; nuts and seeds; sausages and luncheon meats, and beef products. All of these have been published in individual volumes by the USDA. For easier reference we have separated some of the sections—for example dairy and egg products into milk, cream, cheese and eggs—presenting each food type in alphabetical order.

The rest of the nutrient information (except for fast foods) also comes from USDA databases but consists of interim or "provisional" nutrient figures which are the most comprehensive and accurate currently available. We took the figures from two USDA databases. Almost all came from nutrient information used in the USDA's 1985–1986 continuing nationwide food consumption survey. A few items came from the USDA's standard reference listing of nonupdated foods. These two databases were the sources for our nutrient information on lamb, veal, and game; seafood; beverages; legumes; mixed dishes; baked products; grains; candies and sweets, and miscellaneous, such as mustard and olives. This information is the best available at the time, but some is not as thoroughly substantiated as that in the revised *Handbook 8* sections. Some nutrient figures needed for the food consumption surveys are approximations or "best guesses" based on USDA expert knowledge, and may change during the course of the *Handbook 8* update.

Important: New information is regularly added to the USDA's nutrient databases. Because we have used the latest figures available, our charts have some nutrient figures that do not appear in the printed volumes of *Handbook 8*. Also, there may be discrepancies between previously published USDA nutrient figures, for example, in Agriculture's popular *Nutritive Value of Foods* (Home and Garden Bulletin Number 72), 1985 edition, and those used in this book. That is because more current information became available. Notable, for example, are differences in some cholesterol and sodium counts for seafood between previously published USDA information and that from the food consumption survey. According to USDA officials, the food consumption survey figures listed here are more current; they were revised in 1985–1986 on the basis of new data.

The fast-food nutrient information was obtained from fast-food chains directly because the USDA's compilation of such figures for the *Handbook 8* revision is still in progress.

In the future, after the USDA has completed its revision of all of the sections for *Handbook 8,* those sections will be included in updated versions of this book. For now, this is the *last word*—the most current, comprehensive nutrient analysis of America's food supply, compiled by that most impeccable source: the U.S. Department of Agriculture.

Some Cautions on Interpretations

• *Brand names vs. generic.* Most of the figures are generic. Brand names are listed when the products differ so much that it makes no sense to describe them any other way. Thus, cereals are listed by their brand names, as are some candies and all fast foods.

In other cases, agriculture analysts report the average nutritional contents of the brand-name samples from a number of companies—for example, as with baby foods. These, then, are industry averages, and may vary slightly from brand to brand, although the major nutrients should be quite similar. Generic products such as poultry, vegetables, fruits, grains, meat, seafood, nuts, and seeds, of course, carry no brand name nutrient distinctions. Various types of breads are fairly standard among brands because bread must conform to the government's enrichment standards.

• *Salt.* The sodium listed for unprocessed foods (unless otherwise noted) is the amount indigenous to the food and does not take into account extra salt you may add in cooking or preparing. The sodium for processed foods is an average.

• *Fat.* To enable you to see quickly how much of the fat in a food is saturated, we have listed that percentage—and this will usually help you instantly spot foods high in saturated fat, such as cheese, cream, butter. However, be sure to consult the figure on the total amount of fat.

If a food has very little total fat, even though much of it is saturated, such small amounts are not a significant threat. To calculate how much of a food's calories are from fat, simply multiply the number of fat grams by 9. For example, an ounce of blue cheese has 100 calories and 8 grams of fat; thus, 9 times 8, or 72 percent, of the calories come from fat, making cheese a high-fat food. Of that, according to the chart, fully 65 percent of the fat is saturated, so in addition it is a very highly saturated fatty food.

• *Fruit juices and fruit drinks.* Do not confuse the two. Fruit juices are the extracts of fruits; fruit drinks may or may not contain fruit juice. Fruit drinks are often watered-down fruit juices, and usually have added sugar, synthetic vitamins, and coloring. They are not as inherently nutritious as plain fruit juices.

• *Raw vs. cooked and processed fruits and vegetables.* In most cases, cooked or processed foods lose nutrients, so be careful to correctly interpret the charts. For example, ½ cup of raw asparagus contains 80 mg of folacin; compared with 88 mg in ½ cup of cooked asparagus and 115 in ½ cup of canned asparagus spears. This does *not* mean that cooked and processed asparagus somehow *gains* nutrients. The explanation is that it takes more cooked and canned asparagus to make up ½ cup, accounting for the increase in nutrients. To illustrate: ½ cup of raw asparagus weighs 67 grams; ½ cup of cooked asparagus, 98 grams; ½ cup of canned asparagus, 121 grams. Actually, the cooking results in a loss of about 29 micrograms of folacin, and the canning a loss of about 28 micrograms when compared by weight, instead of by volume—a half cup.

• *Carbohydrates.* Government figures do not break down the composition by complex carbohydrates (starch) and simple carbohydrates (sucrose or table sugar).

• *Fiber.* Remember, fiber is found only in plant products. You can assume there is no significant fiber in meat and dairy products. The fiber listed in the charts is "total dietary fiber," not the inaccurate, outmoded "crude fiber." Reliable techniques for analyzing total dietary fiber are fairly new, and figures are not yet available for many foods. The "total dietary fiber" in foods from the Food Consumption Survey, such as mixed dishes, are "best guesses" by USDA experts.

• *Cooking additions.* In the sections taken from USDA's Food Consumption Survey, the figures usually assume that "normal" amounts of salt and, sometimes, fat (margarine or butter) were added during cooking. Thus, in the sections on legumes, pasta, rice, mixed dishes, and seafood, be sure to note that the sodium figures are higher than would be expected in the raw foods. Without added salt, the sodium content of such foods is much lower and is sometimes virtually nonexistent. For example, raw fish contains only 10 to 20 mg of sodium per ounce. A cup of raw rice has a mere 9 to 17 mg of sodium. Uncooked pasta has very little sodium. Even nuts are naturally low in sodium; peanuts and cashews have 4 mg of sodium per ounce, and macadamia nuts, 2 mg per ounce.

• *Cholesterol.* Cholesterol occurs exclusively in animal products. You do not find it in plant products.

• Vitamin B_{12} occurs almost exclusively in animal products.

• Iron is found in both animal and vegetable products; the animal heme iron is more potent. The iron in fortified cereals is poor.

• The protein in animal foods is of higher quality than that in plant foods, but the total protein quality of plants can be greatly enhanced by proper combinations.

Note: A dash means the information was not significant or not available. You will find a number of these in the fiber section because the standards for measuring fiber have changed recently and many foods have not yet been analyzed properly.

What the Measurements Mean

For greater understanding, we have included both the common serving size and the weight of that serving size in grams. There are 28.4 grams in 1 ounce. One hundred grams equals about 3½ ounces. An ounce determined by weight is called an avoirdupois ounce. An ounce measured by volume is a fluid ounce. Here is a conversion table that may help if you need to make additional calculations from the charts:

CONVERSION TABLE
28.4 grams = 1 avoirdupois ounce
100 grams = about 3½ ounces
1 milligram = 1/1000 of a gram or 1/30,000 of an ounce
1 microgram = 1/1,000,000 of a gram or 1/30,000,000 of an ounce

1 tablespoon = 3 teaspoons
2 tablespoons = 1 fluid ounce
4 tablespoons = ¼ cup
5⅓ tablespoons = ⅓ cup
16 tablespoons = 1 cup
1 cup = 8 fluid ounces
1 cup = ½ pint
2 cups = 1 pint
2 pints = 1 quart
1 pound = 16 ounces

Abbreviations Used in Food Charts

all var: all varieties
approx: approximately
blchd: blanched
bld: boiled
bnls: boneless
bns: beans
brd: breaded
brld: broiled
brsd: braised
btld: bottled
btr: butter
bttrmlk: buttermilk
c: cup
cdsd: condensed
chick: chicken
chky: chunky
choc: chocolate
chs: cheese
cinn: cinnamon
conc: concentrate
ckd: cooked
ctl: cocktail
cnd: canned
cstd: custard
cvrd: covered
dehy: dehydrated
dia: diameter
enr: enriched
flav: flavor or flavored
fld: filled
flr: floured
frd: fried
froz: frozen
ftfd: fortified
grl: grilled
grn: grain
hvy: heavy
hlvs: halves
imitn: imitation
ind: individual
jr: junior

lem: lemon
low cal: low calorie
lq: liquid
lt: light
med: medium
Mnhtn: Manhattan
mshd: mashed
mtbls: meatballs
oz: ounce
pk: pack
pkt: packet
prep: prepared
prot: protein
pwdr: powder
rcnstd: reconstituted
reg: regular
rts: ready to serve
stst: substitute
sflwr: safflower
shrd: shredded
sltd: salted
smrd: simmered
st: strained
stfd: stuffed
stmd: steamed
sgr: sugar
swtnd: sweetened
tbsp: tablespoon
tdl: toddler
thk cst: thick crust
thn cst: thin crust
tsp: teaspoon
vac: vacuum
veg: vegetable
vit: vitamin
unblchd: unblanched
unenr: unenriched
unsltd or unstd: unsalted
unswtnd: unsweetened
w: with
whl: whole
wo: without
x-heavy: extra heavy

BABY FOODS

Cereal

	Calories (kcal)	Protein (gm)	Carbohydrates (gm)	Fat (gm)	Percent Saturated Fat	Cholesterol (mg)	Dietary Fiber (gm)	Vitamin A (RE)	Vitamin C (mg)
Barley, dry - ½ oz (14.2gm)	52	1.6	10.7	.5	-	-	-	-	.3
Barley, prep w/whole milk 1 oz (28.4gm)	31	1.3	4.6	.9	-	-	-	-	-
Egg and bacon, jr - 1 jar (213gm)	178	5.4	15.1	11	-	-	-	42.6	2.5
Egg and bacon, st - 1 jar (128gm)	101	3.2	8	6.4	-	-	-	35.8	1.1
Grits & egg yolks, st - 1 jar (128gm)	73	2.3	9.5	2.9	-	-	-	38.4	.6
High-protein, dry - ½ oz (14.2gm)	51	5.1	6.6	.8	-	-	-	-	.3
High-protein, prep w/whole milk - 1 oz (28.4gm)	31	2.5	3.3	1.1	-	-	-	-	-
High-protein, w/apple and orange, dry - ½ oz (14.2gm)	53	3.6	8.2	.9	-	-	-	.7	.4
High-protein w/apple and orange, prep w/whole milk - 1 oz (28.4gm)	32	2	3.8	1.1	-	-	-	8	-
Mixed, dry - ½ oz (14.2gm)	54	1.7	10.4	.6	-	-	-	-	.3
Mixed, prep w/whole milk - 1 oz (28.4gm)	32	1.3	4.5	1	-	-	-	-	-
Mixed, w/applesauce and bananas, jr - 1 jar (220gm)	183	2.6	40.5	.9	-	-	-	4	20
Mixed, w/applesauce and bananas, st - 1 jar (135gm)	111	1.6	24.2	.7	-	-	-	2	34.5
Mixed, w/bananas, dry - ½ oz (14.2gm)	56	1.5	10.9	.7	-	-	-	1.7	.5
Mixed, w/bananas, prep w/whole milk - 1 oz (28.4gm)	33	1.3	4.7	1	-	-	-	8	-
Mixed, w/honey, dry - ½ oz (14.2gm)	55	2	10.4	.7	-	-	-	0	0
Mixed, w/honey, prep w/whole milk - 1 oz (28.4gm)	33	1.4	4.5	1	-	-	-	7	-
Oatmeal, dry - ½ oz (14.2gm)	56	1.9	9.8	1.1	-	-	-	-	.4
Oatmeal, prep w/whole milk - 1 oz (28.4gm)	33	1.4	4.3	1.2	-	-	-	-	-
Oatmeal, w/applesauce and bananas, jr - 1 jar (220gm)	165	2.9	34.6	1.6	-	-	-	6	42.1
Oatmeal, w/applesauce and bananas, st - 1 jar (135gm)	99	1.8	20.8	.9	-	-	-	4	29.4
Oatmeal, w/bananas, dry - ½ oz (14.2gm)	56	1.7	10.4	.9	-	-	-	1	.7
Oatmeal, w/bananas, prep w/whole milk - 1 oz (28.4gm)	33	1.3	4.5	1.1	-	-	-	8	-
Oatmeal, w/honey, dry - ½ oz (14.2gm)	55	1.9	9.8	1	-	-	-	0	0

Thiamin (mg)	Riboflavin (mg)	Niacin (mg)	Vitamin B₆ (mg)	Vitamin B₁₂ (mcg)	Folacin (mcg)	Sodium (mg)	Calcium (mg)	Iron (mg)	Potassium (mg)	Zinc (mg)	Magnesium (mg)
.4	.4	5.1	.1	0	4.1	7	113	10.6	56	.4	16
.1	.2	1.7	0	.1	2.5	14	65	3.5	54	.2	8
0	.1	.3	.1	.2	9.3	97	54	1.1	79	.6	10
.1	.1	.3	0	.1	5.2	62	36	.6	44	.3	6
0	.1	.4	0	.1	3.7	45	36	.6	71	.3	6
.4	.4	4.8	.1	0	27	7	103	10.4	192	.6	32
.1	.2	1.6	0	.1	10	14	62	3.4	99	.3	14
.5	.6	3.4	.1	0	27	15	107	12.4	189	.4	23
.2	.2	1.1	0	.1	7.8	16	63	4.1	98	.2	10
.3	.4	4.9	0	0	6.1	6	104	9	62	.3	14
.1	.2	1.6	0	.1	3.2	13	62	3	56	.2	8
.6	.8	8.9	.3	0	8.1	78	9	12.3	70	.5	16
.4	.5	5.4	.2	0	4.9	3	9	8.9	55	.3	11
.5	.5	2.9	.1	0	2.4	17	99	9.6	95	.2	13
.2	.2	1	0	.1	2	17	61	3.2	67	.2	7
.4	.4	5.3	0	0	6.2	6	168	9.7	38	.4	15
.1	.2	1.8	0	.1	3.2	14	83	3.2	49	.2	8
.4	.4	5.1	0	0	5	5	104	10.4	67	.5	21
.1	.2	1.7	0	.1	2.8	13	62	3.4	58	.3	10
.5	1.1	7.4	.5	0	7.8	69	12	12.1	106	.7	24
.6	.5	6.8	.3	0	4.7	2	11	7.6	63	.5	15
.5	.5	2.9	.1	0	2.7	17	92	9.7	104	.3	17
.2	.2	1	0	.1	2.1	17	58	3.2	70	.2	9
.4	.4	5.2	0	0	5	7	164	9.6	37	.5	21

	Calories (kcal)	Protein (gm)	Carbohydrates (gm)	Fat (gm)	Percent Saturated Fat	Cholesterol (mg)	Dietary Fiber (gm)	Vitamin A (RE)	Vitamin C (mg)
Oatmeal, w/honey, prep w/whole milk - 1 oz (28.4gm)	33	1.4	4.3	1.1	-	-	-	7	-
Rice, dry - ½ oz (14.2gm)	56	1	11	.7	-	-	-	-	.3
Rice, prep w/whole milk - 1 oz (28.4gm)	33	1.1	4.7	1	-	-	-	-	-
Rice, w/honey, prep w/whole milk - 1 oz (28.4gm)	33	1.1	4.9	.9		-	-	7	-
Rice, w/applesauce and bananas, st - 1 jar (135gm)	107	1.6	23.1	.5	-	-	-	3	42.7
Rice, w/bananas, dry - ½ oz (14.2gm)	57	1.2	11.3	.6	-	-	-	.4	.3
Rice, w/bananas, prep w/whole milk - 1 oz (28.4gm)	33	1.2	4.8	1	-	-	-	7	-
Rice, w/honey, dry - ½ oz (14.2gm)	56	1	11.4	.4	-	-	-	0	0
Rice, w/mixed fruit, jr - 1 jar (220gm)	186	2.3	41	.5	-	-	-	3	44.5
w/egg yolks, jr - 1 jar (213gm)	110	4.1	15.1	3.8	34.5	-	-	87.3	1.5
w/egg yolks, st - 1 jar (128gm)	66	2.5	9	2.3	33.9	81.1	-	51.2	.9
w/eggs, st - 1 jar (128gm)	74	2.8	10.2	1.9	33.2	65.8	-	-	1

Desserts

	Calories (kcal)	Protein (gm)	Carbohydrates (gm)	Fat (gm)	Percent Saturated Fat	Cholesterol (mg)	Dietary Fiber (gm)	Vitamin A (RE)	Vitamin C (mg)
Apple betty, jr - 1 jar (220gm)	153	.8	41.7	0	-	-	-	3	59.7
Apple betty, st - 1 jar (135gm)	97	.5	26.5	0	-	-	-	2	46.8
Caramel pudding, jr - 1 jar (213gm)	167	2.9	36.2	1.9	-	-	-	7	4.6
Caramel pudding, st - 1 jar (135gm)	104	1.8	23.2	.9	-	-	-	5	3
Cherry vanilla pudding, jr - 1 jar (220gm)	152	.4	40.5	.4	-	-	-	44	2.4
Cherry vanilla pudding, st - 1 jar (135gm)	91	.3	24.1	.4	-	-	-	27	1.5
Cookies - 1 (6.5gm)	28	.8	4.4	.9	-	-	-	0	.5
Cookies, arrowroot - 1 (6gm)	24	.4	3.9	.8	-	.1	-	-	.3
Cottage cheese w/pineapple, jr - 1 jar (220gm)	172	6.5	35.1	1.5	-	-	-	3	52.4
Cottage cheese w/pineapple, st - 1 jar (135gm)	94	4	17.8	1.1	-	-	-	4	31.4
Custard pudding, chocolate, jr - 1 jar (220gm)	195	4.2	38.3	3.5	-	-	-	10	2.4
Custard pudding, chocolate, st - 1 jar (128gm)	107	2.4	20.6	2.1	-	-	-	6	1.9
Custard pudding, vanilla, jr - 1 jar (220gm)	196	3.5	35.7	5	52	-	-	8	1.8
Custard pudding, vanilla, st - 1 jar (128gm)	109	2	20.6	2.5	51.6	-	-	8	1
Dutch apple, jr - 1 jar (220gm)	151	0	37	2.1	65.2	-	-	11	47.1

Thiamin (mg)	Riboflavin (mg)	Niacin (mg)	Vitamin B_6 (mg)	Vitamin B_{12} (mcg)	Folacin (mcg)	Sodium (mg)	Calcium (mg)	Iron (mg)	Potassium (mg)	Zinc (mg)	Magnesium (mg)
.1	.2	1.7	0	.1	2.8	14	82	3.1	48	.3	10
.4	.3	4.4	.1	0	3.5	5	121	10.5	55	.3	29
.1	.1	1.5	0	.1	2.3	13	68	3.5	54	.2	13
.1	.2	1.7	0	.1	2.4	14	83	3.1	40	.2	13
.4	.6	5.4	0	-	3.4	38	23	9.1	38	.1	4
.6	.5	3.3	1.8	0	-	14	98	9.5	109	.2	20
.2	.2	1.1	0	.1	1.8	16	60	3.1	72	.2	10
.4	.4	5.2	.1	0	3.5	7	166	9.3	12	.3	30
.6	1.3	6	.5	.1	5.9	24	43	10.4	72	.4	10
0	.1	.1	0	.1	7.1	70	51	1.1	75	.6	6
0	.1	.1	0	.1	4.2	42	30	.6	50	.4	4
0	.1	.1	0	.1	12	49	35	.7	56	.4	4
0	.1	.1	0	.1	.9	19	36	.4	117	.1	4
0	.1	.1	0	.1	.5	14	25	.2	68	0	3
0	.1	.1	0	0	1.9	60	116	.3	124	.6	11
0	.1	0	0	0	1.2	37	60	.2	70	.4	7
0	0	.1	0	-	.7	32	11	.4	73	.1	5
0	0	.1	0	-	.4	22	7	.3	46	.1	3
.1	.2	1	.4	.3	.7	12	7	.3	33	.1	3
0	0	.3	0	0	.6	20	2	.2	9	0	1
0	.1	.1	0	.2	11.1	113	68	.3	92	.4	8
0	.1	.1	0	.1	6.1	70	35	.1	58	.2	5
0	.2	.2	0	0	10.6	55	134	.9	196	.7	23
0	.1	.1	0	0	5.8	30	78	.5	110	.4	13
0	.2	.1	0	0	13.6	64	123	.6	136	.6	11
0	.1	.1	0	0	7.7	36	71	.3	85	.4	7
0	0	.1	0	0	1.5	36	10	.4	82	.1	4

	Calories (kcal)	Protein (gm)	Carbohydrates (gm)	Fat (gm)	Percent Saturated Fat	Cholesterol (mg)	Dietary Fiber (gm)	Vitamin A (RE)	Vitamin C (mg)
Dutch apple, st - 1 jar (135gm)	92	0	22.6	1.2	65	-	-	7	28.9
Fruit dessert, jr - 1 jar (220gm)	138	.6	37.9	0	-	-	-	53	6.6
Fruit dessert, st - 1 jar (135gm)	79	.4	21.6	0	-	-	-	33.8	3.4
Fruit pudding, orange, st - 1 jar (135gm)	108	1.5	23.8	1.2	-	-	-	16	12.3
Fruit pudding, pineapple, jr - 1 jar (220gm)	192	3.1	47.4	.9	-	-	-	8.8	58.7
Fruit pudding, pineapple, st - 1 jar (128gm)	104	1.6	26	.4	-	-	-	5	34.8
Peach cobbler, jr - 1 jar (220gm)	147	.7	40.3	0	-	-	-	31	45.1
Peach cobbler, st - 1 jar (135gm)	88	.4	24	0	-	-	-	19	27.7
Peach melba, jr - 1 jar (220gm)	132	.6	36.1	0	-	-	-	43	57.3
Peach melba, st - 1 jar (135gm)	81	.3	22.3	0	-	-	-	25	42.4
Pineapple orange, st - 1 jar (128gm)	89	.3	24.4	0	-	-	-	7	18.3
Tropical Fruit, jr - 1 jar (220gm)	131	.4	36.1	0	-	-	-	4	41.3

Dinners

	Calories (kcal)	Protein (gm)	Carbohydrates (gm)	Fat (gm)	Percent Saturated Fat	Cholesterol (mg)	Dietary Fiber (gm)	Vitamin A (RE)	Vitamin C (mg)
Beef and Rice, tdl - 1 jar (177gm)	146	8.9	15.5	5.1	-	-	-	139.8	6.8
Beef lasagna, tdl - 1 jar (177gm)	137	7.4	17.7	3.8	-	-	-	276.1	3.4
Beef noodle, jr - 1 jar (213gm)	122	5.4	15.7	4	-	-	-	187.4	2.9
Beef noodle, st - 1 jar (128gm)	68	2.9	9	2.2	-	-	-	140.8	1.5
Beef stew, tdl - 1 jar (177gm)	90	9.1	9.6	2.1	49	22.2	-	408.9	5.3
Chicken noodle w/veg, jr - 1 jar (213gm)	137	3.7	19.4	4.8	-	-	-	276.9	1.7
Chicken noodle w/veg, st - 1 jar (128gm)	81	2.6	10.1	3.3	-	-	-	224	1
Chicken noodle, jr - 1 jar (213gm)	109	4.1	16.1	3	-	-	-	227.9	2.6
Chicken noodle, st - 1 jar (128gm)	67	2.7	9.6	1.9	-	-	-	143.4	1.3
Chicken soup, cream, st - 1 jar (128gm)	74	3.2	10.8	2	-	-	-	148.5	1.7
Chicken soup, st - 1 jar (128gm)	64	2	9.2	2.2	-	-	-	282.9	1.2
Chicken stew, tdl - 1 jar (170gm)	132	8.9	10.9	6.4	29.1	48.8	-	205.7	3.2

Thiamin (mg)	Riboflavin (mg)	Niacin (mg)	Vitamin B_6 (mg)	Vitamin B_{12} (mcg)	Folacin (mcg)	Sodium (mg)	Calcium (mg)	Iron (mg)	Potassium (mg)	Zinc (mg)	Magnesium (mg)
0	0	.1	0	0	.9	21	6	.3	44	0	2
0	0	.3	.1	0	7.7	29	19	.5	208	.1	11
0	0	.2	.1	0	4.5	18	11	.3	127	.1	7
.1	.1	.2	0	0	10.5	27	43	.1	117	.2	7
.1	.1	.3	.1	.1	12.2	48	75	.4	198	.4	20
0	.1	.1	.1	.1	6.7	24	40	.2	104	.3	11
0	0	.6	0	0	2.5	20	9	.2	123	.1	4
0	0	.4	0	0	1.5	10	6	.1	73	.4	3
0	.1	.6	0	0	4.2	19	23	.7	205	.6	4
0	0	.5	0	0	2.6	12	13	.4	112	.4	3
0	0	.1	0	.1	3.3	13	14	.2	61	.2	5
0	.1	.2	.1	0	7.3	16	22	.6	128	.1	11
0	.1	2.4	.2	.9	10.6	632	20	1.2	212	1.6	15
.1	.2	2.4	.1	.9	10.6	804	32	1.6	216	1.2	20
.1	.1	1.2	.1	.2	11.7	37	18	.9	99	.9	16
0	.1	.9	.1	.1	6.5	37	12	.5	61	.5	9
0	.1	2.3	.1	.9	10.6	611	16	1.3	251	1.5	20
.1	.1	1.4	0	.2	7.3	54	54	1	126	.7	23
0	.1	.5	0	.1	4.1	26	35	.4	70	.3	13
.1	.1	1.1	.1	.3	11.3	36	36	.8	75	.6	19
0	.1	.6	0	.2	6.9	20	29	.6	50	.4	11
0	.1	.5	.1	.1	7.9	24	44	.4	100	.3	7
0	0	.4	0	.1	6.7	20	47	.4	84	.3	6
.1	.1	2	.1	.2	1.7	683	60	1.1	156	.7	18

	Calories (kcal)	Protein (gm)	Carbohydrates (gm)	Fat (gm)	Percent Saturated Fat	Cholesterol (mg)	Dietary Fiber (gm)	Vitamin A (RE)	Vitamin C (mg)
Lamb and noodles, jr - 1 jar (213gm)	138	4.8	18.6	4.7	-	-	-	223.6	4.1
Macaroni and bacon jr - 1 jar (213gm)	160	5.4	18.2	7.1	-	-	-	340.8	4.5
Macaroni & cheese, jr - 1 jar (213gm)	130	5.5	17.5	4.3	-	-	-	6.4	2.8
Macaroni and cheese, st - 1 jar (128gm)	76	3.3	9.6	2.7	-	-	-	6.4	1.7
Macaroni and ham, jr - 1 jar (213gm)	127	6.8	18	2.9	-	-	-	147	4.8
Macaroni and tomato and beef, jr - 1 jar (213gm)	125	5.3	20.1	2.4	-	-	-	232.2	3.2
Macaroni and tomato and beef, st - 1 jar (128gm)	71	2.9	11.3	1.4	-	-	-	115.2	1.9
Mixed veg, jr - 1 jar (213gm)	71	2.1	16.8	.1	-	-	-	519.7	6.9
Mixed veg, st - 1 jar (128gm)	52	1.5	12.2	.1	-	-	-	349.4	3.5
Spaghetti and tomato and meat, jr - 1 jar (213gm)	135	5.4	21.6	2.7	-	-	-	283.3	4.7
Spaghetti and tomato and meat, tdl - 1 jar (177gm)	133	9.4	19.1	1.8	-	-	-	150.4	7.3
Split pea and ham, jr - 1 jar (213gm)	152	7	24.1	2.8	-	-	-	170.4	4.1
Turkey and rice, jr - 1 jar (213gm)	104	3.8	15.3	2.9	31.7	-	-	315.2	2.5
Turkey and rice, st - 1 jar (128gm)	63	2.4	9.4	1.7	-	12.8	-	121.6	1.5
Veg and bacon, jr - 1 jar (213gm)	150	3.9	16.1	8.2	36.3	-	-	464.3	2.4
Veg and bacon, st - 1 jar (128gm)	88	2	11	4.2	36.2	4.1	-	381.4	1.7
Veg and beef, jr - 1 jar (213gm)	113	5	15.8	3.6	-	-	-	409	3.1
Veg and beef, st - 1 jar (128gm)	67	2.5	9	2.6	-	-	-	218.9	1.5
Veg and chicken, jr - 1 jar (213gm)	106	4	18	2.3	-	-	-	315.2	3.1
Veg and chicken, st - 1 jar (128gm)	55	2.5	8.5	1.4	-	-	-	175.4	1.4
Veg and ham, jr - 1 jar (213gm)	110	5.2	14.9	3.6	-	-	-	172.5	2.7
Veg and ham, st - 1 jar (128gm)	62	2.2	8.8	2.2	-	-	-	121.6	2.1
Veg and ham, tdl - 1 jar (177gm)	128	7.4	13.9	5.2	35.6	13.6	-	83.2	6.6
Veg and lamb, jr - 1 jar (213gm)	108	4.4	15.1	3.7	-	-	-	423.9	3.7
Veg and lamb, st - 1 jar (128gm)	67	2.5	8.9	2.6	-	-	-	362.2	1.5
Veg and liver, jr - 1 jar (213gm)	93	3.9	17.5	1.2	-	-	-	1522.9	3.8

Thiamin (mg)	Riboflavin (mg)	Niacin (mg)	Vitamin B$_6$ (mg)	Vitamin B$_{12}$ (mcg)	Folacin (mcg)	Sodium (mg)	Calcium (mg)	Iron (mg)	Potassium (mg)	Zinc (mg)	Magnesium (mg)
.1	.1	1.4	.1	.4	9.2	39	39	.8	165	.6	17
.1	.2	1.3	0	.1	3.4	166	152	.8	180	.8	17
.1	.1	1.2	0	.1	3.2	163	108	.6	94	.7	14
.1	.1	.6	0	0	1.8	93	69	.4	59	.4	11
.1	.2	1.7	0	.1	4.3	101	159	.8	225	.8	15
.1	.1	1.6	.1	.5	13.8	35	30	.8	153	.8	15
.1	.1	1	.1	.3	25.7	21	21	.6	123	.4	12
0	.1	.9	.2	0	14.2	19	37	.6	240	.5	21
0	0	.6	.1	0	10.2	10	29	.4	155	.2	14
.1	.1	2.3	.1	0	15.1	42	39	1.2	230	.9	17
.1	.2	2.8	.1	.4	10.6	634	39	1.6	289	.9	26
.1	.1	1	.1	.1	27.7	30	49	1.1	291	1.4	-
0	.1	.6	.1	.2	6.7	33	50	.6	71	.5	17
0	0	.4	0	.1	4.1	21	27	.3	53	.3	10
.1	.1	1.2	.1	.2	19.2	96	23	.9	184	.6	17
0	0	.7	.1	.1	11.8	55	17	.4	115	.3	9
.1	.1	1.4	.1	.6	10.4	52	22	1	224	.9	13
0	0	.6	.1	.3	6	27	16	.5	129	.4	7
0	0	.7	.1	.2	8	18	30	.6	54	.7	19
0	0	.2	0	.1	4.1	14	18	.4	38	.3	10
.1	0	.7	.1	.1	11.3	37	16	.5	197	.5	12
0	0	.5	0	.1	6.3	15	11	.4	109	.2	6
.1	.1	1.2	.2	.3	8.9	531	41	1.2	271	.8	30
0	.1	1.2	.1	.3	7.7	28	27	.7	202	.5	16
0	0	.7	.1	.2	4.6	26	15	.4	120	.3	9
0	.5	2.5	.2	17.5	68.1	27	20	3.9	189	.8	26

	Calories (kcal)	Protein (gm)	Carbohydrates (gm)	Fat (gm)	Percent Saturated Fat	Cholesterol (mg)	Dietary Fiber (gm)	Vitamin A (RE)	Vitamin C (mg)
Veg and liver, st - 1 jar (128gm)	50	2.8	8.8	.6	-	-	-	940.8	2.3
Veg and turkey, jr - 1 jar (213gm)	101	3.6	16.4	2.7	-	-	-	244.9	2.3
Veg and turkey, st - 1 jar (128gm)	54	2.1	8.4	1.5	-	-	-	143.4	1.4
Veg and turkey, tdl - 1 jar (177gm)	141	8.5	14.2	6.1	-	-	-	476.1	6.1
Veg and dumplings and beef, jr - 1 jar (213gm)	103	4.4	17	1.7	-	-	-	189.6	1.7
Veg and dumplings and beef, st - 1 jar (128gm)	61	2.6	9.8	1.2	-	-	-	71.7	1
Veg and noodles and turkey, jr - 1 jar (213gm)	110	3.9	16.1	3.2	-	-	-	283.3	1.6
Veg and noodles and turkey, st - 1 jar (128gm)	56	1.5	8.7	1.6	-	-	-	170.2	1
Egg yolks, st - 1 jar (94gm)	191	9.4	.9	16.3	29.9	738.8	-	353	1.3

Dinners, High Meat

Beef and all veg, st - 1 jar (128gm)	96	7.3	5.3	5.3	-	-	-	140.8	2.5
Beef and veg, jr - 1 jar (128gm)	108	8.1	6.7	5.9	-	-	-	125.4	2.4
Chicken and veg, jr - 1 jar (128gm)	117	9	5.4	7	-	-	-	167.7	1.4
Chicken and veg, st - 1 jar (128gm)	100	8	7.6	4.6	-	-	-	106.2	.9
Cottage cheese w/pineapple, st - 1 jar (135gm)	157	8.5	25.4	3	-	-	-	10	1.9
Ham and veg, jr - 1 jar (128gm)	98	8.2	7.9	4.2	34.3	22.6	-	85.8	2.4
Ham and veg, st - 1 jar (128gm)	97	8	7.1	4.4	34.3	-	-	52.5	2.3
Turkey and veg, jr - 1 jar (128gm)	115	7.6	7.5	6.4	-	-	-	142.1	1.7
Turkey and veg, st - 1 jar (128gm)	111	7.2	7.7	6.1	-	-	-	119	2
Veal and veg, jr - 1 jar (128gm)	93	7.8	7.4	4	-	-	-	101.1	2.1
Veal and veg, st - 1 jar (128gm)	89	7.6	7.8	3.4	-	-	-	96	2.4

Fruit

Apple and blueberry, jr - 1 jar (220gm)	137	.4	36.5	.4	-	-	-	8.8	30.6
Apple and blueberry, st - 1 jar (135gm)	82	.3	22	.3	-	-	-	2.7	37.5
Apple and raspberry, jr - 1 jar (220gm)	127	.4	34.1	.4	-	-	-	7	63.6

Thiamin (mg)	Riboflavin (mg)	Niacin (mg)	Vitamin B$_6$ (mg)	Vitamin B$_{12}$ (mcg)	Folacin (mcg)	Sodium (mg)	Calcium (mg)	Iron (mg)	Potassium (mg)	Zinc (mg)	Magnesium (mg)
0	.3	1.5	.1	10.5	36.7	24	9	2.8	120	.5	15
0	0	.5	.1	.2	6.2	36	27	.7	53	.5	19
0	0	.4	0	.1	3.3	17	21	.3	56	.3	10
0	.2	1	.1	.8	5.3	591	82	1.1	294	.6	29
.1	.1	1	.1	.2	15.7	110	30	1	100	.7	14
.1	.1	.7	.1	.1	9.2	62	18	.5	59	.5	8
.1	.1	.6	0	.3	6	37	67	.6	156	.6	20
0	.1	.3	0	.1	3.1	27	41	.3	81	.3	10
.1	.3	0	.1	1.4	86.6	37	72	2.6	73	1.8	6
0	.1	1.7	.1	.6	7.3	46	15	.9	179	1.7	10
0	.1	1.8	.1	.8	8.3	42	15	1	191	1.8	10
0	.1	1.3	.1	.2	1.5	33	56	.9	79	1.3	9
0	.1	1.3	.1	.2	1.4	35	66	1.3	76	1.2	9
.1	.2	.1	.1	.3	5.4	201	88	.1	128	.4	9
.1	.1	1.5	.1	.4	8.3	28	12	.8	208	1.4	12
.1	.1	1.8	.1	.3	8.1	29	14	.8	198	1.3	11
0	.1	1	.1	.6	12.7	56	91	1	137	1.2	10
0	.1	1.3	0	.6	12.3	38	80	.9	153	1.3	10
0	.1	2	.1	.6	7.7	32	14	1.1	201	1.4	12
0	.1	2.1	.1	.6	7.7	30	12	.8	196	1.3	10
0	.1	.2	.1	0	7.8	28	10	.9	143	.1	7
0	0	.2	.1	0	4.7	2	5	.3	93	0	4
0	.1	.2	.1	0	7.3	4	11	.5	158	.1	9

	Calories (kcal)	Protein (gm)	Carbohydrates (gm)	Fat (gm)	Percent Saturated Fat	Cholesterol (mg)	Dietary Fiber (gm)	Vitamin A (RE)	Vitamin C (mg)
Apple and raspberry, st - 1 jar (135gm)	79	.3	21.2	.2	-	-	-	3	36.2
Applesauce and apricots, jr - 1 jar (220gm)	104	.5	27.3	.5	-	-	-	74.8	39.3
Applesauce and apricots, st - 1 jar (135gm)	60	.3	15.7	.3	-	-	-	52.6	25.5
Applesauce and cherries, jr - 1 jar (220gm)	106	.6	28.9	0	-	-	-	9	51
Applesauce and cherries, st - 1 jar (135gm)	65	.4	17.7	0	-	-	-	5	45.3
Applesauce and pineapple, jr - 1 jar (213gm)	83	.2	22.3	.2	-	-	-	4.3	57.1
Applesauce and pineapple, st - 1 jar (128gm)	48	.1	12.9	.1	-	-	-	2.6	36
Applesauce, jr - 1 jar (213gm)	79	.1	21.9	0	-	-	-	2	80.5
Applesauce, st - 1 jar (128gm)	53	.2	14	.2	-	-	-	2	49
Apricot w/tapioca, jr - 1 jar (220gm)	139	.6	38	0	-	-	-	159	39.3
Apricot w/tapioca, st - 1 jar (135gm)	80	.4	22	0	-	-	-	98	29.1
Bananas and pineapple, jr - 1 jar (220gm)	143	.5	39.3	0	-	-	-	9	42.3
Bananas and pineapple, st - 1 jar (135gm)	91	.3	24.8	.1	-	-	-	5	28.6
Bananas, jr - 1 jar (220gm)	147	.8	39.1	.4	-	-	-	10	56.5
Bananas, st - 1 jar (135gm)	77	.5	20.6	.1	-	-	-	6	22.6
Guava and papaya w/tapioca, st - 1 jar (128gm)	80	.3	21.8	.1	-	-	-	23	103.6
Guava w/tapioca, st - 1 jar (128gm)	86	.4	23.4	0	-	-	-	38.4	96.5
Mango w/tapioca, st - 1 jar (135gm)	109	.4	29.2	.3	-	-	-	90.4	167.9
Papaya and applesauce w/tapioca, st - 1 jar (128gm)	89	.3	24.2	.1	-	-	-	10.2	144.8
Peaches, jr - 1 jar (220gm)	157	1.2	41.6	.4	-	-	-	39	41.5
Peaches, st - 1 jar (135gm)	96	.7	25.5	.2	-	-	-	22	42.4
Pears and pineapple, jr - 1 jar (213gm)	93	.6	24.4	.4	-	-	-	7	35.7
Pears and pineapple, st - 1 jar (128gm)	52	.4	13.9	.1	-	-	-	4	35.2
Pears, jr - 1 jar (213gm)	93	.6	24.7	.2	-	-	-	7	46.9
Pears, st - 1 jar (128gm)	53	.4	13.9	.2	-	-	-	4	31.4
Plums w/tapioca, st - 1 jar (135gm))	96	.2	26.6	0	-	-	-	13.5	1.4
Plums w/tapioca, jr - 1 jar (220gm)	163	.3	45	0	-	-	-	19.8	1.7
Prunes w/tapioca, jr - 1 jar (220gm)	155	1.3	41.2	.2	-	-	-	90	1.8

Thiamin (mg)	Riboflavin (mg)	Niacin (mg)	Vitamin B_6 (mg)	Vitamin B_{12} (mcg)	Folacin (mcg)	Sodium (mg)	Calcium (mg)	Iron (mg)	Potassium (mg)	Zinc (mg)	Magnesium (mg)
0	0	.1	0	0	4.6	3	7	.3	108	0	5
0	.1	.3	.1	0	3	6	13	.6	240	.1	8
0	0	.2	0	0	1.8	4	8	.3	162	.1	5
0	.1	.2	.1	0	.8	6	20	.9	214	.1	9
0	.1	.1	.1	0	.5	3	14	.5	130	0	5
0	.1	.2	.1	0	4.2	4	8	.2	162	.1	7
0	0	.1	.1	0	2.4	3	5	.1	100	0	4
0	.1	.1	.1	0	3.7	5	10	.5	164	.1	6
0	0	.1	0	0	2.4	3	5	.3	91	0	4
0	0	.4	.1	0	3.6	14	18	.6	274	.1	9
0	0	.3	0	0	2	11	12	.4	163	.1	5
0	0	.4	.2	0	11.9	13	15	.5	149	.1	14
0	0	.2	.1	0	7.4	10	9	.2	105	0	8
0	0	.5	.3	0	14	21	17	.7	237	.2	25
0	0	.2	.2	0	7.4	12	6	.3	118	.1	14
0	0	.3	0	0	2.6	5	9	.3	95	.1	6
0	.1	.5	.1	0	2.6	2	9	.3	94	.1	3
0	0	.3	.2	0	2.7	6	5	.1	80	.1	5
0	0	.1	0	0	2.6	6	9	.6	101	0	7
0	.1	1.4	0	0	8.5	10	11	.6	342	.1	12
0	0	.8	0	0	5.3	8	8	.3	219	.1	8
.1	0	.4	0	0	6.2	2	21	.4	251	.3	16
0	0	.3	0	0	3.6	5	13	.3	148	.1	9
0	.1	.4	0	0	8.1	4	18	.5	246	.2	19
0	0	.2	0	0	4.6	3	11	.3	166	.1	10
0	0	.3	0	0	1.2	8	8	.3	115	.1	5
0	.1	.5	.1	0	2.1	18	12	.5	182	.2	9
0	.2	1.2	.2	0	.5	5	33	.7	357	.2	21

	Calories (kcal)	Protein (gm)	Carbohydrates (gm)	Fat (gm)	Percent Saturated Fat	Cholesterol (mg)	Dietary Fiber (gm)	Vitamin A (RE)	Vitamin C (mg)
Prunes w/tapioca, st - 1 jar (135gm)	94	.8	25	.1	-	-	-	61	1.1

Juices

	Calories (kcal)	Protein (gm)	Carbohydrates (gm)	Fat (gm)	Percent Saturated Fat	Cholesterol (mg)	Dietary Fiber (gm)	Vitamin A (RE)	Vitamin C (mg)
Apple - 1 jar (130gm)	61	0	15.2	.1	-	-	-	2	75.3
Apple and cherry - 1 jar (130gm)	53	.2	12.9	.3	-	-	-	1	75.8
Apple and grape - 1 jar (130gm)	60	.1	14.8	.2	-	-	-	1	69.6
Apple and peach - 1 jar (130gm)	55	.2	13.6	.1	-	-	-	8	76
Apple and plum - 1 jar (130gm)	63	.1	16	0	-	-	-	5.2	75.6
Apple and prune - 1 jar (130gm)	94	.3	23.4	.2	-	-	-	3	87.8
Mixed fruit - 1 jar (130gm)	61	.2	15.1	.1	-	-	-	5	82.6
Orange - 1 jar (130gm)	58	.8	13.3	.3	-	-	-	7	81.2
Orange and apple - 1 jar (130gm)	56	.5	13.2	.3	-	-	-	9.1	100
Orange and apple and banana - 1 jar (130gm)	61	.5	15	.1	-	-	-	4	41.8
Orange and apricot - 1 jar (130gm)	60	1	14.2	.1	-	-	-	28	111.7
Orange and banana - 1 jar (130gm)	65	.9	15.4	.1	-	-	-	6	44.2
Orange and pineapple - 1 jar (130gm)	63	.7	15.2	.1	-	-	-	4	69.4
Prune and orange - 1 jar (130gm)	91	.8	21.8	.4	-	-	-	17	82.9

Meat

	Calories (kcal)	Protein (gm)	Carbohydrates (gm)	Fat (gm)	Percent Saturated Fat	Cholesterol (mg)	Dietary Fiber (gm)	Vitamin A (RE)	Vitamin C (mg)
Beef heart, st - 1 jar (99gm)	93	12.6	0	4.4	46.8	-	-	37	2.1
Beef, jr - 1 jar (99gm)	105	14.3	0	4.9	52.4	-	-	31	1.8
Beef, st - 1 jar (99gm)	106	13.5	0	5.3	48.1	-	-	55	2.1
Chicken sticks, jr - 1 jar (71gm)	134	10.4	1	10.2	-	-	-	678	1.2
Chicken, jr - 1 jar (99gm)	148	14.6	0	9.5	25.7	-	-	55	1.5
Chicken, st - 1 jar (99gm)	128	13.6	.1	7.8	25.8	-	-	40	1.6
Ham, jr - 1 jar (99gm)	123	14.9	0	6.6	33.5	-	-	9	2.1
Ham, st - 1 jar (99gm)	110	13.7	0	5.7	33.7	-	-	11	2.1
Lamb, jr - 1 jar (99gm)	111	15	0	5.2	48.7	-	-	8	1.7
Lamb, st - 1 jar (99gm)	102	13.9	.1	4.7	48.7	-	-	25	1.2
Liver, st - 1 jar (99gm)	100	14.2	1.4	3.7	36.8	181.5	-	11337	19.1
Meat sticks, jr - 1 jar (71gm)	130	9.5	.8	10.4	39.7	-	-	15	1.7
Pork, st - 1 jar (99gm)	123	13.8	0	7.1	33.4	-	-	11	1.8
Turkey sticks, jr - 1 jar (71gm)	129	9.7	1	10.1	-	-	-	49	1
Turkey, jr - 1 jar (99gm)	128	15.2	0	7	32.7	-	-	169	2.4

Thiamin (mg)	Riboflavin (mg)	Niacin (mg)	Vitamin B$_6$ (mg)	Vitamin B$_{12}$ (mcg)	Folacin (mcg)	Sodium (mg)	Calcium (mg)	Iron (mg)	Potassium (mg)	Zinc (mg)	Magnesium (mg)
0	.1	.7	.1	0	.3	6	20	.5	238	.1	14
0	0	.1	0	0	.1	4	6	.7	118	0	4
0	0	.1	0	0	.4	4	7	.9	127	0	4
0	0	.1	0	0	.4	4	7	.5	118	8	4
0	0	.3	0	0	1.7	1	4	.7	126	0	4
0	0	.3	0	0	.3	1	6	.8	131	0	4
0	0	.4	0	0	.1	7	12	1.2	192	.1	9
0	0	.2	.1	0	8.7	5	10	.4	131	0	7
.1	0	.3	.1	0	34.3	2	16	.2	240	.1	11
0	0	.2	0	0	15.9	4	13	.3	179	0	6
.1	0	.3	.1	0	12.6	6	6	.4	174	0	7
.1	0	.3	.1	0	25.9	7	8	.5	259	0	9
.1	.1	.2	.1	0	31.7	4	22	.1	261	.1	18
.1	0	.3	.1	0	24.2	2	10	.6	183	.1	12
.1	.2	.5	.1	0	17	2	16	1.1	236	.1	10
0	.4	3.8	.1	6.8	5	62	4	2	198	1.8	12
0	.2	3.3	.1	1.5	5.7	65	8	1.6	189	2	9
0	.1	2.8	.1	1.4	5.4	80	7	1.5	218	2.4	17
0	.1	1.4	.1	.3	7.9	340	52	1.1	75	.7	10
0	.2	3.4	.2	.4	11	50	54	1	121	1	11
0	.1	3.2	.2	.4	10.3	47	63	1.4	139	1.2	13
.1	.2	2.8	.2	.1	2.1	66	5	1	208	1.7	11
.1	.2	2.6	.2	.1	1.9	40	6	1	202	2.2	13
0	.2	3.2	.2	2.3	2	73	7	1.6	209	2.6	10
0	.2	2.9	.1	2.2	2.3	62	7	1.5	203	2.7	13
0	1.8	8.2	.3	2.1	334	73	3	5.2	224	2.9	13
0	.1	1.1	.1	.2	6.3	388	24	1	81	1.3	8
.1	.2	2.2	.2	1	1.9	42	5	1	221	2.2	10
0	.1	1.2	.1	.7	8	343	51	.9	65	1.3	11
0	.2	3.4	.2	1.1	12	72	28	1.3	178	1.8	11

	Calories (kcal)	Protein (gm)	Carbohydrates (gm)	Fat (gm)	Percent Saturated Fat	Cholesterol (mg)	Dietary Fiber (gm)	Vitamin A (RE)	Vitamin C (mg)
Turkey, st - 1 jar (99gm)	113	14.1	.1	5.8	32.6	-	-	166	2.2
Veal, jr - 1 jar (99gm)	109	15.1	0	4.9	48.4	-	-	15	2.1
Veal, st - 1 jar (99gm)	100	13.4	0	4.7	48.3	-	-	14	2.3

Vegetables

	Calories (kcal)	Protein (gm)	Carbohydrates (gm)	Fat (gm)	Percent Saturated Fat	Cholesterol (mg)	Dietary Fiber (gm)	Vitamin A (RE)	Vitamin C (mg)
Beets, st - 1 jar (128gm)	43	1.7	9.8	.1	-	-	-	4	3.1
Carrots, buttered, jr - 1 jar (213gm)	70	1.7	14.3	1.2	-	-	-	2095.9	16.2
Carrots, buttered, st - 1 jar (128gm)	46	1.1	9.4	.8	-	-	-	1386.2	11.7
Carrots, jr - 1 jar (213gm)	67	1.7	15.4	.4	-	-	-	2515.5	11.8
Carrots, st - 1 jar (128gm)	34	1	7.7	.2	-	-	-	1466.9	7.3
Corn, creamed, jr - 1 jar (213gm)	138	3.1	34.7	.8	-	-	-	16	4.7
Corn, creamed, st - 1 jar (128gm)	73	1.8	18.1	.5	-	-	-	10	2.7
Garden veg, st - 1 jar (128gm)	48	2.9	8.7	.3	-	-	-	777	7.3
Green beans, buttered, jr - 1 jar (206gm)	67	2.7	12.5	1.8	-	-	-	79	17.7
Green beans, buttered, st - 1 jar (128gm)	42	1.6	8.5	1	-	-	-	58	10.6
Green beans, creamed, st - 1 jar (213gm)	68	2.1	15.3	.9	-	-	-	32	5.8
Green beans, jr - 1 jar (206gm)	51	2.5	11.8	.3	-	-	-	89	17.2
Green beans, st - 1 jar (128gm)	32	1.7	7.6	.1	-	-	-	57.6	6.6
Mix veg, jr - 1 jar (213gm)	88	3.1	17.4	.8	-	-	-	894.6	5.3
Mix veg, st - 1 jar (128gm)	52	1.6	10.2	.6	-	-	-	510.7	2.1
Peas, buttered, jr - 1 jar (206gm)	123	7.3	23.3	2.6	-	-	-	84	26.2
Peas, buttered, st - 1 jar (128gm)	72	4.7	13.6	1.4	-	-	-	42	15.3
Peas, creamed, st - 1 jar (128gm)	68	2.8	11.4	2.4	-	-	-	11	2.1
Peas, st - 1 jar (128gm)	52	4.5	10.4	.4	-	-	-	71.7	8.8
Spinach, creamed, jr - 1 jar (213gm)	90	6.4	13.7	3	-	-	-	783	7.7
Spinach, creamed, st - 1 jar (128gm)	48	3.2	7.3	1.7	-	-	-	533.8	11.1
Squash, buttered, jr - 1 jar (213gm)	63	1.5	13.7	1.3	-	-	-	325.9	16.1
Squash, buttered, st - 1 jar (128gm)	37	.8	8.8	.4	-	-	-	212.5	9.8
Squash, jr - 1 jar (213gm)	51	1.8	12	.4	-	-	-	428.1	16.5
Squash, st - 1 jar (128gm)	30	1.1	7.2	.2	-	-	-	258.6	9.8
Sweet potatoes, buttered, jr - 1 jar (220gm)	126	1.8	26.8	1.6	-	-	-	1328.8	20.5

Thiamin (mg)	Riboflavin (mg)	Niacin (mg)	Vitamin B$_6$ (mg)	Vitamin B$_{12}$ (mcg)	Folacin (mcg)	Sodium (mg)	Calcium (mg)	Iron (mg)	Potassium (mg)	Zinc (mg)	Magnesium (mg)
0	.2	3.6	.2	1	11.2	54	23	1.2	229	1.8	14
0	.2	3.8	.1	1.3	6.6	68	6	1.2	234	2.5	11
0	.2	3.5	.1	1.3	5.8	64	7	1.3	214	2	12
0	.1	.2	0	0	39.4	106	18	.4	233	.2	18
0	.1	1.1	-	-	18.4	34	76	.7	310	-	-
0	.1	.8	-	-	12	24	45	.4	292	-	-
.1	.1	1.1	.2	0	36.8	104	49	.8	429	.4	23
0	.1	.6	.1	0	19.1	48	29	.5	251	.2	12
0	.1	1.1	.1	.1	27.1	111	39	.6	172	.5	17
0	.1	.7	.1	0	14.5	55	25	.4	115	.2	11
.1	.1	1	.1	0	51.5	45	36	1.1	215	.3	27
0	.2	.7	-	-	56.3	4	143	2.4	351	-	-
0	.1	.4	-	-	36.5	4	82	1.6	205	-	-
0	.1	.5	0	.1	84.6	26	68	.6	139	.3	16
0	.2	.7	.1	0	67.4	3	133	2.2	263	.4	46
0	.1	.4	0	0	44.3	2	49	1	202	.3	30
.1	.1	1.4	.2	0	8.7	77	24	.9	362	.6	23
0	0	.4	.1	0	5	16	17	.4	163	.2	13
.1	.2	2.8	-	-	74.5	11	93	2.1	240	-	-
.1	.1	1.8	-	-	44.4	10	49	1.4	124	-	-
.1	.1	1	.1	.1	29.1	18	16	.7	113	.5	20
.1	.1	1.3	.1	0	33.2	5	26	1.2	144	.4	19
0	.2	.6	.1	.1	146.5	117	240	3	471	.7	134
0	.1	.3	.1	.1	77.8	62	113	.8	244	.4	71
0	.1	.7	-	-	25	3	65	.9	288	-	-
0	.1	.5	-	-	15.1	2	42	.5	163	-	-
0	.1	.8	.1	0	32.8	3	50	.7	393	.2	25
0	.1	.5	.1	0	19.7	3	30	.4	229	.2	16
0	.1	.7	-	-	29.4	17	61	.9	474	-	-

	Calories (kcal)	Protein (gm)	Carbohydrates (gm)	Fat (gm)	Percent Saturated Fat	Cholesterol (mg)	Dietary Fiber (gm)	Vitamin A (RE)	Vitamin C (mg)
Sweet potatoes, buttered, st - 1 jar (135gm)	76	1.3	15.9	1	-	-	-	919.4	12.3
Sweet potatoes, jr - 1 jar (220gm)	133	2.4	30.7	.3	-	-	-	1460.8	21.2
Sweet potatoes, st - 1 jar (135gm)	.77	1.5	17.8	.2	-	-	-	869.4	13.4

Baked Goods

Pretzels - 1 (6gm)	24	.7	4.9	.1	-	-	-	0	.2
Teething biscuits - 1 (11gm)	43	1.2	8	.5	-	-	-	1	1
Zwieback - 1 (7gm)	30	.7	5.2	.7	-	1.5	-	.4	.4

BAKED GOODS

Bread

	Calories (kcal)	Protein (gm)	Carbohydrates (gm)	Fat (gm)	Percent Saturated Fat	Cholesterol (mg)	Dietary Fiber (gm)	Vitamin A (RE)	Vitamin C (mg)
Black - 1 slice (26gm)	64	2.4	13.8	.3	13.3	0	1.4	0	0
Bran - 1 slice (36gm)	110	3.4	18.5	2.9	27.5	16.8	1.6	6.7	3
Cheese - 1 slice (26gm)	72	2.5	12.5	1.2	37.8	1.6	.4	3.9	0
Cinnamon - 1 slice (26gm)	70	2.3	13.1	.8	23.7	.3	.4	0	0
Corn and molasses - 1 slice (32gm)	85	2.1	14.8	1.9	-	2	.5	5.7	.1
Cracked wheat - 1 slice (26gm)	68	2.3	13.5	.6	-	0	1	0	0
Egg, chalah - 1 slice (23gm)	75	1.9	10.9	2.6	18.3	28.4	.3	8.7	0
French, vienna - 1 slice (25gm)	72	2.3	13.8	.8	-	0	.4	0	0
Garlic - 1 slice (29gm)	100	2.4	14.1	3.8	20	0	.4	40.6	.1
Gluten - 1 slice (26gm)	69	6.8	8.1	1	-	5.4	.2	1.5	0
Italian, Grecian, Armenian - 1 slice (20gm)	55	1.8	11.3	.2	-	.2	.3	0	0
Low sodium - 1 slice (26gm)	70	2.2	12.8	.8	-	.3	.4	0	0
Oatmeal - 1 slice (25gm)	66	2.2	11.7	1.1	-	.7	.7	2	0
Pita - 1 small (6½″ dia) (60gm)	165	5.7	33.7	.5	-	0	1.3	0	0
Pita whole wheat - 1 small (6½″ dia) (60gm)	190	6.1	30.4	6.1	14.8	0	5.6	0	0
Potato - 1 slice (26gm)	70	2.3	13.1	.8	-	.3	.4	0	0
Pumpernickel - 1 slice (26gm)	64	2.4	13.8	.3	-	0	1.4	0	0
Raisin - 1 slice (26gm)	68	1.7	13.9	.7	-	0	1	0	0
Rye - 1 slice (26gm)	63	2.4	13.5	.3	-	0	1.1	0	0
Sour dough - 1 slice (25gm)	72	2.3	13.8	.8	-	0	.4	0	0
Sprouted wheat - 1 slice (26gm)	63	2.4	12.8	.7	-	0	2.9	0	0
Triticale - 1 slice (25gm)	61	2.4	12.5	.5	-	0	1.9	0	0
Wheat germ - 1 slice (28gm)	78	2.7	13.6	1.4	-	.4	.6	.9	.1

Thiamin (mg)	Riboflavin (mg)	Niacin (mg)	Vitamin B$_6$ (mg)	Vitamin B$_{12}$ (mcg)	Folacin (mcg)	Sodium (mg)	Calcium (mg)	Iron (mg)	Potassium (mg)	Zinc (mg)	Magnesium (mg)
0	.1	.4	-	-	17.7	11	28	.6	281	-	-
.1	.1	.8	.2	0	22.6	49	35	.9	535	.2	26
0	0	.5	.1	0	13.2	27	21	.5	355	.3	18

Thiamin (mg)	Riboflavin (mg)	Niacin (mg)	Vitamin B$_6$ (mg)	Vitamin B$_{12}$ (mcg)	Folacin (mcg)	Sodium (mg)	Calcium (mg)	Iron (mg)	Potassium (mg)	Zinc (mg)	Magnesium (mg)
0	0	.2	0	0	1.2	16	1	.2	8	0	2
0	.1	.5	0	0	2.2	40	29	.4	35	.1	4
0	0	.1	0	0	1.4	16	1	0	21	0	1

Source: USDA Revised *Handbook 8*

Thiamin (mg)	Riboflavin (mg)	Niacin (mg)	Vitamin B$_6$ (mg)	Vitamin B$_{12}$ (mcg)	Folacin (mcg)	Sodium (mg)	Calcium (mg)	Iron (mg)	Potassium (mg)	Zinc (mg)	Magnesium (mg)
.1	.1	.5	0	0	6	147.9	21.8	.8	118	.3	12.7
.2	.2	2.1	.1	.4	14.6	162.1	16.8	1.4	88.4	.6	24.6
.1	.1	.8	0	0	10.6	133.3	39	.7	27.2	.2	6.5
.1	.1	.9	0	0	10.9	131.8	31.2	.7	27.3	.2	6.5
.1	.1	.8	0	0	9.8	260.8	31.6	1	82.5	.2	10.1
.1	.1	.8	0	0	7	137.5	22.9	.7	34.8	.4	12.7
.1	.1	.7	0	.1	10.7	119.8	27.6	.7	22.4	.2	4
.1	.1	.8	0	0	7.5	145	22.5	.7	22.5	.2	5
.1	.1	.8	0	0	7.5	180.4	23.8	.7	26.8	.2	5.2
.1	.1	.8	0	0	4	23.6	7.5	.7	13.1	.1	2.5
.1	0	.7	0	0	5.2	117	16	.6	14.8	.2	4.8
.1	.1	1	0	0	10.9	9.6	31.2	.7	33.8	.1	4.2
.1	.1	.6	0	0	8.1	99.1	11.1	.7	35.9	.2	9.2
.2	.2	2.5	.1	0	34.5	205.3	49.2	2.1	68.3	.4	13.2
.2	.1	2.1	.2	0	42.5	83	18.8	2	181.3	1.1	62.3
.1	.1	.9	0	0	10.9	131.8	31.2	.7	27.3	.2	6.5
.1	.1	.5	0	0	6	147.9	21.8	.8	118	.3	12.7
.1	.1	.6	0	0	8.1	94.9	27.3	.8	60.6	.2	6
.1	.1	.7	0	0	10.1	144.8	19.5	.7	37.7	.3	8.8
.1	.1	.8	0	0	7.5	145	22.5	.7	22.5	.2	5
.1	0	.7	0	0	14.3	137.8	21.8	.8	66.6	.5	25.2
.1	0	.7	0	0	12.1	135.5	21.8	.7	52.3	.4	17.1
.1	.1	.9	0	0	14.5	200.1	8.4	.9	46.4	.5	12.1

	Calories (kcal)	Protein (gm)	Carbohydrates (gm)	Fat (gm)	Percent Saturated Fat	Cholesterol (mg)	Dietary Fiber (gm)	Vitamin A (RE)	Vitamin C (mg)
White - 1 slice (26gm)	70	2.3	13.1	.8	-	.3	.4	0	0
Whole wheat - 1 slice (26gm)	63	2.7	12.4	.8	-	0	2.9	0	0
Breadsticks - 1 (10gm)	43	1.3	6.4	1.3	-	0	.2	0	0
Bread, stuffing - 1 cup, moist type (200gm)	599	14.3	79.1	26	20.1	1.1	1.7	293.7	0
Croutons - 8 cubes (2gm)	6	.2	1.2	.1	-	0	0	0	0

Biscuits

	Calories (kcal)	Protein (gm)	Carbohydrates (gm)	Fat (gm)	Percent Saturated Fat	Cholesterol (mg)	Dietary Fiber (gm)	Vitamin A (RE)	Vitamin C (mg)
Baking pwdr/btrmilk-1 (2" dia) (30gm)	101	2.2	16.4	2.9	23.4	.4	.4	6.7	.1
Baking pwdr/btrmlk from mix - 1 (2" dia) (30gm)	102	2.2	16.4	2.9	23.4	.4	.4	6.7	.1

Muffins

	Calories (kcal)	Protein (gm)	Carbohydrates (gm)	Fat (gm)	Percent Saturated Fat	Cholesterol (mg)	Dietary Fiber (gm)	Vitamin A (RE)	Vitamin C (mg)
Bran w/raisin and nuts - 1 (2⅝" dia) (50gm)	126	4.7	19.6	5.1	29.7	47.6	5.2	19	.1
Oatmeal - 1 (2⅝" dia) (47gm)	112	3.2	17.4	3.2	32.1	23	.7	11.7	.1
English - 1 (58gm)	132	4.6	25.3	1.2	-	0	1.2	0	0
English, cracked wheat - 1 (58gm)	158	5.2	31.2	1.3	-	0	2.3	0	0
English, w/raisins - 1 (61gm)	146	4.5	29.5	1.1	-	0	1.6	.1	.2
English, whole wheat - 1 (58gm)	130	5.4	25.8	1.6	-	0	4.9	0	0
Fruit and/or nuts - 1 (2⅝" dia) (58gm)	165	4.2	25.3	5.2	30.3	49.2	.7	20	.3

Bagels

	Calories (kcal)	Protein (gm)	Carbohydrates (gm)	Fat (gm)	Percent Saturated Fat	Cholesterol (mg)	Dietary Fiber (gm)	Vitamin A (RE)	Vitamin C (mg)
Plain - 1 (3" dia) (55gm)	164	5.5	32.8	.8	-	19.4	1.1	5.5	0
Pumpernickel - 1 med (3" dia) (55gm)	152	5	31.5	.5	-	0	1.9	.1	0
Whole wheat - 1 (3" dia) (55gm)	152	5.5	31.5	.6	-	0	2.4	0	0

Rolls

	Calories (kcal)	Protein (gm)	Carbohydrates (gm)	Fat (gm)	Percent Saturated Fat	Cholesterol (mg)	Dietary Fiber (gm)	Vitamin A (RE)	Vitamin C (mg)
Cinnamon bun - 1 (55gm)	174	4.7	27.1	5	-	18.1	.9	11.5	0
Cracked wheat - 1 (36gm)	95	3.1	18.8	.8	-	0	1.4	0	0
Diet - 1 (28gm)	81	2.5	15.5	.8	-	0	.4	0	0
Croissants - 1 (56gm)	205	4.5	22.4	10.8	22	39	.7	139.5	.1
French or Vienna - 1 (45gm)	130	4.1	24.9	1.3	-	0	.7	0	0
Hoagie, submarine, sandwich - 1 (100gm)	290	9.1	55.4	3	-	0	1.6	0	0
Rye - 1 (36gm)	87	3.3	18.8	.4	-	0	1.5	0	0
Sour dough - 1 (45gm)	130	4.1	24.9	1.3	-	0	.7	0	0
Sweet - 1 (55gm)	174	4.7	27.1	5	27.6	18.1	.9	11.5	0
Sweet w/fruit and nuts, frosted - 1 (55gm)	174	3.1	33	3.8	17.6	.1	1.7	17.9	.1
Sweet w/fruit, frosted - 1 (55gm)	167	3	33.9	2.6	21.9	.1	1.6	18.3	0

Thiamin (mg)	Riboflavin (mg)	Niacin (mg)	Vitamin B_6 (mg)	Vitamin B_{12} (mcg)	Folacin (mcg)	Sodium (mg)	Calcium (mg)	Iron (mg)	Potassium (mg)	Zinc (mg)	Magnesium (mg)
.1	.1	.9	0	0	10.9	131.8	31.2	.7	27.3	.2	6.5
.1	0	.7	0	0	15.1	137	25.7	.8	71	.5	26.8
.1	.1	.6	0	0	1.1	58.3	8.2	.4	21.6	.1	4.7
.3	.3	3.9	0	0	39.2	1709.8	145.9	3.5	199.1	.8	29.1
0	0	.1	0	0	1	11.8	2.8	.1	2.4	0	.6
.1	.1	.9	0	0	1.9	305.8	19.8	.8	36.7	.2	7
.1	.1	.9	0	0	1.9	305.8	19.8	.8	36.7	.2	7
.1	.1	2.9	.1	.2	16.7	178	116.4	2.3	242.1	1.3	83.8
.1	.1	.9	0	.1	4.8	161.4	69.5	.9	56.8	.3	9.7
.2	.2	2.2	.1	0	50.2	159.2	93.8	1.8	73	.4	12.4
.2	.2	1.9	0	0	16.2	317.3	52.8	1.7	80.4	.8	29.4
.2	.2	2.1	.1	0	47.1	149.8	115.1	1.8	118.2	.4	14
.2	.1	2.1	.2	0	61.5	170.9	64.2	1.9	173.4	1	54.5
.1	.1	1.2	0	.1	7.9	311.3	72.6	1.2	69	.4	9.8
.2	.2	2.2	.1	0	28.2	459.5	23.1	2	62.4	.4	12.7
.2	.2	1.9	.1	0	33.3	539.5	13.5	1.9	72.9	.4	21.3
.2	.2	2.3	.1	0	33.9	524.8	14.9	2	98.5	.6	28.5
.2	.2	1.2	.1	0	17	213.9	57.7	1.2	68.2	.3	9.9
.1	.1	1.2	0	0	9.7	190.4	31.7	1	48.2	.5	17.6
.1	.1	.9	0	0	8.4	162.4	25.2	.8	25.2	.2	5.6
.1	.2	1.4	0	.1	17.4	270.3	28.4	1.4	67.6	.4	9.8
.2	.1	1.5	0	0	13.5	261	40.5	1.3	40.5	.3	9
.4	.2	3.3	0	0	30	580	90	2.8	90	.6	20
.1	.1	1	0	0	14	200.5	27	1	52.2	.4	12.2
.2	.1	1.5	0	0	13.5	261	40.5	1.3	40.5	.3	9
.2	.2	1.2	.1	0	17	213.9	57.7	1.2	68.2	.3	9.9
.1	.3	1.7	0	0	14	183.9	46.2	1.3	112.2	.3	13
.1	.3	1.7	0	0	13.2	190.7	46	1.3	105.9	.3	9.9

	Calories (kcal)	Protein (gm)	Carbohydrates (gm)	Fat (gm)	Percent Saturated Fat	Cholesterol (mg)	Dietary Fiber (gm)	Vitamin A (RE)	Vitamin C (mg)
Sweet, cinnamon bun, frosted - 1 (55gm)	185	3.6	30.9	5.2	25.7	14.1	.7	27.2	0
Sweet, w/fruit - 1 (55gm)	151	3.8	31	1.6	23.4	0	2.1	0	0
White, hard - 1 (50gm)	156	4.9	29.8	1.6	21.9	0	.8	0	0
White, soft, hamburger, frankfurter - 1 (43gm)	128	3.5	22.8	2.4	24.5	0	.7	0	0
Whole wheat - 1 (36gm)	93	3.6	18.8	1	21.8	0	2.1	0	0

Scones

Scones - 1 (42gm)	151	3.8	18.4	6.7	31.9	64.3	.5	81.5	.1
Scones, whole wheat - 1 (42gm)	145	4.5	17.7	6.8	31.2	63.1	2.8	79.9	0

Doughnuts

Cake type - 1 (42gm)	164	1.9	21.6	7.8	24.9	16.4	.5	4.2	0
Cake type, choc covered - 1 (53gm)	205	2.3	29	9.3	29.3	16.6	.8	10.8	0
Cake type, choc covered w/peanuts - 1 (53gm)	190	2.6	26.5	8.6	29.3	16.6	.7	11.2	.1
Raised or yeast - 1 (50gm)	202	2.7	22.3	11.4	37.6	17.5	.5	1	0
Raised or yeast, choc - 1 (50gm)	203	3.4	19.2	13.2	45.7	19.5	1.4	1.5	0
Choc w/choc icing - 1 (53gm)	207	2.4	28.6	9.9	32	16.1	1.1	10.5	0
Choc creme filled - 1 (65gm)	239	3.8	22.9	14.9	44.6	23.6	.6	4.9	.1
Jelly - 1 (65gm)	253	3.4	28.3	14.3	45.2	21.9	.6	1.7	.1
Custard filled - 1 (65gm)	239	3.8	22.6	15	45.5	23.8	.6	4.3	.1
Oriental - 1 (18gm)	75	1.2	9.6	3.6	26.2	17.1	.2	5.5	0
Whole wheat - 1 (42gm)	171	2.7	21.6	8.6	25	17.5	1.3	6.2	.1

Cake

Angel food - 1/12 of 10" dia (57gm)	146	3.2	33.7	.1	-	0	.1	0	0
Angel food w/icing - 1/12 of 10" dia (77gm)	210	3.4	49.8	.1	-	0	.1	0	0
Angel food, choc - 1/12 of 10" dia (57gm)	146	3.4	33.5	.3	-	0	.9	0	0
Applesauce - 1/12 of 10" dia (87gm)	314	3.1	52.1	11.5	25.1	28.9	2	8.7	.9
Applesauce w/icing - 1/12 of 10" dia (108gm)	399	2.9	69.9	13.3	24.2	26.5	1.8	47.6	.9
Banana - 1/12 of 10" dia (87gm)	247	3.1	43.3	7.5	21.9	38.2	1.2	99.1	3.4
Banana, w/icing - 1/12 of 10" dia (108gm)	310	3.5	58.4	7.8	21.9	39.9	1.2	103.5	3.5
Boston cream pie - 1/12 of 8" dia (69gm)	207	3.8	34.5	6.2	26.8	64.3	.4	78.3	.2
Carrot - 1/12 of 10" dia (111gm)	478	5.2	53.2	28.1	13.5	91.8	1.6	642.7	1.8

Thiamin (mg)	Riboflavin (mg)	Niacin (mg)	Vitamin B$_6$ (mg)	Vitamin B$_{12}$ (mcg)	Folacin (mcg)	Sodium (mg)	Calcium (mg)	Iron (mg)	Potassium (mg)	Zinc (mg)	Magnesium (mg)
.2	.1	.9	0	0	13.2	192.8	46	.9	54.7	.2	7.8
.2	.3	2.2	0	0	17	211.2	57.7	1.7	134.7	.4	12.6
.2	.1	1.7	0	0	18	312.5	50	1.4	48.5	.6	12
.2	.1	1.4	0	0	16.3	217.6	43	1.2	40.8	.3	9
.1	0	1.1	0	0	19.8	203	38.2	.9	105.1	.6	34.9
.1	.1	1	0	.2	7.9	247.5	63.8	1.2	47.9	.3	7.1
.1	.1	.9	.1	.1	12.7	174.6	58	1.2	182.2	.7	33.4
.1	.1	.7	0	0	3.4	210.4	16.8	.8	37.8	.2	9.7
.1	.1	.7	0	0	3.7	213.5	23.1	.9	59.8	.3	16.3
.1	.1	.7	0	.1	3.7	196.2	22.4	.9	62	.3	15.4
.1	.1	.8	0	.1	11	100	16	.9	34.5	.5	11
.1	.1	.9	0	.2	13.3	111.9	21	1.3	75.6	.7	24.7
.1	.1	.7	0	0	3.7	207.1	23.5	1	70.9	.3	21
.1	.1	1	0	.2	14.6	141.1	31.4	1.2	57.9	.7	16.4
.1	.1	1	0	.2	14	129.5	21.1	1.2	50.4	.6	14.5
.1	.1	1.1	0	.2	14.8	142.7	31	1.2	56.7	.7	15.5
0	0	.3	0	0	2.3	49.1	19.5	.4	14.8	.1	2.3
.1	.1	.8	0	.1	7.1	187.8	19.8	.9	70.8	.4	16.7
0	.1	.3	0	0	3.5	73	41.7	.3	42.7	.1	4.4
0	.1	.3	0	0	3.7	99.1	41.8	.3	46.5	.1	4.8
0	.1	.4	0	0	4	70.9	42.5	.6	70.1	.2	13.8
.1	.1	1	.1	.1	5.1	206.1	18.3	1.4	144.3	.3	11
.1	.1	.9	.1	.1	4.8	221.4	21.1	1.3	136.8	.2	10.4
.1	.1	1	.2	.1	11.9	180.5	22.7	1	190.5	.3	16.6
.1	.1	1	.3	.1	12.7	211.9	24.2	1	202.7	.3	17.6
.1	.1	.9	0	.3	11	175.1	62.5	1	66.7	.3	8
.2	.1	1.3	.1	.2	15.9	170.5	58.9	1.7	145.3	.6	19.1

	Calories (kcal)	Protein (gm)	Carbohydrates (gm)	Fat (gm)	Percent Saturated Fat	Cholesterol (mg)	Dietary Fiber (gm)	Vitamin A (RE)	Vitamin C (mg)
Carrot w/icing - 1/12 of 10" dia (134gm)	548	5.2	70.9	28.2	18.5	102.1	1.4	690.5	1.8
Cheesecake - 1/12 of 9" dia (128gm)	406	11.3	36.6	24.9	40.6	100.5	.3	301.1	.8
Cheesecake w/fruit - 1/12 of 9" dia (142gm)	384	9	46	19.3	40.6	78	.5	257	1.3
Cheesecake, choc - 1/12 of 9" dia (128gm)	500	8.3	48.4	32.2	48.1	136.4	2	340.9	.1
Cheesecake, low-cal - 1 individual cake (113gm)	241	6.8	33	10.1	51.4	22.8	.6	90	.1
Chiffon - 1/12 of 10" dia (66gm)	254	2.9	36.9	10.8	18	105.9	.4	36.5	.2
Chiffon, w/icing - 1/12 of 10" dia (92gm)	314	3.9	48.1	12.3	18.4	91	.4	72.2	2
Chiffon, choc - 1/12 of 10" dia (66gm)	226	4.1	29.9	10.8	29.3	91.5	1.1	34.3	.1
Chiffon, choc, w/icing - 1/12 of 10" dia (92gm)	325	4.8	45.8	15.3	32.6	94.9	1.8	62.6	.1
Choc, devil's food - 1/10 of 8" or 9" dia (42gm)	131	2.1	23.4	4.1	31.9	29.2	.8	8.3	0
Choc devil's food, w/icing 1/12 of 2-layer, 8" or 9" dia (109gm)	378	3.7	70.8	11.2	27.7	43.3	2.1	77	0
Choc devil's food, pudding mix - 1/10 of 8" or 9" dia (53gm)	194	2.6	26.1	9.8	24.1	55	.8	15.7	0
Choc devil's food, pudding mix w/icing - 1/12 of 2-layer, 8" or 9" dia (139gm)	524	5	82.8	21.8	23.8	92.4	2.3	95.8	0
Coffeecake - 1/12 of 9" sq (58gm)	137	2.8	22	4.2	26.4	52.1	.2	14.8	0
Cupcake, w/icing - 1 (48gm)	169	1.4	30.7	5.1	24.2	18.7	.5	33.2	0
Cupcake - 1 (33gm)	107	1.4	17.9	3.4	25.3	22.2	.2	6.3	0
Cupcake, choc 1 (33gm)	100	1.6	17.8	3.1	30.5	23.1	1.1	9.3	0
Cupcake, choc, w/icing - 1 (46gm)	157	1.5	29.5	4.6	26.9	18.3	1.2	34.6	0
Dobos torte - 1/12 of 8½" dia (123gm)	501	7.5	57.2	28.3	31.7	243	1.3	287.4	0
Fruitcake - 1/12 of 7" dia (113gm)	433	6.3	71.1	15.6	19	37.9	3.5	12.3	1.1
German choc - 1/12 of 2-layer, 8" or 9" dia (109gm)	379	5.3	43	21.6	28.3	90.2	1.3	197.7	.4
Lemon, made w/pudding - 1/10 of 8" or 9" dia (53gm)	203	2.4	26.2	10.1	21.7	55	.3	15.7	0
Marble - 1/10 of 8" or 9" dia (40gm)	134	2.1	22.5	4.6	29.7	28.6	.6	8.2	0
Marble, w/icing - 1/12 of 2-layer, 8" or 9" dia (87gm)	301	4	51.6	10.6	36.6	44.7	1.7	27.5	.1
Plum pudding - 1½ oz (42gm)	129	1.7	18.7	5.7	41.2	21,7	.9	7.1	.4
Gingerbread - 1/10 of 8" dia (69gm)	214	2.9	34.4	7.4	25.2	34.6	.5	9.9	.1

Thiamin (mg)	Riboflavin (mg)	Niacin (mg)	Vitamin B_6 (mg)	Vitamin B_{12} (mcg)	Folacin (mcg)	Sodium (mg)	Calcium (mg)	Iron (mg)	Potassium (mg)	Zinc (mg)	Magnesium (mg)
.1	.2	1.3	.1	.2	14.6	279.5	31	1.7	131.7	.5	11.3
0	.3	.6	.1	.4	15.7	531.4	69.3	1.2	156.5	.6	12.7
0	.2	.5	.1	.3	14.7	414.6	57.4	1.4	154.2	.5	11.9
.1	.2	1.1	.1	.3	14.7	405.4	72.8	2.2	183.1	.9	38.1
0	.3	1.1	.1	.3	12.6	365.7	60.3	1.8	192.5	.6	17.2
.1	.1	.8	0	.2	10	261.7	59.3	1.1	38.2	.3	5.6
.1	.1	.7	0	.2	10.6	280.9	54.3	1	57.6	.3	6.4
.1	.1	.6	0	.2	10.3	208.3	59.9	1.1	95.1	.5	21
.1	.2	.7	0	.2	11.2	255.5	69.5	1.4	136.4	.7	34.8
.1	.1	.5	.1	.1	4.9	146.1	27.5	.8	43.6	.3	15
.1	.1	.8	.1	.1	8.3	314.1	49.3	1.6	129	.6	33.4
0	.1	.4	.1	.1	6.9	237.6	28	.9	48.8	.4	15.8
.1	.1	.8	.1	.2	12.8	504.7	56.5	1.9	151.5	.8	38.7
.1	.1	.8	0	.1	6.2	187.5	16.1	.8	37	.2	4.2
.1	.1	.4	0	.1	4.4	126.1	32.8	.6	49	.2	7.3
.1	.1	.5	0	.1	4.7	99.5	34.7	.5	25.1	.1	2.9
0	0	.1	0	.1	4.9	94.8	37.4	.5	78.2	.3	13.7
0	0	.3	0	.1	3.5	116.8	33.2	.7	89	.3	15.6
.1	.2	.6	.1	.6	23.6	351.2	38.5	1.9	135.1	1	31.2
.2	.2	1.6	.1	.1	11.8	170.1	97.9	2.7	420.3	.8	47.3
.1	.2	.7	0	.2	13.5	275.3	62	1.3	139.4	.8	22.5
.1	.1	.5	0	.1	6.6	224.4	43.8	.7	39.5	.2	6
.1	.1	.6	0	.1	4.8	120.6	41.8	.8	62.5	.2	6.1
.1	.1	1	0	.2	11	198.9	78.3	1.5	145.6	.5	24.6
0	.1	.4	0	.1	3.7	56	45.3	.9	170.2	.2	12.6
.1	.1	1	.1	.1	5.4	97.4	55.9	1.9	214.4	.3	14.5

	Calories (kcal)	Protein (gm)	Carbohydrates (gm)	Fat (gm)	Percent Saturated Fat	Cholesterol (mg)	Dietary Fiber (gm)	Vitamin A (RE)	Vitamin C (mg)
Ice cream roll - ⅒ of roll (34gm)	100	1.4	14.9	4	40.3	18.3	.1	18.5	.1
Ice cream roll, choc - ⅒ of roll (34gm)	101	1.4	13.7	5	43.9	18.3	.4	18.3	.1
Jelly roll - ⅒ of roll (51gm)	148	3.3	28.5	2.5	29.6	119.9	.2	34.3	1.3
Pound - ⅒ of loaf (91gm)	351	5.7	49.5	14.7	22.4	149.8	.6	195.3	.1
Pound, choc, - ⅒ of loaf (91gm)	381	5.1	48.1	20.1	28.4	87.2	1.6	220.7	.1
Shortcake, biscuit type w/fruit - 1 (162gm)	364	6.1	57.1	13.3	24.7	.6	2.6	21.1	35.9
Shortcake, sponge type w/fruit - 1 (156gm)	296	5.7	61.8	4.1	28.9	189.5	2	55.8	37.1
Spice - ⅒ of 8″ or 9″ dia (42gm)	146	2	23.8	5	34.9	30.4	.5	8.6	0
Spice, w/icing - 1/12 of 2-layer, 8″ or 9″ dia (109gm)	374	4.3	65.1	11.4	33.9	61.5	1.1	36.1	.1
Sponge - 1/12 of 10″ dia (66gm)	193	4.8	35.7	3.6	29.6	172.2	.3	49.2	.9
Sponge, w/icing - 1/12 of 10″ dia (92gm)	281	4.5	55.3	5.2	30.9	158.1	.3	67.4	.9
Sponge, w/whpd cr and fruit - 1 (163gm)	314	5.8	58.9	7.3	45.2	186.3	1.8	84.7	34.3
Torte - 1/12 (76gm)	224	2.6	28.9	11.3	37.9	81	.9	135	2.3
Upside down (all fruits) - 1/12 of 9″ dia (121gm)	374	3.1	59.1	14.7	22.2	45.4	.9	115.4	4.8
White - ⅒ of 8″ or 9″ dia (42gm)	141	1.7	25.1	3.8	31.1	0	.3	0	0

Pies

	Calories (kcal)	Protein (gm)	Carbohydrates (gm)	Fat (gm)	Percent Saturated Fat	Cholesterol (mg)	Dietary Fiber (gm)	Vitamin A (RE)	Vitamin C (mg)
Apple - ⅛ of 9″ dia (151gm)	457	3.9	62.6	22	24.8	0	2	1.8	1.7
Apple, indiv size - 1 (117gm)	378	3.4	48.8	19.3	24.8	0	1.6	1.2	1.2
Apricot - ⅛ of 9″ dia (151gm)	428	4.8	57.5	20.6	24.6	0	2.3	171.3	6.2
Apricot, indiv size - 1 (117gm)	354	4	45.4	17.9	24.6	0	1.8	120.9	4.4
Banana cream - ⅛ of 9″ dia (145gm)	311	5.9	42	13.8	31	84.8	1.2	43.1	3.3
Banana cream, indiv size - 1 (117gm)	262	4.7	33.2	12.6	29.5	57.9	1	29.5	2.3
Berry - ⅛ of 9″ dia (151gm)	415	3.8	56.4	20.2	24.1	0	2.4	34.8	8.7
Berry indiv size - 1 (117gm)	342	3.3	44.6	17.5	24.2	0	1.8	24.9	6.2
Blackberry - ⅛ of 9″ dia (151gm)	413	3.8	55.5	20.3	24	0	4.3	38.5	13.3
Blackberry, indiv size - 1 (117gm)	341	3.3	43.9	17.5	24.1	0	3.2	27.5	9.5
Blueberry - ⅛ of 9″ dia (151gm)	406	4	49.2	22.4	32.8	10.8	2	77.2	7.5
Blueberry, indiv size - 1 (117gm)	343	3.3	44.6	17.5	24.2	0	1.8	24.9	6.2
Cherry - ⅛ of 9″ dia (151gm)	407	3.8	54.1	20.3	24.3	0	1.2	38.4	1.3

Thiamin (mg)	Riboflavin (mg)	Niacin (mg)	Vitamin B$_6$ (mg)	Vitamin B$_{12}$ (mcg)	Folacin (mcg)	Sodium (mg)	Calcium (mg)	Iron (mg)	Potassium (mg)	Zinc (mg)	Magnesium (mg)
0	.1	.3	0	.1	2.2	61.2	45.8	.3	43.4	.2	4.2
0	.1	.2	0	.1	2.2	70	43.9	.4	55	.3	9.4
.1	.1	.4	0	.3	12	91.9	14.7	.9	44.3	.4	5.2
.2	.2	1.3	0	.4	16.7	271	55	1.8	79.5	.6	10.6
.1	.2	1.1	0	.2	10.9	447.6	38.4	1.6	119.8	.6	29.6
.2	.2	2.4	.1	.1	19	417	176.1	2.4	180.8	.5	19.3
.1	.2	1	.1	.4	31.7	137.2	32.4	1.9	149.2	.6	13.9
.1	.1	.5	0	.1	4.9	124	26.4	.6	37.9	.2	4.2
.1	.2	1.1	0	.2	10	270.4	78.2	1.7	150.5	.4	13.2
.1	.1	.6	0	.4	17	113.3	20.7	1.2	58	.5	7.1
.1	.1	.6	0	.4	15.6	120.1	24.7	1.2	60.6	.5	7
.1	.2	1	.1	.4	29.6	147.1	46.2	1.7	161.4	.7	14.5
.1	.1	.4	0	.2	10	103.2	27.5	.7	71.9	.3	7
.1	.1	1	.1	.1	9.6	298.2	91.9	1.5	157.2	.3	15.2
.1	.1	.6	0	0	2	125.5	48.8	.6	33.3	.2	4
.2	.1	1.8	0	0	4.3	355	10.8	1.7	88	.3	10.7
.2	.1	1.6	0	0	3.7	356.9	9.3	1.5	68	.2	9.2
.2	.2	2.1	.1	0	8	303.3	18.1	2	239.8	.4	14.7
.2	.1	1.8	0	0	6.3	318.8	14.5	1.7	175.3	.4	12
.1	.2	1.1	.3	.3	15.9	196.2	85.4	1.3	270.6	.6	25.8
.1	.2	1	.2	.2	11.5	171.5	59.8	1.1	190.5	.5	19.1
.2	.1	1.7	0	0	6.6	295.2	12.1	1.5	92.5	.3	11.4
.2	.1	1.5	0	0	5.3	304.5	10.2	1.3	71.2	.2	9.6
.2	.1	1.7	.1	0	18.4	291.8	29.9	1.8	161.4	.4	22.1
.2	.1	1.5	0	0	13.8	301.4	22.8	1.5	120.5	.3	17.3
.2	.2	1.5	0	0	7.7	265.1	38.7	1.3	113.8	.3	12.4
.2	.1	1.5	0	0	5.3	304.5	10.2	1.3	71.2	.2	9.6
.2	.1	1.7	0	0	5.4	319.9	15.8	1.7	120	.3	14.4

	Calories (kcal)	Protein (gm)	Carbohydrates (gm)	Fat (gm)	Percent Saturated Fat	Cholesterol (mg)	Dietary Fiber (gm)	Vitamin A (RE)	Vitamin C (mg)
Cherry, indiv size - 1 (117gm)	338	3.3	42.7	17.8	24.4	0	1	27.4	1
Cherry, w/crm cheese, sour crm - ⅛ of 9″ dia (160gm)	457	5.5	62.9	21.4	47.9	91	.8	198.4	1.2
Chiffon w/liqueur - ⅛ of 9″ dia (99gm)	350	4.6	32.7	19.7	36.3	125	.4	98.5	.1
Chiffon, choc - ⅛ of 9″ dia (99gm)	321	6.1	40.1	16.1	31.4	138.1	1.3	58.8	0
Chiffon - ⅛ of 9″ dia (99gm)	297	6.4	39.7	12.9	26.3	177	.4	50.6	4.8
Choc cream - ⅛ of 9″ dia (145gm)	406	6.9	52.1	20.6	38	97.5	2.1	54	.5
Choc cream, indiv size - 1 (117gm)	356	5.8	43.8	18.8	35.3	70.4	1.7	39	.3
Coconut cream - ⅛ of 9″ diam (145gm)	570	9.2	55.4	35.7	49.8	205.3	5.1	58.5	1.3
Coconut cream, indiv size - 1 (117gm)	303	6.1	28.3	18.9	46.8	86.8	2.1	40.6	.9
Custard - ⅛ of 9″ dia (136gm)	283	7.1	30.3	14.9	33	122.9	.4	58.9	.5
Custard, indiv size - 1 (117gm)	223	6.6	30.2	8.4	36.6	101.1	.5	48.5	.4
Lemon meringue - ⅛ of 9″ dia (137gm)	341	4.7	48	14.9	25.1	122.3	.5	57.9	4
Lemon meringue, indiv size - 1 (117gm)	329.1	4.4	43	15.8	25.5	95.5	.5	27.3	3.1
Lemon (not cream or meringue) - ⅛ of 9″ dia (99gm)	386	5	56.5	16.1	24.8	96.9	.7	55	6.1
Mince - ⅛ of 9″ dia (151gm)	431.5	4.1	62.9	19.3	24.9	0	2.8	.6	1.6
Mince, indiv size - 1 (117gm)	357	3.6	49.4	16.9	24.9	0	2.1	.4	1.1
Peach - ⅛ of 9″ dia (151gm)	410	4.1	55.9	19.5	24.8	0	2	37	4.3
Peach, indiv size - 1 (117gm)	345.7	3.5	43.9	17.8	24.8	0	1.5	26.1	3
Pear - ⅛ of 9″ dia (151gm)	407	3.6	57.3	19	24.6	0	2.7	1.1	2.2
Pear, indiv size - 1 (117gm)	339	3.1	45	16.9	24.6	0	2	.8	1.5
Pecan - ⅛ of 9″ dia (115gm)	488	5.4	60.9	26.3	15.6	74.9	2	24.1	.4
Pecan, indiv size - 1 (57gm)	248	2.8	29.9	13.7	16.9	33.2	1	10.7	.2
Pumpkin - ⅛ of 9″ dia (155gm)	333	7.8	31.7	20	32.3	93.7	1.7	1426.7	2.8
Raisin - ⅛ of 9″ dia (151gm)	420	4.3	60.7	19	24.9	0	2.6	.3	1.6
Raisin, indiv size - 1 (117gm)	373	3.9	50	18.4	24.9	0	2.1	.2	1.2
Raspberry, one crust - ⅛ of 9″ dia (137gm)	333	2.7	51.1	14	23.2	0	4.1	43.6	16.6
Raspberry cream - ⅛ of 9″ dia (145gm)	294	3.5	33.5	17.2	46	36.4	3.4	114.5	8.4
Rhubarb - ⅛ of 9″ dia (151gm)	428	4.6	50.8	23.3	24.8	0	2.2	5.6	2.3
Shoo-fly - ⅛ of 9″ dia (114gm)	393	4.5	66.1	12.7	25.3	47.2	.9	13.5	0
Strawberry-rhubarb - ⅛ of 9″ dia (151gm)	431	4.6	52	23.2	24.7	0	2.3	4.3	17.9

Thiamin (mg)	Riboflavin (mg)	Niacin (mg)	Vitamin B6 (mg)	Vitamin B12 (mcg)	Folacin (mcg)	Sodium (mg)	Calcium (mg)	Iron (mg)	Potassium (mg)	Zinc (mg)	Magnesium (mg)
.1	.1	1.5	0	0	4.4	319.1	12.8	1.4	90.7	.2	11.7
.1	.2	.7	.1	.2	14.1	126.6	59.5	1.9	138.4	.5	11.6
.1	.1	.5	0	.3	14.2	390	32.3	1	60.2	.5	11.4
.1	.1	.8	0	.3	14.6	186.6	22.4	1.6	91.3	.7	23.8
.1	.2	.8	0	.4	18.6	181.9	22.9	1.4	71.9	.6	8.6
.2	.3	1.3	.1	.3	12.8	271.9	111.7	1.9	215	1	44.8
.2	.2	1.3	0	.2	10.1	276.9	82.5	1.7	163	.8	34.3
.2	.2	1.7	.1	.5	32.4	390.5	34.1	3.2	223.7	1.2	25.4
.1	.2	1	0	.3	15.4	230.7	84.3	1.5	180.2	.7	19
.1	.3	.9	.1	.4	15.3	302.1	120.9	1.2	176.3	.7	18.7
.1	.2	1.1	0	.3	13.4	313.2	101	1.3	151.6	.7	17
.1	.1	.9	0	.3	13.9	289.8	19.7	1.4	59.8	.5	8.7
.1	.1	1.1	0	.2	11.6	274	16.4	1.4	52.9	.4	8.4
.2	.1	1.3	0	.2	12.7	234.4	18.4	1.6	65.1	.4	9.2
.2	.2	1.9	.1	0	4.4	495.1	38.5	2.7	296.3	.3	21.9
.2	.1	1.6	.1	0	3.8	242.6	27.7	2.2	216.9	.3	16.5
.2	.2	2.3	0	0	5.5	290.3	11.3	1.6	175.9	.3	13.8
.2	.1	1.9	0	0	4.5	304.3	9.6	1.4	129.5	.3	11.3
.2	.1	1.6	0	0	6.5	304.5	14.6	1.6	106.7	.3	11.9
.2	.1	1.4	0	0	5.3	310.3	11.9	1.4	81.2	.2	9.9
.3	.1	1.1	.1	.2	15.8	211.5	21.5	1.9	133.4	1.6	35.7
.1	.1	.7	0	.1	7.4	126.7	10.4	1	62.7	.7	16.7
.1	.3	1.2	.1	.2	18.9	227.7	160.5	2.2	323.7	.8	33.7
.2	.1	1.8	.1	0	4.4	321.9	21.5	2	217.7	.3	17.6
.2	.1	1.6	.1	0	4	343.6	17.7	1.8	168.5	.3	14.8
.1	.1	1.5	0	0	14.3	209.7	21.5	1.3	127.6	.5	18.6
.1	.1	1.1	.1	0	12.5	134.8	30.7	1	122.5	.3	16.6
.2	.2	2	0	0	7.4	347.1	134.1	2	104.8	.3	22
.2	.2	1.6	.1	.1	7.9	140.2	79.3	3.4	395.2	.5	26.3
.2	.2	2.1	0	0	10.4	344.5	75.9	2	126.5	.4	19.1

	Calories (kcal)	Protein (gm)	Carbohydrates (gm)	Fat (gm)	Percent Saturated Fat	Cholesterol (mg)	Dietary Fiber (gm)	Vitamin A (RE)	Vitamin C (mg)
Strawberry, one crust - ⅛ of 9″ dia (168gm)	387	3.8	56	17.3	24.4	0	2.9	2.8	49.3
Sweet potato - ⅛ of 9″ dia (155gm)	323	6.5	35.6	17.4	30.1	83.1	1.7	791.5	7.7
Squash - ⅛ of 9″ dia (155gm)	299	6.4	39.7	13.3	31.1	87.1	2	242.4	3.1
Vanilla cream - ⅛ of 9″ dia (145gm)	383	7.8	47.4	18.2	31.5	111.2	.6	55.6	.4
Yogurt - ⅛ of 9″ dia (145gm)	355	4.6	41.4	20.2	51.7	2.9	.6	154.6	6.3
Pie shell - 9″ dia (172gm)	958	11.7	84.5	63.7	24.8	0	2.6	0	0

Crackers

	Calories (kcal)	Protein (gm)	Carbohydrates (gm)	Fat (gm)	Percent Saturated Fat	Cholesterol (mg)	Dietary Fiber (gm)	Vitamin A (RE)	Vitamin C (mg)
Cheese - 4 (12gm)	57	1.3	7.2	2.6	34.2	5.3	0	5.5	0
Graham, plain - 2 (28gm)	107	2.2	20.5	2.6	23.7	0	.5	0	0
Graham, sugar/honey coated - 2 (28gm)	115	1.9	21.4	3.2	23.8	0	.5	0	0
Low-sodium thins - 1 (2gm)	9	.2	1.4	.4	-	0	0	.3	0
Matzo - 1 (30gm)	120	3.1	25.4	.4	-	0	.5	0	0
Milk - 2 (22gm)	100	1.7	15.1	3.6	34.2	12.1	.1	0	0
Oatmeal - 2 (22gm)	101	1.6	15.1	3.8	25	0	.6	.3	0
Oyster - 4 (4gm)	18	.4	2.8	.5	-	0	.1	0	0
Rice - 4 (12gm)	46	.7	9	.6	-	0	.1	0	0
Rye wafers - 3 (21gm)	72	2.7	16	.3	-	0	1.9	0	0
Saltines - 4 (12gm)	52	1.1	8.6	1.4	-	4.1	.2	0	0
Saltines, low-sodium - 4 (12gm)	52	1.1	8.6	1.4	-	4.1	.2	0	0
Soda - 4 (8gm)	35	.7	5.6	1	-	0	.2	0	0
Whole wheat - 4 (16gm)	64	1.3	10.9	2.2	-	0	.5	0	0

BEVERAGES

Fruit Drinks

	Calories (kcal)	Protein (gm)	Carbohydrates (gm)	Fat (gm)	Percent Saturated Fat	Cholesterol (mg)	Dietary Fiber (gm)	Vitamin A (RE)	Vitamin C (mg)
Apple drink - 1 cup (250gm)	117	0	30	0	0	0	0	0	.3
Apple drink, w/vit C - 1 cup (250gm)	117	0	30	0	0	0	0	0	27.7
Apple cherry drink - 1 cup (250gm)	116	.1	29.9	0	0	0	.1	.6	.3
Apricot-pineapple juice drink - 1 cup (250gm)	128	.4	32.4	.1	-	0	.4	45.5	9.9
Banana orange - 1 cup (250gm)	126	.2	32.3	0	0	0	.1	2	7.9
Black cherry drink - 1 cup (250gm)	117	.2	30.1	0	0	0	.2	3.3	.6
Black cherry drink w/vit C - 1 cup (250gm)	117	.2	30.1	0	0	0	.2	3.3	80.6
Cherry drink w/vit C - 1 cup (250gm)	117	.2	30.1	0	0	0	.2	3.3	80.6

Thiamin (mg)	Riboflavin (mg)	Niacin (mg)	Vitamin B$_6$ (mg)	Vitamin B$_{12}$ (mcg)	Folacin (mcg)	Sodium (mg)	Calcium (mg)	Iron (mg)	Potassium (mg)	Zinc (mg)	Magnesium (mg)
.2	.2	1.6	.1	0	14.8	248.4	20.7	1.7	190.3	.3	17.8
.1	.3	1.2	.2	.3	16.5	199.6	101.3	1.4	222	.7	19.7
.1	.2	1.1	.1	.3	15.8	242.8	91.3	1.4	242.2	.6	21.7
.2	.3	1.3	.1	.3	14.8	289	121.1	1.6	181.8	.8	20.2
0	.2	.7	0	.3	10.2	265.3	103.1	.8	212	.6	18.3
.6	.4	5.3	0	0	12.4	932.5	24.4	4.9	105.6	.7	26.4
0	0	.4	0	.1	3	124.7	40.3	.4	13.1	.1	2.5
0	.2	1	0	.1	4.8	187.6	11.2	1	107.5	.2	12
0	.1	.7	0	.1	3.9	141.1	24.6	.9	75.6	.2	7.8
0	0	.1	0	0	.5	5	.6	.1	4.3	0	1
.1	.1	1.2	0	0	3.3	.6	5.7	.9	36	.2	6
.1	.1	1	0	0	5.5	131.6	37.6	.7	25.3	.2	4.6
.1	0	.6	0	0	1.9	122.3	10	.7	43.5	.2	8.9
0	0	.2	0	0	2.3	44	.9	.2	4.8	0	1.3
0	0	.2	0	0	1.1	93.6	3.3	.1	10.3	.1	4.1
.1	.1	.3	.1	0	9.4	185.2	11.1	.8	126	.6	25.2
.1	0	.5	0	0	3.8	132	2.5	.6	14.4	.1	2.8
.1	0	.5	0	0	3.8	3.6	2.5	.6	14.4	.1	2.8
0	0	.4	0	0	4.6	88	1.8	.3	9.6	0	2.6
.1	0	.7	0	.2	4.2	87.5	3.7	.5	19.2	.2	9.9

Source: USDA Food Consumption Survey

Thiamin (mg)	Riboflavin (mg)	Niacin (mg)	Vitamin B$_6$ (mg)	Vitamin B$_{12}$ (mcg)	Folacin (mcg)	Sodium (mg)	Calcium (mg)	Iron (mg)	Potassium (mg)	Zinc (mg)	Magnesium (mg)
0	.1	0	0	0	5	12.5	17.5	.7	47.5	.3	5
0	.1	0	0	0	5	12.5	17.5	.7	47.5	.3	5
0	0	0	0	0	.2	6.6	6.7	.1	31.4	0	3.2
.1	0	.3	.1	0	21.4	5.2	20.4	.4	161.2	.2	14.6
0	0	.1	0	0	9.4	6	6.6	.1	61.4	.1	5.6
0	0	.1	0	0	1.1	6.6	8.2	.2	34.1	.1	5
0	0	.1	0	0	1.1	6.6	8.2	.2	34.1	.1	5
0	0	.1	0	0	1.1	6.6	8.2	.2	34.1	.1	5

	Calories (kcal)	Protein (gm)	Carbohydrates (gm)	Fat (gm)	Percent Saturated Fat	Cholesterol (mg)	Dietary Fiber (gm)	Vitamin A (RE)	Vitamin C (mg)
Citrus drink w/vit C - 1 cup (250gm)	126	.1	32.4	0	0	0	0	1.8	78.9
Citrus fruit juice drink - 1 cup (247gm)	113	.8	28.1	.1	-	0	.1	10.4	66.4
Cranberry juice cktl, w/vit C - 1 cup (253gm)	147	0	37.4	0	0	0	0	0	89.8
Cranberry juice cktl, low-cal, w/vit C - 1 cup (240gm)	46	0	11.3	0	0	0	0	0	77.3
Cranberry-apple juice drink w/vit C - 1 cup (253gm)	169	.3	43.3	0	0	0	0	0	81
Fruit ades, punches - 1 cup (248gm)	112	0	28.3	0	0	0	0	2.5	2
Fruit ades, punches w/vit C - 1 cup (247gm)	111	0	28.1	0	0	0	0	2.5	78.5
Fruit drink, low-cal - 1 cup (240gm)	43	0	11.3	0	0	0	0	2.4	77.5
Grapefruit juice drink - 1 cup (250gm)	128	.4	32.3	.1	-	0	.1	.8	21.9
Grapefruit juice drink w/vit C - 1 cup (250gm)	128	.4	32.3	.1	-	0	.1	.8	79.4
Grape drink w/vit C - 1 cup (250gm)	112	0	28.5	0	0	0	0	0	85
Grape drink, low-cal - 1 cup (240gm)	43	0	11.3	0	0	0	0	2.4	77.5
Grape juice drink - 1 cup (250gm)	135	.3	34.5	0	0	0	0	0	40
Grapeade, grape drink - 1 cup (250gm)	112	0	28.5	0	0	0	0	0	0
Lemon-limeade - 1 cup (248gm)	105	.1	27.7	.1	0	0	.2	1.4	11.6
Lemonade - 1 cup (248gm)	108	.1	28.2	.1	0	0	.2	2.8	16.6
Limeade - 1 cup (248gm)	103	.1	27.2	.1	0	0	.2	0	6.6
Orange brkfst drink from froz conc - 1 cup (250gm)	116	.2	29.2	.2	-	0	.2	.7	154.1
Orange drink, orangeades - 1 cup (249gm)	124	0	32.1	0	0	0	0	5	8.5
Orange drink, ade w/vit C - 1 cup (249gm)	124	0	32.1	0	0	0	0	5	85.6
Orange apricot juice drink - 1 cup (249gm)	124	.7	31.6	.2	6	0	.2	144.4	39.8
Orange-lemon drink - 1 cup (249gm)	124	.1	32	0	0	0	0	3.7	8.1
Pineapple-grape juice drink - 1 cup (250gm)	117	.5	29	.3	-	0	.3	10	115
Pineapple-grapefruit juice drink - 1 cup (250gm)	117	.5	29	.3	-	0	.3	10	115
Pineapple-orange juice drink w/vit C - 1 cup (250gm)	125	3	29.5	0	0	0	.3	132.5	56.3
Strawberry drink - 1 cup (250gm)	125	0	32.3	0	0	0	0	0	0

Thiamin (mg)	Riboflavin (mg)	Niacin (mg)	Vitamin B$_6$ (mg)	Vitamin B$_{12}$ (mcg)	Folacin (mcg)	Sodium (mg)	Calcium (mg)	Iron (mg)	Potassium (mg)	Zinc (mg)	Magnesium (mg)
0	0	.1	0	0	.8	6.5	7.9	.5	48.1	.1	4.5
0	0	.4	.1	0	4.9	7.1	21.5	2.7	273.9	.1	15.7
0	.1	.1	0	0	0	5.1	7.6	.4	48.1	.4	7.6
0	0	.1	0	0	0	7.2	21.6	.1	52.8	0	4.8
0	.1	.2	0	0	0	5.1	17.7	.2	68.3	.1	5.1
0	0	0	0	0	5	52.1	17.4	.7	52.1	.3	5
0	0	0	0	0	4.9	51.9	17.3	.7	51.9	.3	4.9
0	0	0	0	0	4.8	50.4	16.8	.6	50.4	.3	4.8
0	0	.2	0	0	7.8	5.2	8.7	.2	115.7	.1	9
0	0	.2	0	0	7.8	5.2	8.7	.2	115.6	.1	9
0	0	.1	0	0	0	15	2.5	.4	12.5	.3	2.5
0	0	0	0	0	4.8	50.4	16.8	.6	50.4	.3	4.8
0	0	.3	0	0	2.5	2.5	7.5	.3	87.5	0	7.5
0	0	.1	0	0	0	15	2.5	.4	12.5	.3	2.5
0	0	0	0	0	5.2	6	7	.2	35.7	.1	4.4
0	0	0	0	0	8.3	6.5	6.7	.4	38.8	.1	4.7
0	0	.1	0	0	2.2	5.4	7.2	.1	32.6	.1	4.1
.3	1.3	.3	.1	0	40.1	22.9	476.3	.2	321.4	.1	14.8
0	0	.1	0	0	0	39.8	14.9	.7	44.8	.2	5
0	0	.1	0	0	0	39.8	14.9	.7	44.8	.2	5
0	0	.5	.1	0	14.9	0	12.4	.2	234.1	.1	10
0	0	.1	0	0	4.1	7.2	6.7	.1	41	.1	4.5
.1	0	.7	.1	0	25	35	17.5	.8	152.5	.1	15
.1	0	.7	.1	0	25	35	17.5	.8	152.5	.1	15
.1	0	.5	.1	0	27.5	7.5	12.5	.7	115	.1	15
0	0	0	0	0	0	6.4	5.1	0	1.2	0	2.2

	Calories (kcal)	Protein (gm)	Carbohydrates (gm)	Fat (gm)	Percent Saturated Fat	Cholesterol (mg)	Dietary Fiber (gm)	Vitamin A (RE)	Vitamin C (mg)
Strawberry drink w/vit C - 1 cup (250gm)	89	0	22.7	0	0	0	0	0	20.1
Tang - 1 tbsp dry (14gm)	54	0	13.8	0	0	0	0	87.9	57.3

Soft Drinks

	Calories (kcal)	Protein (gm)	Carbohydrates (gm)	Fat (gm)	Percent Saturated Fat	Cholesterol (mg)	Dietary Fiber (gm)	Vitamin A (RE)	Vitamin C (mg)
Club soda - 12 fl oz (355gm)	0	0	0	0	0	0	0	0	0
Choc flavored - 12 fl oz (369gm)	155	0	39.5	0	0	0	0	0	0
Choc-flavored, sugar-free - 12 fl oz (355gm)	7	0	0	.7	-	0	0	0	0
Cola - 12 fl oz (369gm)	151	0	38.4	0	0	0	0	0	0
Cola, sugar-free - 12 fl oz (355gm)	7	0	0	.7	-	0	0	0	0
Cream - 12 fl oz (371gm)	189	0	49.3	0	0	0	0	0	0
Cream, sugar-free - 12 fl oz (355gm)	7	0	0	.7	35	0	0	0	0
Ginger ale - 12 fl oz (366gm)	113	0	29.3	0	0	0	0	0	0
Ginger ale, sugar-free - 12 fl oz (355gm)	7	0	0	.7	-	0	0	0	0
Fruit flavored - 12 fl oz (372gm)	156	0	40.2	0	0	0	0	0	0
Fruit flavored, sugar-free - 12 fl oz (355gm)	7.1	0	0	.7	-	0	0	0	0
Pepper-type - 12 fl oz (369gm)	151	0	38.4	0	0	0	0	0	0
Pepper-type, sugar-free - 12 fl oz (355gm)	7	0	0	.7	-	0	0	0	0
Root beer - 12 fl oz (369gm)	151	0	39.1	0	0	0	0	0	0
Root beer, sugar-free - 12 fl oz (355gm)	7	0	0	.7	-	0	0	0	0

Alcoholic Beverages

	Calories (kcal)	Protein (gm)	Carbohydrates (gm)	Fat (gm)	Percent Saturated Fat	Cholesterol (mg)	Dietary Fiber (gm)	Vitamin A (RE)	Vitamin C (mg)
Alexander - 1 (74gm)	179	.4	7.6	1.8	-	5.6	0	16.3	.1
Bacardi - 1 (63gm)	118	0	6	0	0	0	0	.3	1
Beer, ale - 12 fl oz (360gm)	151	1.1	13.7	0	0	0	.7	0	0
Beer, light - 12 fl oz (360gm)	101	.7	4.7	0	0	0	0	0	0
Black Russian - 1 (90gm)	255	0	14	.1	-	0	0	0	0
Bloody Mary - 1 (148gm)	123	.8	4.8	.1	-	0	.8	51.2	20.4
Bourbon or scotch w/soda - 1 (116gm)	105	0	0	0	0	0	0	0	0
Brandy - 1 fl oz (28gm)	65	0	0	0	0	0	0	0	0
Cordial or liqueur - 1 cordial glass (20gm)	74	0	8.3	.1	0	0	0	0	0
Daiquiri - 1 (61gm)	113	0	4.1	0	0	0	0	.3	1
Gibson - 1 (71gm)	158	.1	.2	0	0	0	0	0	0
Gimlet - 1 (71gm)	132	0	1	0	0	0	0	.3	1

Thiamin (mg)	Riboflavin (mg)	Niacin (mg)	Vitamin B$_6$ (mg)	Vitamin B$_{12}$ (mcg)	Folacin (mcg)	Sodium (mg)	Calcium (mg)	Iron (mg)	Potassium (mg)	Zinc (mg)	Magnesium (mg)
0	0	0	0	0	0	7.3	41.2	.1	1.1	.1	2.5
0	0	0	0	0	0	2.4	5.5	.1	23.2	0	.3
0	0	0	0	0	0	74.5	17.7	0	7.1	.4	3.5
0	0	0	0	0	0	324.7	14.8	.4	184.5	.6	3.7
0	0	0	0	0	0	31.9	10.6	.4	7.1	.3	0
0	0	0	0	0	0	14.8	11.1	0	3.7	0	3.7
0	0	0	0	0	0	31.9	10.6	.4	7.1	.3	0
0	0	0	0	0	0	44.5	18.5	.4	3.7	.2	3.7
0	0	0	0	0	0	31.9	10.6	.4	7.1	.3	0
0	0	0	0	0	0	25.6	11	.7	3.7	.2	3.7
0	0	0	0	0	0	31.9	10.6	.4	7.1	.3	0
0	0	0	0	0	0	52.1	11.2	.4	11.2	.4	3.7
0	0	0	0	0	0	31.9	10.6	.4	7.1	.3	0
0	0	0	0	0	0	14.8	11.1	0	3.7	0	3.7
0	0	0	0	0	0	31.9	10.6	.4	7.1	.3	0
0	0	0	0	0	0	0	0	0	0	.3	3.7
0	0	0	0	0	0	31.9	10.6	.4	7.1	.3	0
0	0	0	0	.1	.4	7.4	15.9	0	20.5	.1	1.5
0	0	0	0	0	1.2	9	2	.1	13.4	0	1.2
0	.1	1.8	.2	.7	25.2	25.2	18	0	90	.1	21.6
0	.1	1.4	.1	.2	25.2	21.6	18	.1	64.8	.1	18
0	0	0	0	0	0	2.2	0	0	1.1	0	0
0	0	.6	.1	0	19.6	331.9	9.9	.5	216.4	.2	11.2
0	0	0	0	0	0	16	3.7	0	2.3	.1	.7
0	0	0	0	0	0	.3	0	0	.6	0	0
0	0	0	0	0	0	1	0	0	0	0	0
0	0	0	0	0	1.2	2.9	1.9	0	12.6	0	1.1
0	0	0	0	0	.1	1.6	1.3	.1	14	0	1.5
0	0	0	0	0	1.2	3	1.8	0	12.6	0	1.1

	Calories (kcal)	Protein (gm)	Carbohydrates (gm)	Fat (gm)	Percent Saturated Fat	Cholesterol (mg)	Dietary Fiber (gm)	Vitamin A (RE)	Vitamin C (mg)
Gin - 1 jigger (42gm)	110	0	0	0	0	0	0	0	0
Gin 'n tonic - 1 (225gm)	171	0	15.8	0	0	0	0	.3	1
Gin Rickey - 1 (205gm)	114	.1	1.4	0	0	0	0	.2	4.5
Glug - 4 fl oz (116gm)	112	.5	10.6	0	0	0	0	0	0
Gold Cadillac - 1 (125gm)	394	.8	41.3	3.6	60.7	10.6	0	30.7	.2
Grasshopper - 1 (64gm)	164	.9	15.3	3.6	61.7	11.2	0	32.5	.3
Mai Tai - 1 (126gm)	310	0	28.5	.1	0	0	0	.3	1
Manhattan - 1 (57gm)	127	0	1.8	0	0	0	0	0	0
Margarita - 1 (77gm)	170	0	10	.1	0	0	0	.3	1
Martini - 1 (71gm)	158	.1	.2	0	0	0	0	0	0
Mint Julep - 1 (65gm)	156	0	4	0	0	0	0	0	0
Near beer - 12 fl oz (360gm)	32	1.1	5	0	0	0	0	0	0
Old fashioned - 1 (60gm)	155	0	4.1	0	0	0	0	0	0
Pina colada - 1 (133gm)	231	.6	30	2.5	87.2	0	.4	0	6.5
Rum - 1 jigger (42gm)	97	0	0	0	0	0	0	0	0
Rum and carbonated beverage - 1 (211gm)	160	.1	16.4	.1	-	0	.1	.6	2
Rum, hot buttered - 1 (251gm)	317	.2	4.5	11.9	62.5	31	0	107.1	0
Screwdriver - 1 (213gm)	182	1.2	18.4	0	12.5	0	.2	13.7	66.5
Singapore sling - 1 (225gm)	228	.1	11.9	.1	0	0	0	.3	3.8
Sloe gin fizz - 1 (222gm)	121	.1	3	0	0	0	0	.3	3.8
Stinger - 1 (92gm)	282	0	20.9	0	0	0	0	0	0
Tequila sunrise - 1 (172gm)	189	.6	14.7	.2	12.4	0	.1	17.2	33.2
Tom Collins - 1 (222gm)	121	.1	3	0	0	0	0	.3	3.8
Vodka - 1 jigger (42gm)	97	0	0	0	0	0	0	0	0
Whiskey - 1 jigger (42gm)	105	0	0	0	0	0	0	0	0
Whiskey sour - 1 (90gm)	122	.2	5	.1	0	0	.1	.9	11.4
White Russian - 1 (100gm)	268	.3	14.5	1.3	-	3.7	0	10.7	.1
Wine, cooking - 1 fl oz (29gm)	2	.1	.3	0	0	0	0	0	0
Wine cooler - 7 fl oz (210gm)	101	.5	11.5	0	0	0	0	.3	3.8
Wine, light - 1 fl oz (29gm)	14	.1	.3	0	0	0	0	0	0
Wine spritzer - 1 (146gm)	61	.4	1	0	0	0	0	0	0
Wine, Chinese - 3½ fl oz (100gm)	70	.5	1.1	0	0	0	0	0	0
Wine, dessert - 3½ fl oz (100gm)	153	.2	11.8	0	0	0	0	0	0
Wine, table - 3½ fl oz (100gm)	70	.5	1.1	0	0	0	0	0	0

Coffee and Tea

Coffee, ground - 6 fl oz (180gm)	2	0	0	0	0	0	0	0	0
Coffee, instant - 6 fl oz (180gm)	1.3	0	.4	0	0	0	0	0	0

Thiamin (mg)	Riboflavin (mg)	Niacin (mg)	Vitamin B_6 (mg)	Vitamin B_{12} (mcg)	Folacin (mcg)	Sodium (mg)	Calcium (mg)	Iron (mg)	Potassium (mg)	Zinc (mg)	Magnesium (mg)
0	0	0	0	0	0	.4	0	0	.8	0	0
0	0	0	0	0	1.2	9.6	3.5	0	12.4	.2	1.1
0	0	0	0	0	1.3	31.6	8.8	0	20.5	.2	2.4
0	0	.1	0	0	1	7.6	9.6	.4	94.4	.1	10.7
0	.1	0	0	.1	.7	16.5	30.1	.1	37.2	.1	2.9
0	.1	0	0	.1	.8	14	31.8	0	39.3	.2	3.1
0	0	0	0	0	1.2	10.3	3.1	.1	18.4	.1	1.9
0	0	0	0	0	0	1.6	1.2	0	14.6	0	1.3
0	0	0	0	0	1.2	275.4	3.6	.1	12.5	0	1.9
0	0	0	0	0	.1	1.6	1.3	.1	14	0	1.5
0	0	0	0	0	0	.7	.1	0	1.3	0	0
0	.1	1.6	.2	0	25.2	18	25.2	0	90	0	32.4
0	0	0	0	0	0	.6	0	0	1.2	0	0
0	0	.2	.1	0	15.5	8.1	10.1	.2	94.2	.2	10
0	0	0	0	0	0	.4	0	0	.8	0	0
0	0	.1	0	0	2.4	10.9	7.8	.1	25.3	1	3.5
0	0	0	0	0	1.1	6.8	8.8	.1	9.5	.1	3.8
.1	0	.3	.1	0	74.9	2.1	15.4	.2	325.6	.1	17.1
0	0	0	0	0	1.5	32.6	8.3	0	19.4	.2	2.5
0	0	0	0	0	1.5	37.8	9.8	0	19.7	.2	2.8
0	0	0	0	0	0	2.9	0	0	.8	0	0
.1	0	.3	.1	0	18.2	6.7	9.7	.5	178.4	.1	11.6
0	0	0	0	0	1.5	37.8	9.8	0	19.7	.2	2.8
0	0	0	0	0	0	.4	0	0	.8	0	0
0	0	0	0	0	0	.4	0	0	.8	0	0
0	0	.1	0	0	4.6	10.1	5	.1	47.7	0	3.7
0	0	0	0	0	.3	6.3	10.5	0	14.1	.1	1
0	0	0	0	0	.3	181.5	2.6	.1	25.5	0	2.9
0	0	.1	0	0	2.4	16.8	12.7	.6	93.1	.1	11
0	0	0	0	0	.3	2	2.6	.1	25.5	0	2.9
0	0	.1	0	0	.9	18.5	10.8	.3	77.7	.1	9.3
0	0	.1	0	0	1	7	9	.4	88	.1	10
0	0	.2	0	0	0	8	8	.2	92	.1	9
0	0	.1	0	0	1	7	9	.4	88	.1	10
0	0	.4	0	0	0	1.8	3.6	.1	124.2	0	10.8
0	0	.3	0	0	0	5.4	5.6	0	36.2	0	5.1

	Calories (kcal)	Protein (gm)	Carbohydrates (gm)	Fat (gm)	Percent Saturated Fat	Cholesterol (mg)	Dietary Fiber (gm)	Vitamin A (RE)	Vitamin C (mg)
Coffee, espresso - 2 fl oz (60gm)	1	0	0	0	0	0	0	0	0
Coffee, Turkish - 4 fl oz (120gm)	45	0	11.4	0	0	0	0	0	0
Tea - 6 fl oz (180gm)	2	0	.5	0	0	0	0	0	0
Tea, herb - 6 fl oz (180gm)	2	0	.4	0	0	0	0	0	0
Tea, instant, w/lem and sgr - 6 fl oz (184gm)	63	.1	15.9	0	0	0	0	0	0
Tea, instant w/aspartame - 6 fl oz (184gm)	4	0	.7	0	0	0	0	0	0
Tea, Russian - 6 fl oz (184gm)	111	0	28.5	0	0	0	0	76	49.6

CANDIES AND SWEETS

Candy

	Calories (kcal)	Protein (gm)	Carbohydrates (gm)	Fat (gm)	Percent Saturated Fat	Cholesterol (mg)	Dietary Fiber (gm)	Vitamin A (RE)	Vitamin C (mg)
Almonds, choc-covered - 5 (15gm)	85	1.8	5.9	6.6	27.6	1.6	1.3	.9	0
Almonds, sugar-coated - 4 (14gm)	64	1.1	9.8	2.6	8	0	.7	0	0
Baby Ruth - 1 (34gm)	162	3.8	20.5	7.4	37.6	11.2	1.9	0	0
Butterfinger - 1 (45gm)	211	3.8	31.5	8.2	42.1	0	1.7	0	0
Caramel w/nuts, choc-covered - 2 oz (50.8gm)	277	5.3	36	11.8	37.6	0	2.4	0	.8
Caramels, plain or choc - 1 oz (28.4gm)	115	1	22	3	64.9	1	.1	.7	0
Caramel, choc roll - ½ oz (14.2gm)	55	.3	11.6	1.1	-	.1	.4	.8	0
Caramel sucker - 1 (59gm)	235	2.4	45.2	6	70	1.2	0	1.2	0
Chocolate, milk, plain - 1 oz (28.4gm)	145	2.2	15.8	9	59.4	6	.7	3	0
Chocolate, semisweet - 1 oz (28.4gm)	142	1.2	16	10	58.6	0	1.8	.6	0
Chocolate, sweet or dark - 1 oz (28.4gm)	147	1.2	16	10	60.7	.3	1.4	.5	0
Chocolate, milk, w/almonds - 1 piece (1.4gm)	150	3	15	10	44.4	5	1.8	8	0
Chocolate, milk, w/peanuts - 1 piece (43gm)	155	4	13	11	39.7	5	1.1	8	0
Chocolit - 1 bar (32gm)	172	1.6	19.9	9.6	59.4	5.8	.8	3.5	0
Coconut, choc-covered - 1 oz (28.4gm)	114	.8	18.7	4.9	61.7	.6	1.6	.3	0
Coconut, plain - 1 bar (40gm)	146	.5	24.8	5.7	88.7	0	.8	0	.1
Fruit bar - 1 oz (28.4gm)	104	1	16.5	4.8	8.5	0	2.2	2.3	.7
Fruit leather - 1 oz (28.4gm)	82	.1	21.1	.6	13	0	.6	.3	.0

Thiamin (mg)	Riboflavin (mg)	Niacin (mg)	Vitamin B_6 (mg)	Vitamin B_{12} (mcg)	Folacin (mcg)	Sodium (mg)	Calcium (mg)	Iron (mg)	Potassium (mg)	Zinc (mg)	Magnesium (mg)
0	0	.1	0	0	0	.6	1.2	0	41.4	0	3.6
0	0	.2	0	0	0	1.2	2.2	.1	75.3	0	6.5
0	0	0	0	0	9	0	0	0	28.8	0	1.8
0	0	0	0	0	3.6	1.8	3.6	.1	19.8	.1	1.8
0	0	.1	0	0	6.8	14.1	4.4	0	35.5	0	3.5
0	0	.1	0	0	7.4	29.4	0	.2	69.9	0	3.7
0	0	.1	0	0	3.2	7	5.9	.1	63.5	.1	3.5

Source: USDA Food Consumption Survey

Thiamin (mg)	Riboflavin (mg)	Niacin (mg)	Vitamin B_6 (mg)	Vitamin B_{12} (mcg)	Folacin (mcg)	Sodium (mg)	Calcium (mg)	Iron (mg)	Potassium (mg)	Zinc (mg)	Magnesium (mg)
0	.1	.3	0	0	4.9	6.3	30.4	.4	86.2	.3	26.8
0	0	.1	0	0	2.7	2.8	14	.3	35.7	.1	13.7
1.1	2.1	5.7	.1	.1	15	80.9	1.7	2.2	94.2	1	30.6
.9	2.6	7.7	.1	.1	23.4	104.8	1.3	2.9	110.7	.5	29.7
0	.1	2.7	.1	0	51.5	13.4	43.7	1	249.2	1	45.4
0	0	0	0	0	1	64	42	.4	54	.1	5.4
0	0	0	0	0	.4	27.6	4.1	.3	29.3	.1	4.5
0	.1	.1	0	0	2.9	155.2	97.3	.8	155.8	.3	4.7
0	.1	.1	0	.2	1.9	22	55	.4	105	.3	17
0	0	.1	0	0	.8	3.9	8.4	1	97.7	.5	30.8
0	.1	.1	0	0	.8	4	7.2	.6	81	.4	31
0	.2	.2	0	.2	4	23	65	.5	125	.4	27
.1	.1	1.4	0	.2	15.6	19	49	.4	138	.5	28
0	.1	.1	0	.2	2.2	26.2	54.7	.3	119.7	.3	15.4
0	0	0	0	0	.6	51.8	3.9	.5	43.4	.2	12.3
0	0	.1	0	0	1.3	59.9	4.3	.8	63.8	.3	9.4
.1	0	.3	0	0	3.9	3	15.5	.5	155.7	.4	16.4
0	0	.4	.1	0	0	3.4	12	1.1	24.6	0	25.8

	Calories (kcal)	Protein (gm)	Carbohydrates (gm)	Fat (gm)	Percent Saturated Fat	Cholesterol (mg)	Dietary Fiber (gm)	Vitamin A (RE)	Vitamin C (mg)
Fruit peel, candied - 3 pieces (9gm)	28	0	7.3	0	9	0	.3	.4	0
Fruit, choc-covered - ½ oz (14.2gm)	55	.3	11	1.3	57	.9	.1	.4	0
Fudge, choc - 1½ cubic in (30gm)	120	.8	22.5	3.7	63.4	.3	.4	0	0
Fudge, choc w/nuts - 1½ cubic in (30gm)	128	1.2	20.7	5.2	47.7	0	.5	0	0
Fudge, choc, choc-coated - 1½ cubic in (30gm)	129	1.1	21.9	4.8	64.2	1.8	.5	.9	0
Fudge, divinity - 2 cubic in (24gm)	95	1	19.9	1.8	6.4	0	.2	.9	.1
Fudge, peanut butter - 1½ cubic in (30gm)	134	2.8	18.1	6.3	36	.5	.6	0	0
Fudge, peanut butter w/nuts - 1½ cubic in (30gm)	140	3.1	16.7	7.5	30.2	.5	.7	.2	0
Fudge, vanilla - 1½ cubic in (30gm)	119	.9	22.4	3.3	65.3	.6	0	0	0
Fudge, brown sugar (panuchi) - 1½ cubic in (30gm)	121	.6	22.9	3.6	14.1	1.1	.4	11	.1
Fudge, choc-coated, choc w/nuts - 1½ cubic in (30gm)	136	1.5	20.2	6.2	47.9	.6	.6	1.2	0
Fudge, vanilla, w/nuts - 1½ cubic in (30gm)	127	1.3	20.6	4.9	44.1	.6	.1	.3	0
Gumdrops - 1 oz (28.4gm)	97	0	24.5	.2	12.9	0	0	0	0
Halvah, plain - 1 oz (28.4gm)	141	2.9	15.8	8.2	17.4	0	.3	.7	0
Halvah, choc-covered - 1 oz (28.4gm)	142	2.7	15.8	8.5	30	1.7	.4	1.4	0
Kitkat - 1 (43gm)	217	3.1	25.5	11.4	65.3	2.6	.6	8.6	0
Licorice - 1 box (51gm)	187	0	47.5	.3	66	0	0	0	0
M&M plain - 1 pkg. (42gm)	207	2.7	28.6	9	59.8	5.5	.2	5	0
Mars Bar - 1 (50gm)	242	4.5	30.3	11.4	59.6	3	.8	5	0
Marshmallows - 2 (14gm)	45	.3	11.3	0	0	.1	0	0	0
Marshmallows, candy-coated - 1 oz (28.4gm)	96	.4	24.4	0	0	.2	0	0	0
Marshmallow rabbit choc-covered - ½ oz (14.2gm)	53	.4	10.3	1.5	60.7	.1	.2	.1	0
Milky Way - 1 (54gm)	247	2.5	39.5	8	53.7	3.2	.1	3.2	.2
Nougat, choc-covered - 1 bar (53gm)	216	2.1	39.1	7	65.7	3.3	.5	4.7	0
Nougat w/caramel, choc-covered - 1 bar (57gm)	237	2.3	41.5	7.9	50.6	2.8	.9	3.4	0
Nuts, carob-coated - 1 oz (28.4gm)	127	5.1	13.6	6.3	15.5	0	2.5	4.5	0
Nuts, choc-covered - 1 oz (28.4gm)	161	3.1	10.5	13	33.3	3.1	1	1.8	.1
$100,000 Bar - 1 (43gm)	205	1.5	31.2	8.3	59.6	2.6	.4	1.7	0

Thiamin (mg)	Riboflavin (mg)	Niacin (mg)	Vitamin B$_6$ (mg)	Vitamin B$_{12}$ (mcg)	Folacin (mcg)	Sodium (mg)	Calcium (mg)	Iron (mg)	Potassium (mg)	Zinc (mg)	Magnesium (mg)
0	0	0	0	0	0	0	0	0	0	0	.5
0	0	0	0	0	.3	6.7	8.2	.1	15.2	.1	2.5
0	0	.1	0	.1	.9	57	23.1	.3	44.1	.1	4.8
0	0	.1	0	.1	2.7	51.3	23.7	.4	53.1	.2	9.3
0	0	.1	0	.1	1.2	68.4	30.3	.4	57.9	.2	8.7
0	0	0	0	0	2.4	16.3	2.3	.1	21.3	.1	6.6
0	0	1	0	.1	7	81.8	27.7	.2	79.6	.3	16.6
0	0	1	0	.1	8.4	77.1	27.5	.3	76.7	.3	20
0	0	0	0	.1	1.2	62.4	33.6	.1	38.1	.1	4.8
0	0	.1	0	0	1.9	36.3	30.9	.6	106.4	.3	10.9
0	0	.1	0	.1	3	61.5	30.3	.4	65.7	.2	12.9
0	0	0	0	.1	3	56.1	33.3	.2	34.2	.2	9.3
0	0	0	0	0	0	9.8	1.7	.1	1.4	0	.3
.1	0	.5	0	0	0	4.5	14.3	.9	44.9	1.1	37.9
.1	0	.4	0	0	.6	9.6	25.5	.7	61.7	.9	32.1
0	.1	.1	0	.1	3	38.7	64.5	.6	129	.4	19.3
0	0	0	0	0	0	12.7	1.5	.6	18.9	0	1
0	.1	.2	0	.3	2.9	36.1	69.3	.7	150.4	.5	26.5
0	.2	.5	0	.1	6	75.5	83	.5	165	.6	36
0	0	0	0	0	0	12.3	.7	.2	.8	0	.4
0	0	0	0	0	0	15.9	.9	.3	1.4	0	.5
0	0	0	0	0	.1	9.3	1.6	.2	12.7	.1	5
0	.1	.2	0	.2	3.8	102.6	70.7	.4	141.5	.4	18.4
0	.1	.3	0	.1	3.3	92.2	31.1	.4	67.9	.2	11.5
0	.1	.2	0	.2	4	118.6	68.4	.5	150.5	.4	18.2
0	.1	.7	.1	0	21	9	47.6	4.5	95.8	.5	19.3
.1	.1	.2	.1	.1	6	12.1	47.8	.8	130.1	.8	43.4
0	.1	.1	0	.1	3.4	75.7	33.1	.2	70.5	.3	11.6

	Calories (kcal)	Protein (gm)	Carbohydrates (gm)	Fat (gm)	Percent Saturated Fat	Cholesterol (mg)	Dietary Fiber (gm)	Vitamin A (RE)	Vitamin C (mg)
Peanut bar - 1 oz (28.4gm)	144	4.9	13.2	9	17.4	0	1.7	0	0
Peanut brittle - 1 oz (28.4gm)	118	1.6	22.7	2.9	17.4	0	.5	0	0
Peanut butter morsels - 90 (28.4gm)	148	5.8	12.6	8.3	20.3	0	1.5	1.4	0
Peanut butter, choc-covered - 1.2 oz (34.08gm)	171	4.3	18.8	9.9	33.2	2.6	1.2	1.3	0
Peanuts, choc-covered - 1 oz (28.4gm)	157	4.6	10.9	11.6	39.7	2.8	1.7	1.7	0
Peanuts, sugar-coated - 1 oz (28.4gm)	144	4.9	13.2	9	17.4	0	1.7	0	0
Peanuts, yogurt-covered - 1 oz (28.4gm)	127	2.5	10.6	8.6	19.3	.8	1.2	6.7	.6
Planter's Peanut Bar - 1 (16gm)	84	2.6	7.4	5.4	17.3	0	1	0	0
Pralines - 1 cubic in (21gm)	85	.4	16	2.5	14.1	.8	.3	7.7	.1
Raisins, choc-covered - 28 (28.4gm)	119	1.5	19.7	4.8	52.7	2.8	1.3	1.7	0
Raisins, carob-covered - 28 (28gm)	111	2	18.7	4	80.5	0	1.8	1.3	.5
Reese's Peanut Butter Cups - 1 pkg (45gm)	243	5.3	23	13.9	34.7	3.6	2.2	1.8	0
Reese's Pieces - 1 oz (28.4gm)	134	3.8	15.4	5.7	34.6	2.2	.7	1.4	0
Rolo - 9 pieces (27gm)	134	1.3	18.3	6.2	59.6	1.6	.2	3	0
Royals - 1.5 oz (42.6gm)	211	2.9	29.5	9.1	59.7	5.6	.2	7.7	0
Sesame crunch - 5 pieces (10gm)	54	1.5	3.6	3.4	14.1	0	1	.4	0
Skittles - 1 (35gm)	142	.1	32.4	1	-	0	0	0	0
Snickers - 1 (57gm)	276	5.8	33.6	12.7	39.7	9.1	1.4	2.8	0
Special Dark - 1 (41gm)	221	2.3	25.3	12.2	59.6	0	2.7	.8	0
Summit - 1 (39gm)	211	4	22	11.9	59.7	2.3	.6	7.8	.4
Taffy, plain - 1 oz (28.4gm)	100	0	23.9	.8	-	0	0	11.4	0
Toffee, plain - 1 oz (28.4gm)	113	1.1	21.8	2.9	70	.6	0	.6	0
3 Musketeers - 1 (23gm)	100	.8	17.5	2.9	52.4	2.3	.4	0	.1
Twix Caramel - 1 pkg (54gm)	268	3.1	35.4	12.6	59.6	3.2	.1	10.8	0
Twix Peanut Butter - 1 pkg (54gm)	288	6.2	29.9	16	59.6	3.2	1.3	0	0
Whatchamacallit - 1 (40gm)	216	4	22.9	11.8	41.6	4.4	1.6	2.4	0

Jellies and Jams

	Calories (kcal)	Protein (gm)	Carbohydrates (gm)	Fat (gm)	Percent Saturated Fat	Cholesterol (mg)	Dietary Fiber (gm)	Vitamin A (RE)	Vitamin C (mg)
Fruit butters, all flavors - 1 tbsp (18gm)	33	.1	8.4	.1	-	0	.2	0	.4
Jam, preserves, all flavors - 1 tbsp (20gm)	54	.1	14	0	0	0	.5	.1	1.7
Jam, preserves, marmalade - ½ tbsp (10gm)	14	0	3.7	0	0	0	.1	.1	1.5
Jams, preserves, diet, all flavors - 1 tbsp (20gm)	2.2	.1	10.7	.1	-	0	10	0	0

Thiamin (mg)	Riboflavin (mg)	Niacin (mg)	Vitamin B_6 (mg)	Vitamin B_{12} (mcg)	Folacin (mcg)	Sodium (mg)	Calcium (mg)	Iron (mg)	Potassium (mg)	Zinc (mg)	Magnesium (mg)
.1	0	2.4	.1	0	42.3	60.5	12.3	.5	113.7	.8	29.1
0	0	1	0	0	14	28.3	9.8	.6	42.3	.3	10.6
0	.1	2.3	.1	.2	41.4	54.6	30.8	.5	141.4	.6	30.8
0	.1	1.6	.1	.1	10.6	65.6	27	.4	126.4	.5	28.2
.1	.1	2.1	.1	.1	34.7	16.8	32.5	.4	141.1	.6	30.2
.1	0	2.4	.1	0	42.3	60.5	12.3	.5	113.7	.8	29.1
0	0	1.6	0	.1	31.6	9.5	10.9	.3	70.6	.6	16.5
.1	0	1.4	0	0	24.2	34.6	7	.3	65.1	.4	16.6
0	0	0	0	0	1.3	25.4	21.6	.4	74.4	.2	7.6
0	.1	.1	0	.1	1.4	12.9	34.2	.5	157.6	.2	13.4
0	.1	.3	.1	.1	.5	1.9	62.1	.4	227.8	.1	10.7
0	.1	2.1	.1	.1	44.5	137.2	38.2	.6	180	.6	38.2
0	0	1.5	0	.2	21.3	36.4	23.2	.3	107.8	.5	23.8
.1	0	.1	0	0	1.6	41.8	70.2	.3	70.2	.2	8.1
0	.1	.2	0	.3	3	36.1	70.1	.6	156.9	.5	25.4
0	0	.4	0	0	6.3	2.6	8.6	.4	26.9	.4	22.8
0	0	0	0	0	0	9.4	1	0	8	0	.3
0	.1	1.7	.1	.2	29.1	144.8	66.1	.5	189.2	.6	36.5
0	0	.1	0	0	1.2	2	12.3	1.2	137.3	.6	47.1
0	.1	.8	0	.1	2.7	57.7	49.9	.5	131.8	.5	25
0	0	0	0	0	0	139.5	1.8	.1	3.2	0	.8
0	0	.1	0	0	1.4	74.8	46.9	.4	75	.1	2.3
0	0	.1	0	.1	1.4	47.8	17.7	.2	41.4	.1	6.4
0	.1	.2	0	.1	3.8	105.8	62.6	.4	113.4	.4	15.7
.1	.1	1.7	.1	.1	12.4	157.7	69.7	1.3	174.4	.8	41.6
0	.1	1.2	0	.1	26.8	131.2	51.2	.4	130	.6	24.8
0	0	0	0	0	.2	.4	2.5	.1	45.4	0	1.8
0	0	0	0	0	3.3	3.3	4	.1	17.6	0	1
0	0	0	0	0	.6	1.7	.6	0	5.9	0	.4
0	0	0	0	0	1.8	0	1.8	.1	13.8	0	1

	Calories (kcal)	Protein (gm)	Carbohydrates (gm)	Fat (gm)	Percent Saturated Fat	Cholesterol (mg)	Dietary Fiber (gm)	Vitamin A (RE)	Vitamin C (mg)
Jellies, all flavors - 1 tbsp (19gm)	51.9	0	13.4	0	0	0	.1	.2	.2
Jellies, diet, all flavors - 1 tbsp (19gm)	6	.1	10.9	0	0	0	9.4	0	0
Marmalade, all flavors - 1 tbsp (20gm)	51	.1	14	0	0	0	1	1	1.2

Sugar

	Calories (kcal)	Protein (gm)	Carbohydrates (gm)	Fat (gm)	Percent Saturated Fat	Cholesterol (mg)	Dietary Fiber (gm)	Vitamin A (RE)	Vitamin C (mg)
Brown - 2 tsp, packed (9gm)	34	0	8.7	0	0	0	0	0	0
Caramelized - 2 tbsp (30gm)	112	0	28.9	0	0	0	.1	0	0
Cinnamon sugar - 2 tsp (8gm)	30	0	7.9	0	0	0	.1	.1	.1
Maple - 1 tsp (3gm)	10	0	2.7	0	0	0	0	0	0
Raw sugar - 1 indiv packet (41gm)	153	0	39.5	0	0	0	.2	0	0
White, confectioner's - 1 cup (120gm)	462	0	119.4	0	0	0	0	0	0
White, granulated - 2 tsp (8gm)	31	0	8	0	0	0	0	0	0

Syrup

	Calories (kcal)	Protein (gm)	Carbohydrates (gm)	Fat (gm)	Percent Saturated Fat	Cholesterol (mg)	Dietary Fiber (gm)	Vitamin A (RE)	Vitamin C (mg)
Buttered blends - 2 tbsp (39gm)	116	0	28.5	.6	62.3	1.7	0	5.9	0
Cane - 2 tbsp (41gm)	108	0	27.9	0	0	0	0	0	0
Chocolate, thin - 2 tbsp (38gm)	83	.9	22.3	.3	60	0	.7	.4	0
Corn - 2 tbsp (41gm)	119	0	30.7	0	0	0	0	0	0
Dietetic - 2 tbsp (30gm)	12	.2	14.8	0	0	0	0	0	0
Fruit - 2 tbsp (39gm)	103	0	26.5	0	0	0	0	0	0
Grenadine - 2 tbsp (40gm)	105	0	27.2	0	0	0	0	0	0
Honey - 2 tbsp (42gm)	128	.1	34.6	0	0	0	.1	0	.4
Maple - 2 tbsp (39gm)	98	0	25.3	0	0	0	0	0	0
Molasses - 2 tbsp (41gm)	103	0	26.6	0	0	0	0	0	0
Molasses, Blackstrap - 1 cup (328gm)	699	0	180.4	0	-	0	-	0	0
Reduced calorie - 2 tbsp (30gm)	51	0	12.9	0	0	0	.1	0	0
Sorghum - 2 tbsp (41gm)	105	0	27.9	0	0	0	0	0	0

Toppings

	Calories (kcal)	Protein (gm)	Carbohydrates (gm)	Fat (gm)	Percent Saturated Fat	Cholesterol (mg)	Dietary Fiber (gm)	Vitamin A (RE)	Vitamin C (mg)
Butterscotch or caramel - 2 tbsp (42gm)	124	.1	29.9	.9	90.6	.1	0	1.2	0
Dietetic - 2 tbsp (28gm)	15	.6	3.8	.4	58.2	0	1.2	.1	.1
Chocolate - 2 tbsp (34gm)	132	.4	26.1	3.7	22.8	.3	.6	46.3	0
Chocolate fudge - 2 tbsp (42gm)	139	2.1	22.7	5.8	61.2	5	1.3	11.8	0
Fruit - 2 tbsp (42gm)	114	.3	29.4	0	0	0	.9	0	.8
Marshmallow - 2 tbsp (38gm)	108	.7	27.3	0	0	.3	0	0	0

Thiamin (mg)	Riboflavin (mg)	Niacin (mg)	Vitamin B$_6$ (mg)	Vitamin B$_{12}$ (mcg)	Folacin (mcg)	Sodium (mg)	Calcium (mg)	Iron (mg)	Potassium (mg)	Zinc (mg)	Magnesium (mg)
0	0	0	0	0	.2	7	1.3	.1	12.5	0	.9
0	0	0	0	0	.2	.2	1.3	0	12.5	0	.9
0	0	0	0	0	7.2	11.2	7	0	6.6	0	.4
0	0	0	0	0	0	2.7	7.6	.2	31	0	1.8
0	0	0	0	0	0	9	25.5	.7	103.2	.1	6
0	0	0	0	0	.1	.2	6.3	.2	2.8	0	.3
0	0	0	0	0	0	.4	4.3	0	7.3	0	.4
0	0	0	0	0	0	12.3	34.8	.9	141	.1	8.2
0	0	0	0	0	0	1.2	0	.1	3.6	0	0
0	0	0	0	0	0	.1	0	0	.2	0	0
0	0	0	0	0	0	117.4	1.8	.2	7.4	0	1
.1	0	0	0	0	0	23.8	5.3	1.5	25.8	.1	4.1
0	0	.2	0	0	1.5	36.5	6.5	.8	85.1	.3	24.7
0	0	0	0	0	0	37.7	1.2	.2	7.8	0	.8
0	0	0	0	0	0	6.3	0	0	0	0	0
.1	0	0	0	0	0	22.6	5.1	1.4	24.6	.1	3.9
.1	0	0	0	0	0	23.2	5.2	1.4	25.2	.1	4
0	0	.1	0	0	0	2.1	2.1	.2	26	.2	.8
.1	0	0	0	0	0	3.9	40.6	.5	68.6	0	3.5
0	0	.1	.1	0	0	6.1	67.6	1.8	376	.1	18.9
.4	.6	6.6	-	-	-	314.9	2243.5	52.8	9600	-	-
0	0	0	0	0	0	57.9	.9	0	.6	0	.6
.1	0	0	0	0	0	4.1	70.5	5.1	72.2	0	.8
0	0	0	0	0	.1	35.1	3.7	.2	10.4	0	1
0	0	.1	0	0	1.2	23.7	7.1	.5	104.4	.2	16.1
0	0	0	0	0	.8	71.7	6.5	.3	46.6	.1	8.2
0	.1	.1	0	.2	2.5	48.3	42	.5	90.3	.3	20.2
0	0	.1	0	0	0	5	8.4	.4	37	0	2.5
0	0	0	0	0	0	29.9	1.7	.5	2	0	1

	Calories (kcal)	Protein (gm)	Carbohydrates (gm)	Fat (gm)	Percent Saturated Fat	Cholesterol (mg)	Dietary Fiber (gm)	Vitamin A (RE)	Vitamin C (mg)
Nut, wet - 2 tbsp (42gm)	172	2.3	20.4	10.1	9	0	.9	2	.5
White - 2 tbsp (40gm)	161	.1	31.7	4.3	20.5	.4	0	57.7	0

CEREALS

Ready To Serve

	Calories (kcal)	Protein (gm)	Carbohydrates (gm)	Fat (gm)	Percent Saturated Fat	Cholesterol (mg)	Dietary Fiber (gm)	Vitamin A (RE)	Vitamin C (mg)
All-Bran - ⅓ c (28.4gm)	71	4	21.1	.5	-	0	8.5	375	15
Alpha-Bits - 1 c (28.4gm)	111	2.2	24.6	.6	-	0	.3	375	0
Apple Jacks - 1 c (28.4gm)	110	1.5	25.7	.1	-	0	.2	375	15
Bran, wheat unprocessed 1 cup (58 gm)	124	9.3	35.9	2.7	16.1	0	23.3	0	0
Bran Buds - ⅓ c (28.4gm)	73	3.9	21.6	.7	-	0	7.9	375	15
Bran Chex - ⅔ c (28.4gm)	91	2.9	22.6	.8	-	0	4.6	6	15
C.W. Post, plain - 1 oz (28.4gm)	126	2.6	20.3	4.4	75.2	.1	.7	375	0
C.W. Post, w/raisins - 1 oz (28.4gm)	123	2.4	20.3	4	75.5	.1	.5	375	0
Cap'n Crunch - ¾ c (28.4gm)	119	1.5	22.9	2.6	65.8	0	.3	4	0
Cap'n Crunch's Crunchberries - ¾ c (28.4gm)	118	1.5	23.1	2.4	65	.1	.3	4	0
Cap'n Crunch's Peanut Butter - ¾ c (28.4gm)	124	2	21.5	3.7	41.6	0	.3	4	0
Cheerios - 1¼ c (28.4gm)	111	4.3	19.6	1.8	18.9	0	1.1	375	15
Cocoa Krispies - ¾ c (28.4 gm)	110	1.5	25.2	.4	-	0	.1	375	15
Cocoa Pebbles - ⅞ c (28.4gm)	116	1.3	24.3	1.5	-	0	.1	375	0
Cookie-Crisp, choc chip and van - 1 c (28.4gm)	114	1.4	24.8	1	-	0	.2	375	15
Corn bran - 1 oz (28.4gm)	98	1.9	23.9	1	-	0	5.4	6	0
Corn Chex - 1 c (28.4gm)	111	2	24.9	.1	-	0	.5	14	15
Corn Flakes, Kellogg's - 1 c (28.4gm)	110	2.3	24.4	.1	-	0	.3	375	15
Corn flakes, low-sodium - 1 c (28.4gm)	113	2.2	25.2	.1	-	0	.5	11	0
Corn Flakes, Ralston Purina - 1 c (28.4gm)	111	2.2	24.6	.1	-	0	.6	11	0
Cracklin' Bran - ½ c (28.4gm)	108	2.6	19.4	4.1	-	0	4.3	375	15
Crisp rice, low-sodium - 1 c (28.4gm)	114	1.6	25.8	.1	-	0	.2	0	0
Crispy Rice - 1 c (28.4gm)	112	1.8	25.1	.1	-	0	.4	0	1
Crispy Wheats 'n Raisins - ¾ c (28.4gm)	99	2	23.1	.5	-	0	1.3	375	0
Fortified oat flakes - ⅔ c (28.4gm)	105	5.3	20.5	.4	-	0	.7	375	0

Thiamin (mg)	Riboflavin (mg)	Niacin (mg)	Vitamin B$_6$ (mg)	Vitamin B$_{12}$ (mcg)	Folacin (mcg)	Sodium (mg)	Calcium (mg)	Iron (mg)	Potassium (mg)	Zinc (mg)	Magnesium (mg)
.1	0	.2	.1	0	10.8	16.5	18.7	1.3	98.4	.5	30.2
0	0	0	0	0	.2	89.1	5	0	7.2	0	.6

Source: USDA Food Consumption Survey and "nonupdated" database

Thiamin (mg)	Riboflavin (mg)	Niacin (mg)	Vitamin B$_6$ (mg)	Vitamin B$_{12}$ (mcg)	Folacin (mcg)	Sodium (mg)	Calcium (mg)	Iron (mg)	Potassium (mg)	Zinc (mg)	Magnesium (mg)
.4	.4	5	.5	0	100	320	23	4.5	350	3.7	106
.4	.4	5	.5	1.5	100	219	8	1.8	110	1.5	17
.4	.4	5	.5	0	100	125	3	4.5	23	3.7	6
.4	.2	12.2	.2	0	63.8	5.2	69	6.3	650	4.8	348
.4	.4	5	.5	0	100	174	19	4.5	474	3.7	90
.4	.1	5	.5	1.5	100	263	17	4.5	228	1.2	73
.4	.4	5	.5	1.5	100	49	14	4.5	58	.5	20
.4	.4	5	.5	1.5	100	44	14	4.5	72	.4	20
.5	.6	6.6	.8	1.8	182	213	5	7.5	36	3.1	12
.5	.5	6.6	.8	2	103	197	9	7.3	40	2.9	11
.5	.6	7.3	.8	1.9	197	217	6	7.4	46	3.1	15
.4	.4	5	.5	1.5	6	307	48	4.5	101	.8	39
.4	.4	5	.5	0	100	217	5	1.8	42	1.5	9
.4	.4	5	.5	1.5	100	136	5	1.8	47	1.5	12
.4	.4	5	.5	1.5	3	195	5	4.5	28	.3	8
.3	.6	8.6	.7	1.1	183	244	33	9.6	55	3.1	14
.4	.1	5	.5	1.5	100	271	3	1.8	23	.1	4
.4	.4	5	.5	0	100	351	1	1.8	26	.1	3
0	.1	.1	0	0	2	3	12	.6	21	.1	4
.1	0	1.2	0	0	2	271	2	.7	25	.1	3
.4	.4	5	.5	0	100	230	19	1.8	168	1.5	55
0	.1	.4	0	0	3	3	19	.9	22	.4	11
.1	0	2	0	.1	3	208	5	.7	27	.5	12
.4	.4	5	.5	1.5	10	135	47	4.5	115	.3	23
.4	.4	5	.5	1.5	100	253	40	8.1	203	.9	34

	Calories (kcal)	Protein (gm)	Carbohydrates (gm)	Fat (gm)	Percent Saturated Fat	Cholesterol (mg)	Dietary Fiber (gm)	Vitamin A (RE)	Vitamin C (mg)
Froot Loops - 1 c (28.4gm)	111	1.7	25	.5	-	0	.2	375	15
Frosted Mini-Wheats - abt 4 biscuits (28.4gm)	102	2.9	23.4	.3	-	0	2.1	375	15
Frosted Rice Krinkles - ⅞ c (28.4gm)	109	1.4	25.8	.1	-	0	0	375	0
Frosted Rice Krispies - 1 c (28.4gm)	109	1.3	25.7	.1	-	0	.1	375	15
Fruity Pebbles - ⅞ c (28.4gm)	115	1.1	24.4	1.5	-	0	0	375	0
Golden Grahams - ¾ c (28.4gm)	109	1.6	24.1	1.1	-	.1	.5	375	15
Graham Crackos - 1 oz (28.4gm)	102	2.1	24.5	.2	-	0	1.7	375	15
Granola, homemade - ⅓ c (28.4gm)	138	3.5	15.6	7.7	17.7	0	-	-	0
Grape-Nuts Flakes - ⅞ c (28.4gm)	102	3	23.2	.3	-	0	1.8	375	0
Grape-Nuts - ¼ c (28.4gm)	101	3.3	23.2	.1	-	0	1.4	375	0
Heartland Natural, plain - 1 oz (28.4gm)	123	2.9	19.4	4.4	-	0	1.3	-	0
Heartland Natural, w/coconut - 1 oz (28.4gm)	125	3	19.2	4.6	-	0	1.4	-	0
Heartland Natural, w/raisins - 1 oz (28.4gm)	120	2.8	19.6	4	-	0	1.3	-	0
Honey & Nut Corn Flakes - ¾ c (28.4gm)	113	1.8	23.3	1.5	-	0	.3	375	15
Honey Nut Cheerios - ¾ c (28.4gm)	107	3.1	22.8	.7	-	0	-	375	15
Honeybran - 1 oz (28.4gm)	97	2.5	23.2	.6	-	0	3.1	375	15
Honeycomb - 1⅓ c (28.4gm)	111	1.6	25.3	.5	-	0	.4	375	0
Kix - 1½ c (28.4gm)	110	2.5	23.4	.7	-	0	.4	375	15
Life, plain and cinn - ⅔ c (28.4gm)	104	5.2	20.3	.5	-	0	.9	-	-
Lucky Charms - 1 c (28.4gm)	110	2.6	23.2	1.1	-	0	.6	375	15
Nature Valley Granola - 1 oz (28.4gm)	126	2.9	18.9	4.9	66.7	0	1	-	0
Nutri-Grain, Barley - ½ c (28.4gm)	106	3.1	23.5	.2	-	0	1.7	375	15
Nutri-Grain, Corn - ½ c (28.4gm)	108	2.3	23.9	.7	-	0	1.8	375	15
Nutri-Grain, Rye - 1 oz (28.4gm)	102	2.5	24	.2	-	0	1.8	375	15
Nutri-Grain, Wheat - ⅔ c (28.4gm)	102	2.5	24	.3	-	0	1.8	375	15
Product 19 - ¾ c (28.4gm)	108	2.8	23.5	.2	-	0	.3	1502	60
Quisp - 1⅙ c (28.4gm)	117	1.4	23.6	2.1	-	0	.4	4	0
Raisin Bran, Kellogg's - ¾ c (36.9gm)	115	4	27.9	.7	-	0	4	375	0

Thiamin (mg)	Riboflavin (mg)	Niacin (mg)	Vitamin B$_6$ (mg)	Vitamin B$_{12}$ (mcg)	Folacin (mcg)	Sodium (mg)	Calcium (mg)	Iron (mg)	Potassium (mg)	Zinc (mg)	Magnesium (mg)
.4	.4	5	.5	0	100	145	3	4.5	26	3.7	7
.4	.4	5	.5	0	100	8	9	1.8	97	1.5	23
.4	.4	5	.5	1.5	100	179	4	1.8	14	1.5	8
.4	.4	5	.5	0	100	240	1	1.8	21	.3	5
.4	.4	5	.5	1.5	100	157	3	1.8	21	1.5	8
.4	.4	5	.5	1.5	4	346	17	4.5	63	.3	12
.4	.4	5	.5	0	100	185	13	1.8	102	1.5	24
.2	.1	.5	.1	0	23	3	18	1.1	142	1	33
.4	.4	5	.5	1.5	100	218	11	4.5	99	.6	31
.4	.4	5	.5	1.5	100	197	11	1.2	95	.6	19
.1	0	.4	0	0	16	72	19	1.1	95	.8	36
.1	0	.5	0	0	15	57	18	1.4	104	.7	37
.1	0	.4	.1	0	11	58	17	1	107	.7	36
.4	.4	5	.5	0	100	225	3	1.8	36	.1	6
.4	.4	5	.5	1.5	18	257	20	4.5	99	.7	33
.4	.4	5	.5	1.5	19	164	13	4.5	122	.7	37
.4	.4	5	.5	1.5	100	213	5	1.8	91	1.5	10
.4	.4	5	.5	1.5	3	339	35	8.1	44	.3	12
.6	.6	7.5	.1	0	24	148	99	7.5	127	.9	9
.4	.4	5	.5	1.5	6	201	32	4.5	59	.5	24
.1	.1	.2	0	0	21	58	18	.9	98	.6	29
.4	.4	5	.5	1.5	100	192	8	1	75	3.7	22
.4	.4	5	.5	1.5	100	187	1	.6	66	3.7	18
.4	.4	5	.5	1.5	100	193	6	.8	51	3.7	22
.4	.4	5	.5	1.5	100	193	8	.8	77	3.7	22
1.5	1.7	20	2	6	400	325	3	18	44	.4	11
.5	.7	5.5	.9	2.4	8	228	9	6	42	.2	12
.4	.4	5	.5	1.5	100	269	13	4.5	192	3.8	48

	Calories (kcal)	Protein (gm)	Carbohydrates (gm)	Fat (gm)	Percent Saturated Fat	Cholesterol (mg)	Dietary Fiber (gm)	Vitamin A (RE)	Vitamin C (mg)
Raisin Bran, Post - ½ c (28.4gm)	87	2.6	21.4	.5	-	0	3	375	0
Raisin Bran, Ralston Purina - ¾ c (37.8gm)	120	3	31.4	.2	-	0	4.8	375	1
Raisins, Rice & Rye - 1.3 oz (36.9gm)	124	2.1	31.5	.1	-	0	-	375	0
Rice Chex - 1⅛ c (28.4gm)	112	1.5	25.3	.1	-	0	.2	2	15
Rice Krispies - 1 c (28.4gm)	112	1.9	24.8	.2	-	0	.1	375	15
Rice, puffed - 1 c (14.2gm)	57	.9	12.8	.1	-	0	.1	0	0
Special K - 1 c (28.4gm)	111	5.6	21.3	.1	-	0	.2	375	15
Sugar Corn Pops - 1 c (28.4gm)	108	1.4	25.6	.1	-	0	.2	375	15
Sugar Frosted Flakes, Kellogg's - ¾ c (28.4gm)	108	1.4	25.7	.1	-	0	.3	375	15
Sugar Frosted Flakes, Ralston Purina - ¾ c (28.4gm)	111	1.5	25.5	.4	-	0	.4	375	15
Sugar Smacks - ¾ c (28.4gm)	106	2	24.7	.5	-	0	.4	375	15
Super Sugar Crisp - ⅞ c (28.4gm)	106	1.8	25.6	.3	-	0	.4	375	0
Tasteeos - 1 oz (28.4gm)	111	3.6	22.4	.8	-	0	1	375	15
Team - 1 oz (28.4gm)	111	1.8	24.3	.5	-	0	.3	375	15
Toasties - 1 oz (28.4gm)	110	2.3	24.3	.1	-	0	.5	375	-
Total - 1 c (28.4gm)	100	2.8	22.3	.6	-	0	2	1502	60
Trix - 1 c (28.4gm)	109	1.5	25.2	.4	-	0	.1	375	15
Waffelos - 1 oz (28.4gm)	115	1.6	24.5	1.2	-	0	.3	375	15
Wheat 'n Raisin Chex - 1⅓ oz (37.8gm)	130	3.5	30.1	.3	-	0	2.5	0	1
Wheat Chex - ⅔ c (28.4gm)	104	2.8	23.3	.7	-	0	2.1	0	15
Wheat germ tstd, plain - ¼ c (28.4gm)	108	8.3	14.1	3	-	0	-	0	2
Wheat germ, tstd, w/brn sgr and honey - ¼ c (28.4gm)	107	6.2	17.2	2.3	-	0	-	0	-
Wheat, puffed - 1 c (14.2gm)	52	2.1	11.3	.2	-	0	.5	0	0
Wheat, shredded, large - 1 biscuit (23.6gm)	83	2.6	18.8	.3	-	0	2.2	0	0
Wheat, shredded, small - 1 oz (28.4gm)	102	3.1	22.6	.6	-	0	2.6	0	0
Wheaties - 1 c (28.4gm)	99	2.7	22.6	.5	-	0	2	375	15
100% Bran - ⅓ c (28.4gm)	76	3.5	20.7	1.4	-	0	8.4	0	27
100% Natural, plain - ¼ c (28.4gm)	133	3.3	17.8	6.1	67.2	.2	1	-	0
100% Natural, w/apple and cinn - ¼ c (28.4gm)	130	2.9	19	5.3	79.6	.3	1.3	-	0
100% Natural, w/raisins and dates - ¼ c (28.4gm)	128	2.9	18.7	5.2	67.9	.2	1.1	-	0
40% Bran Flakes, Kellogg's - ¾ c (28.4gm)	93	3.6	22.2	.5	-	0	4	375	0

Thiamin (mg)	Riboflavin (mg)	Niacin (mg)	Vitamin B$_6$ (mg)	Vitamin B$_{12}$ (mcg)	Folacin (mcg)	Sodium (mg)	Calcium (mg)	Iron (mg)	Potassium (mg)	Zinc (mg)	Magnesium (mg)
.4	.4	5	.5	1.5	100	185	13	4.5	175	1.5	48
.4	.4	5	.5	1.5	100	328	18	4.5	194	1.1	57
.4	.4	5	.5	1.5	100	280	8	4.5	115	3.8	16
.4	0	5	.5	1.5	100	237	4	1.8	33	.4	7
.4	.4	5	.5	0	100	340	4	1.8	30	.5	10
.4	.3	5	0	0	3	0	1	4.5	16	.1	3
.4	.4	5	.5	0	100	265	8	4.5	49	3.7	16
.4	.4	5	.5	0	100	103	1	1.8	17	1.5	2
.4	.4	5	.5	0	100	230	1	1.8	18	0	2
.4	.4	5	.5	1.5	2	184	3	.7	18	.6	2
.4	.4	5	.5	0	100	75	3	1.8	42	.3	13
.4	.4	5	.5	1.5	100	25	6	1.8	105	1.5	17
.4	.4	5	.5	1.5	11	216	13	4.5	84	.8	31
.4	.4	5	.5	1.5	5	175	4	1.7	48	.4	13
.4	.4	5	.5	1.5	100	297	1	.8	33	.1	4
1.5	1.7	20	2	6	400	352	48	18	106	.7	32
.4	.4	5	.5	1.5	3	181	6	4.5	27	.1	6
.4	.4	5	.5	1.5	3	118	8	4.5	25	.2	6
.4	.4	5	.5	1.5	100	214	17	5.4	159	.8	37
.4	.1	5	.5	1.5	100	190	11	4.5	107	.8	36
.5	.2	1.6	.3	0	100	1	13	2.6	268	4.7	91
.4	.2	1.2	.2	0	75	1	9	1.9	201	3.5	68
.4	.3	5	0	0	5	1	4	4.5	49	.3	21
.1	.1	1.1	.1	0	12	0	10	.7	77	.6	40
.1	.1	1.5	.1	0	14	3	11	1.2	102	.9	37
.4	.4	5	.5	1.5	9	354	43	4.5	106	.6	31
.7	.8	9	.9	2.7	20	196	20	3.5	354	2.5	134
.1	.1	.6	.1	0	9	12	49	.8	140	.6	34
.1	.2	.5	0	.1	5	14	43	.8	140	.6	19
.1	.2	.5	0	0	12	12	41	.8	139	.5	32
.4	.4	5	.5	1.5	100	264	14	8.1	180	3.7	52

	Calories (kcal)	Protein (gm)	Carbohydrates (gm)	Fat (gm)	Percent Saturated Fat	Cholesterol (mg)	Dietary Fiber (gm)	Vitamin A (RE)	Vitamin C (mg)
40% Bran Flakes, Post - ¾ c (28.4gm)	92	3.2	22.5	.5	-	0	3.9	375	0
40% Bran Flakes, Ralston Purina - ¾ c (28.4gm)	92	3.3	22.6	.4	-	0	3.5	375	15

Cooked Cereals

	Calories (kcal)	Protein (gm)	Carbohydrates (gm)	Fat (gm)	Percent Saturated Fat	Cholesterol (mg)	Dietary Fiber (gm)	Vitamin A (RE)	Vitamin C (mg)
Corn grits, instant, plain - 1 pkt (22.7gm)	82	2.1	17.8	.2	-	0	-	0	0
Corn grits, instant, w/art cheese flavor - 1 pkt (28.4gm)	107	2.8	21.3	.9	-	.9	-	3	0
Corn grits, instant, w/imitn bacon bits - 1 pkt (28.4gm)	104	3	21.5	.5	-	0	-	0	0
Corn grits, instant, w/imtn ham bits - 1 pkt (28.4gm)	103	2.9	21.4	.4	-	0	-	0	0
Corn grits reg and quick - 1 c ckd w/salt (242gm)	146	3.5	31.4	.5	-	0	.6	0	0
Corn grits, reg and quick, - 1 c ckd wo/salt (242gm)	146	3.5	31.4	.5	-	0	.6	0	0
Corn grits, reg and quick - 1 c dry (156gm)	579	13.7	124.1	1.8	-	0	2.5	0	0
Cream of Rice - 1 c ckd w/salt (244gm)	126	2.1	28.1	.1	-	0	-	0	0
Cream of Rice - 1 c ckd wo/salt (244gm)	126	2.1	28.1	.1	-	0	-	0	0
Cream of Rice - 1 c dry (173gm)	641	10.8	142.6	.8	-	0	-	0	0
Cream of Wheat, instant - 1 c dry (178gm)	651	18.9	134.3	2.5	-	0	-	0	0
Cream of Wheat, instant - 1 c ckd w/salt (241gm)	153	4.4	31.6	.6	-	0	-	0	0
Cream of Wheat, instant - 1 c ckd wo/salt (241gm)	153	4.4	31.6	.6	-	0	-	0	0
Cream of Wheat, Mix 'n Eat (appl, ban, mapl flav) - 1 pkt (35.4gm)	132	2.5	28.9	.4	-	0	-	375	0
Cream of Wheat, Mix 'n Eat, plain - 1 pkt (28.4gm)	102	2.8	21.4	.3	-	0	-	375	0
Cream of Wheat, quick - 1 c ckd w/salt (239gm)	129	3.6	26.7	.5	-	0	-	0	0
Cream of Wheat, quick - 1 c ckd w/o salt (239gm)	129	3.6	26.7	.5	-	0	-	0	0
Cream of Wheat, quick, dry - 1 c (175gm)	632	17.8	131.2	2.3	-	0	-	0	0
Cream of Wheat, regular - 1 c ckd w/salt (251gm)	134	3.8	27.7	.5	-	0	-	0	0
Cream of Wheat, regular - 1 c ckd wo/salt (251gm)	134	3.8	27.7	.5	-	0	-	0	0
Cream of Wheat, regular - 1 c dry (173gm)	640	18.2	132.4	2.5	-	0	-	0	0

Thiamin (mg)	Riboflavin (mg)	Niacin (mg)	Vitamin B$_6$ (mg)	Vitamin B$_{12}$ (mcg)	Folacin (mcg)	Sodium (mg)	Calcium (mg)	Iron (mg)	Potassium (mg)	Zinc (mg)	Magnesium (mg)
.4	.4	5	.5	1.5	100	260	12	4.5	151	1.5	61
.4	.4	5	.5	1.5	100	264	13	4.5	166	1.2	68
.2	.1	1.3	0	0	1	344	7	1	29	.1	5
.2	.1	1.4	0	0	1	481	14	1.2	40	.1	7
.2	.1	1.6	0	0	8	531	6	1.3	60	.2	9
.3	.2	1.7	0	0	10	657	7	1.5	52	.2	9
.2	.1	2	.1	0	1	540	1	1.6	54	.2	11
.2	.1	2	.1	0	1	0	1	1.6	54	.2	11
1	.6	7.7	.2	0	7	1	3	6.1	213	.6	42
.1	0	1	.1	0	8	422	8	.4	49	.4	8
.1	0	1	.1	0	8	2	8	.4	49	.4	8
.3	.2	5.2	.3	0	51	10	42	2.2	247	1.9	40
.9	.4	7.5	.2	0	61	27	251	50.9	205	1.7	61
.2	.1	1.8	0	0	11	364	59	12	48	.4	14
.2	.1	1.8	0	0	11	6	59	12	48	.4	14
.4	.2	5	.5	0	100	241	40	8.1	55	.2	9
.4	.3	5	.5	0	100	241	20	8.1	38	.2	8
.2	.1	1.5	0	0	9	464	50	10.2	46	.3	12
.2	.1	1.5	0	0	9	139	50	10.2	46	.3	12
.9	.4	7.4	.2	0	60	684	247	50	228	1.7	58
.2	.1	1.5	0	0	9	336	50	10.3	43	.3	10
.2	.1	1.5	0	0	9	2	50	10.3	43	.3	10
.9	.4	7.3	.2	0	59	11	244	49.4	208	1.5	46

	Calories (kcal)	Protein (gm)	Carbohydrates (gm)	Fat (gm)	Percent Saturated Fat	Cholesterol (mg)	Dietary Fiber (gm)	Vitamin A (RE)	Vitamin C (mg)
Farina - 1 c ckd w/salt (233gm)	116	3.4	24.6	.2	-	0	-	0	0
Farina - 1 c ckd wo/salt (233gm)	116	3.4	24.6	.2	-	0	-	0	0
Farina - 1 c dry (176gm)	649	18.6	137.2	.9	-	0	-	0	0
Malt-O-Meal, plain and choc - 1 c dry (165 mg)	607	17.3	128.3	1.4	-	0	-	0	0
Malt-O-Meal, plain and choc - 1 c ckd w/salt (240gm)	122	3.5	25.8	.3	-	0	-	0	0
Malt-O-Meal, plain and choc - 1 c ckd wo/salt (240gm)	122	3.5	25.8	.3	-	0	-	0	0
Maltex - 1 c ckd w/salt (249gm)	180	5.7	39.5	1.1	-	0	-	0	0
Maltex - 1 c ckd wo/salt (249gm)	180	5.7	39.5	1.1	-	0	-	0	0
Maltex - 1 c dry (151gm)	531	16.9	116.7	3.2	-	0	-	0	0
Maypo - 1 c ckd w/salt (240gm)	170	5.8	31.8	2.4	-	0	-	702	28
Maypo - 1 c ckd wo/salt (240gm)	170	5.8	31.8	2.4	-	0	-	702	28
Maypo - 1 c dry (94gm)	362	12.4	67.7	5	-	0	-	1494	60
Oats, instant, plain - 1 pkt (28.4gm)	104	4.4	18.1	1.7	-	0	-	455	0
Oats, instant w/apples and cinn - 1 pkt (35.4gm)	135	3.9	26.3	1.6	-	0	-	435	0
Oats, instant w/bran and rsns - 1 pkt (42.5gm)	158	4.9	30.4	1.9	-	0	-	479	0
Oats, instant w/cinn and spice - 1 pkt (46.1gm)	177	4.8	35.1	1.9	-	0	-	475	0
Oats, instant w/maple and brn sug flav - 1 pkt (42.5gm)	163	4.6	31.9	1.9	-	0	-	451	0
Oats, instant w/raisins and spice - 1 pkt (42.5gm)	161	4.3	31.8	1.8	-	0	-	440	0
Oats, reg and quick and instant - 1 c ckd w/salt (234gm)	145	6	25.2	2.4	-	0	2.1	-	0
Oats, reg and quick and instant - 1 c ckd wo/salt (234gm)	145	6	25.2	2.4	-	0	2.1	-	0
Oats, reg and quick and instant - 1 c dry (81gm)	311	13	54.2	5.1	-	0	4.6	-	0
Ralston - 1 c ckd w/salt (253gm)	134	5.5	28.2	.8	-	0	-	0	0
Ralston - 1 c ckd wo/salt (253gm)	134	5.5	28	.8	-	0	-	0	0
Ralston - 1 c dry (118gm)	402	16.7	85.1	2.5	-	0	11.2	0	0
Roman Meal - 1 c ckd w/salt (240gm)	169	7.2	34.1	2	-	0	-	-	0
Roman Meal w/oats - 1 c ckd wo/salt (240gm)	169	7.2	34.1	2	-	0	-	-	0

Thiamin (mg)	Riboflavin (mg)	Niacin (mg)	Vitamin B_6 (mg)	Vitamin B_{12} (mcg)	Folacin (mcg)	Sodium (mg)	Calcium (mg)	Iron (mg)	Potassium (mg)	Zinc (mg)	Magnesium (mg)
.2	.1	1.3	0	0	6	767	4	1.2	30	.2	4
.2	.1	1.3	0	0	6	1	4	1.2	30	.2	4
1	.6	7.1	.1	0	42	5	25	6.5	165	.9	23
2.1	1.5	29	.1	0	40	17	23	47.2	155	.9	22
.4	.3	5.9	0	0	6	324	5	9.5	31	.2	4
.4	.3	5.9	0	0	6	2	5	9.5	31	.2	4
.3	.1	2.4	.1.	0	22	189	18	1.8	266	1.9	57
.3	.1	2.4	.1	0	22	9	18	1.8	266	1.9	57
.8	.3	7	.2	0	86	26	54	5.3	787	5.5	168
.7	.8	9.4	.9	2.8	9	259	125	8.4	211	1.5	51
.7	.8	9.4	.9	2.8	9	9	125	8.4	211	1.5	51
1.5	1.7	19.9	2	5.9	25	18	265	17.9	449	3.1	108
.5	.3	5.5	.7	0	150	286	163	6.3	100	.9	42
.5	.3	5.1	.7	0	137	222	158	6.1	107	.7	34
.6	.6	8.1	.8	0	155	247	173	7.6	236	1.4	57
.6	.3	5.7	.8	0	153	280	172	6.6	104	1	51
.5	.3	5.4	.7	0	145	280	162	6.4	102	.9	42
.5	.4	5.5	.7	0	150	225	165	6.6	150	.7	35
.3	.1	.3	0	0	9	374	20	1.6	132	1.1	56
.3	.1	.3	0	0	9	1	20	1.6	132	1.1	56
.6	.1	.6	.1	0	26	3	42	3.4	284	2.5	120
.2	.2	2.1	.1	.1	18	476	14	1.6	153	1.4	59
.2	.2	2.1	.1	.1	18	4	14	1.6	153	1.4	59
.6	.6	6.2	.3	.3	71	12	42	4.9	462	4.3	179
.3	.2	3.3	.4	0	24	540	27	1.4	256	1.9	75
.3	.2	3.3	.4	0	24	10	27	1.4	256	1.9	75

	Calories (kcal)	Protein (gm)	Carbohydrates (gm)	Fat (gm)	Percent Saturated Fat	Cholesterol (mg)	Dietary Fiber (gm)	Vitamin A (RE)	Vitamin C (mg)
Roman Meal w/oats - 1 c dry (100gm)	340	14.5	68.5	4	-	0	-	-	0
Roman Meal, plain - 1 c ckd w/salt (241gm)	147	6.6	33	1	-	0	-	0	0
Roman Meal, plain - 1 c ckd wo/salt (241gm)	147	6.6	33	1	-	0	-	0	0
Roman Meal, plain - 1 c dry (94gm)	302	13.5	67.6	2	-	0	-	0	0
Wheatena - 1 c ckd wo/salt (243gm)	135	5	28.7	1.1	-	0	-	0	0
Wheatena - 1 c ckd w/salt (243gm)	135	5	28.7	1.1	-	0	-	0	0
Wheatena - 1 c dry (141gm)	503	18.4	106.6	4	-	0	-	0	0
Whole Wheat Natural - 1 c ckd w/salt (242gm)	151	4.9	33.2	.9	-	0	-	0	0
Whole Wheat Natural - 1 c ckd wo/salt (242gm)	151	4.9	33.2	.9	-	0	-	0	0
Whole Wheat Natural - 1 c dry (94gm)	321	10.5	70.7	1.9	-	0	-	0	0

CHEESE

Cheese: Natural

	Calories (kcal)	Protein (gm)	Carbohydrates (gm)	Fat (gm)	Percent Saturated Fat	Cholesterol (mg)	Dietary Fiber (gm)	Vitamin A (RE)	Vitamin C (mg)
Blue - 1 oz (28.4gm)	100	6.1	.7	8.1	65	21.3	0	64.6	0
Brick - 1 oz (28.4gm)	90	5.6	.7	7.1	63.2	22.7	0	73	0
Brie - 1 oz (28.4gm)	95	5.9	.1	7.8	62.9	28.4	0	51.6	0
Camembert, domestic - 1 oz (28.4gm)	85	5.6	.1	6.9	62.9	20.4	0	71.4	0
Caraway - 1 oz (28.4gm)	107	7.1	.9	8.3	63.7	26.4	0	81.9	0
Cheddar, domestic - 1 oz (28.4gm)	114	7.1	.4	9.4	63.7	29.7	0	85.9	0
Cheshire - 1 oz (28.4gm)	110	6.6	1.4	8.7	63.6	29.2	0	69.5	0
Colby - 1 oz (28.4gm)	95	5.7	.4	7.7	63	22.8	0	66	0
Cottage, creamed - 4 oz (113.6gm)	117	14.1	3	5.1	63.3	16.8	0	54.2	0
Cottage, creamed, w/fruit - 4 oz (113.6gm)	140	11.2	15	3.8	63.2	12.7	0	40.7	0
Cottage, lowfat, 1% fat - 4 oz (113.6gm)	82	14	3.1	1.2	-	5	0	12.4	0
Cottage, lowfat, 2% fat - 4 oz (113.6gm)	101	15.5	4.1	2.2	-	9.5	0	22.6	0
Cottage, dry - 4 oz (113.6gm)	96	19.5	2.1	.5	-	7.6	0	9	0
Cream - 1 oz (28.4gm)	99	2.1	.8	9.9	63	31.1	0	123.9	0
Edam - 1 oz (28.4gm)	101	7.1	.4	7.9	63.2	25.3	0	71.7	0
Feta - 1 oz (28.4gm)	75	4	1.2	6	70.2	25.2	0	36.3	0

Thiamin (mg)	Riboflavin (mg)	Niacin (mg)	Vitamin B$_6$ (mg)	Vitamin B$_{12}$ (mcg)	Folacin (mcg)	Sodium (mg)	Calcium (mg)	Iron (mg)	Potassium (mg)	Zinc (mg)	Magnesium (mg)
.6	.4	6.5	.8	0	70	20	55	2.8	513	3.9	150
.2	.1	3.1	.1	0	24	198	30	2.1	302	1.8	109
.2	.1	3.1	.1	0	24	3	30	2.1	302	1.8	109
.5	.2	6.3	.2	0	66	6	61	4.4	620	3.7	223
0	.1	1.3	0	0	17	5	11	1.4	187	1.7	49
0	.1	1.3	0	0	17	578	11	1.4	187	1.7	49
.1	.2	5	.2	0	83	18	40	5	693	6.2	183
.2	.1	2.1	.2	0	26	564	17	1.5	171	1.2	54
.2	.1	2.1	.2	0	26	1	17	1.5	171	1.2	54
.4	.3	4.6	.4	0	74	2	37	3.2	365	2.5	115

Source: USDA Revised *Handbook 8*

0	.1	.3	0	.3	10.3	395.6	149.6	.1	72.7	.8	6.5
0	.1	0	0	.3	4.9	135	162	.1	32.8	.6	6
0	.1	.1	.1	.5	18.4	178.4	52.2	.1	43.1	.7	5.7
0	.1	.2	.1	.4	17.6	238.6	109.9	.1	52.9	.7	5.7
0	.1	.1	0	.1	5.2	195.6	190.9	.2	26.4	.8	6.3
0	.1	0	0	.2	5.2	175.9	204.5	.2	27.9	.9	7.9
0	.1	0	0	.2	5.2	198.4	182.3	.1	26.9	.8	5.9
0	.1	0	0	.1	4.3	145	165	.1	30.5	.7	6.2
0	.2	.1	.1	.7	13.8	457.4	67.8	.2	95.3	.4	5.9
0	.1	.1	.1	.6	11	457.4	53.8	.1	75.6	.3	4.7
0	.2	.1	.1	.7	14	458.8	68.8	.2	96.6	.4	6
0	.2	.2	.1	.8	14.8	458.8	77.4	.2	108.7	.5	6.8
0	.2	.2	.1	.9	16.7	14.5	35.8	.3	36.6	.5	4.5
0	.1	0	0	.1	3.7	83.8	22.7	.3	33.9	.2	1.8
0	.1	0	0	.4	4.6	273.6	207.2	.1	53.2	1.1	8.4
0	.2	.3	.1	.5	9.1	316.4	139.6	.2	17.5	.8	5.4

	Calories (kcal)	Protein (gm)	Carbohydrates (gm)	Fat (gm)	Percent Saturated Fat	Cholesterol (mg)	Dietary Fiber (gm)	Vitamin A (RE)	Vitamin C (mg)
Fontina - 1 oz (28.4gm)	110	7.3	.4	8.8	61.6	32.9	0	82.2	0
Gjetost - 1 oz (28.4gm)	132	2.7	12.1	8.4	64.9	26.6	0	77.7	0
Gouda - 1 oz (28.4gm)	101	7.1	.6	7.8	64.2	32.3	0	49.3	0
Gruyere - 1 oz (28.4 gm)	117	8.5	.1	9.2	58.5	31.2	0	85.3	0
Limburger - 1 oz (28.4gm)	93	5.7	.1	7.7	61.5	25.5	0	89.6	0
Monterey - 1 oz (28.4gm)	106	6.9	.2	8.6	63	25.2	0	71.7	0
Mozzarella, part skim - 1 oz (28.4gm)	72	6.9	.8	4.5	63.5	16.4	0	50.2	0
Mozzarella, part skim, low moisture -1 oz (28.4gm)	80	8	1	5	63.5	15	0	54	0
Mozzarella, whole milk - 1 oz (28.4gm)	80	5.5	.6	6.1	60.9	22.2	0	68.3	0
Muenster - 1 oz (28.4gm)	104	6.6	.3	8.5	63.6	27.1	0	89.6	0
Neufchatel - 1 oz (28.4gm)	74	2.8	.8	6.6	63.2	21.6	0	74.8	0
Parmesan, grated -1 tbsp (5gm)	23	2.1	.2	1.5	-	3.9	0	8.6	0
Parmesan - 1 oz (28.4gm)	111	10.1	.9	7.3	63.5	19.2	0	42.2	0
Port de Salut - 1 oz (28.4gm)	98	6.7	.2	8	59.2	34.9	0	105.5	0
Provolone - 1 oz (28.4gm)	100	7.3	.6	7.5	64.2	19.5	0	74.8	0
Ricotta, part skim -½ c (124gm)	171	14.1	6.4	9.8	62.3	38.2	0	140.1	0
Ricotta, whole milk - ½ c (124gm)	216	14	3.8	16.1	63.9	62.7	0	166.2	0
Romano - 1 oz (28.4gm)	110	9	1	7.6	63.5	29.5	0	40	0
Roquefort - 1 oz (28.4gm)	105	6.1	.6	8.7	62.9	25.5	0	84.8	0
Swiss - 1 oz (28.4gm)	83	6.4	.5	6	64.8	20	0	56	0
Tilsit - 1 oz (28.4gm)	96	6.9	.5	7.4	64.6	28.9	0	82.5	0

Cheese: Processed

	Calories (kcal)	Protein (gm)	Carbohydrates (gm)	Fat (gm)	Percent Saturated Fat	Cholesterol (mg)	Dietary Fiber (gm)	Vitamin A (RE)	Vitamin C (mg)
American - 1 oz (28.4gm)	105	6	.3	9	63	27	0	82	0
Swiss - 1 oz (28.4gm)	95	7	.4	7	64.2	24	0	65	0
Cheese food; cold pack, American - 1 oz (28.4gm)	94	5.6	2.4	6.9	62.8	18	0	57.3	0
Cheese food; pasteurized American - 1 oz (28.4gm)	93	5.6	2.1	7	62.8	18.1	0	62.1	0
Cheese food, Swiss - 1 oz (28.4gm)	92	6.2	1.3	6.8	64.2	23.2	0	68.9	0
Cheese spread; American - 1 oz (28.4gm)	82	4.7	2.5	6	62.8	15.6	0	53.6	0

COOKIES

	Calories (kcal)	Protein (gm)	Carbohydrates (gm)	Fat (gm)	Percent Saturated Fat	Cholesterol (mg)	Dietary Fiber (gm)	Vitamin A (RE)	Vitamin C (mg)
Almond - 1 (10gm)	52	.9	5.1	3.2	16.5	5.9	.2	27.9	0
Applesauce - 1 (13gm)	48	.7	8.2	1.6	20.2	4.1	.5	19.6	.1

Thiamin (mg)	Riboflavin (mg)	Niacin (mg)	Vitamin B$_6$ (mg)	Vitamin B$_{12}$ (mcg)	Folacin (mcg)	Sodium (mg)	Calcium (mg)	Iron (mg)	Potassium (mg)	Zinc (mg)	Magnesium (mg)
0	.1	0	0	.5	1.7	226.8	155.9	.1	18	1	4
.1	.4	.2	.1	.7	1.3	170.1	113.4	.1	399.5	.3	19.8
0	.1	0	0	.4	5.9	232.3	198.4	.1	34.2	1.1	8.2
0	.1	0	0	.5	2.9	95.3	286.6	0	23	1.1	10.2
0	.1	0	0	.3	16.3	226.8	140.8	0	36.3	.6	6
0	.1	0	0	.2	5.2	152	211.6	.2	22.9	.9	7.7
0	.1	0	0	.2	2.5	132.1	183.1	.1	23.7	.8	6.6
0	.1	0	0	.2	1.7	150	207	.1	27	.8	6.4
0	.1	0	0	.2	2	105.8	146.6	.1	19	.6	5.3
0	.1	0	0	.4	3.4	178	203.4	.1	38.1	.8	7.8
0	.1	0	0	.1	3.2	113.2	21.3	.1	32.3	.1	2.2
0	0	0	0	.1	.4	93.1	68.8	0	5.4	.2	2.5
0	.1	.1	0	.3	2	454	335.5	.2	26.1	.8	12.4
0	.1	0	0	.4	5.2	151.4	184.2	.1	38.5	.7	6.9
0	.1	0	0	.4	2.9	248.2	214.3	.1	39.2	.9	7.8
0	.2	.1	0	.4	16.2	154.6	337.3	.5	155	1.7	18.3
0	.2	.1	.1	.4	15.1	104.3	256.7	.5	129.7	1.4	14
0	.1	0	0	.3	1.9	340.2	301.6	.2	24.5	.7	11.6
0	.2	.2	0	.2	13.9	512.9	187.6	.2	25.7	.6	8.4
0	.1	0	0	.4	1.5	58	213	0	24.5	.9	8
0	.1	.1	0	.6	5.7	213.5	198.4	.1	18.3	1	3.7
0	.1	0	0	.1	2	406	174	.1	46	.7	5.8
0	0	0	0	.2	1.7	388	219	.1	61	.9	7.7
0	.1	0	0	.4	1.5	273.9	141	.2	102.9	.9	8.4
0	.1	0	0	.3	2.1	337.2	162.8	.2	79.1	.8	8.7
0	.1	0	0	.7	1.6	440	205.1	.2	80.5	1	7.9
0	.1	0	0	.1	2	381.4	159.3	.1	68.6	.7	8.1

Source: USDA Revised *Handbook 8*

0	0	.2	0	0	1.9	35.9	7.5	.2	20.9	.1	7.1
0	0	.1	0	0	1.1	39.4	7.9	.3	27.3	.1	4.1

	Calories (kcal)	Protein (gm)	Carbohydrates (gm)	Fat (gm)	Percent Saturated Fat	Cholesterol (mg)	Dietary Fiber (gm)	Vitamin A (RE)	Vitamin C (mg)
Bar w/choc and graham crackers - 1 (25gm)	117	1.4	14	6.7	38.5	4.1	.5	35.7	.2
Brownies, wo/icing - 1 (34gm)	129	1.5	21.3	4.6	24.3	13.4	.9	4.3	0
Brownies, w/icing - 1 (42gm)	176	2.1	25.5	8.7	37.9	22.7	1.5	30.2	.1
Butterscotch brownie - 1 (34gm)	149	1.6	21.6	6.6	18.7	22.8	.3	74.4	.1
Butterscotch chip - 1 (10gm)	47	.5	6.6	2.2	19.4	5.5	.1	23.7	0
Carob - 1 (13gm)	51	1.2	8.2	2.3	18.1	10	.8	2.9	0
Carob and honey brownie - 1 (34gm)	143	1.9	16.2	9.3	15.5	27.6	1.4	70.3	.2
Chocolate chip - 1 (2" dia) (10gm)	47	.5	7	2.1	33.3	1.2	.5	3.5	0
Chocolate chip w/raisins - 1 (10gm)	46	.5	7	2	33.3	1.1	.5	3.3	0
Chocolate, choc-cvrd or fudge sandwich - 1 (11gm)	54	.5	7.6	2.5	24.6	0	.1	0	0
Chocolate-covered, marsh-mallow pie - 1 (34gm)	139	1.4	24.6	4.5	34.3	8.8	.1	25.8	.1
Chocolate fudge - 1 (13gm)	58	.9	9.3	2	28.7	3.4	.3	6	0
Date bar - 1 (16gm)	57	.6	12.1	.9	29.6	7.7	.4	1.8	0
Dietetic, apple pastry - 1 (24gm))	115	1	12.5	7	49.1	0	.2	0	0
Dietetic, fruit type - 1 (11gm)	51	.5	6.5	2.6	24.4	.4	.1	0	0
Dietetic, sand type - 1 (11gm)	50	.5	6.1	2.7	24.6	0	.1	0	0
Fig bars - 1 (16gm)	57	.6	12.1	.9	29.6	7.7	.4	1.8	0
Fruit-filled bars - 1 (16gm)	57	.6	12.1	.9	29.6	7.7	.4	1.8	0
Granola - 1 (13gm)	60	1.1	8.7	2.2	86.2	0	.6	.1	.1
Lady fingers - 1 (14gm)	50	1.1	9	1.1	42.6	1.4	.1	27.3	0
Lebkuchen - 1 (16gm)	61	1	12.8	.9	11.7	3.5	.3	1.1	0
Lemon bar - 1 (16gm)	70	.8	10	3	20.7	16	.1	40.4	.6
Macaroons - 1 (14gm)	66	.7	9.3	3.2	44.2	0	.8	0	0
Marshmallow w/coconut - 1 (18gm)	74	.7	13	2.4	34.3	4.7	0	13.7	0
Molasses - 1 (15gm)	63	1	11.4	1.6	27.8	0	.2	3.6	0
Oatmeal w/choc chips - 1 (15gm)	68	.9	9.9	3	37	2	.5	1.3	0
Oatmeal w/nuts - 1 (13gm)	54	.8	6.4	2.9	23.3	5.4	.2	13.2	0
Oatmeal, w/raisins, dates, nuts - 1 (13gm)	59	.8	9.6	2	24.8	1.9	.3	3	0
Oatmeal sandwich - 1 (15gm)	73	.7	10.2	3.3	25.2	1.8	.3	1.1	0
Peanut - 1 (16gm)	76	1.6	10.7	3.1	29.3	3.5	.2	9.6	0
Peanut butter - 1 (16gm)	78	1.6	9.4	3.9	18.9	6.6	.4	31.2	0
Peanut butter w/oatmeal - 1 (16gm)	69	1.9	11.1	2.1	19.1	13.3	.6	4.2	0
Pumpkin - 1 (11gm)	43	.5	6.4	1.9	18.5	5.4	.3	78.1	.2
Raisins - 1 (16gm)	61	.7	12.9	.8	26.4	5.3	.1	9.8	0

Thiamin (mg)	Riboflavin (mg)	Niacin (mg)	Vitamin B$_6$ (mg)	Vitamin B$_{12}$ (mcg)	Folacin (mcg)	Sodium (mg)	Calcium (mg)	Iron (mg)	Potassium (mg)	Zinc (mg)	Magnesium (mg)
0	.1	.1	0	0	2.3	55.9	35	.3	77.7	.3	11.7
.1	.1	.5	0	.1	3.6	50.1	12.1	.8	60.5	.2	12.4
.1	.1	.5	0	.1	4.6	84	16.8	1	75.2	.3	15.1
0	0	.4	0	.1	3.8	94.6	24.2	.8	79.2	.2	8.3
0	0	.1	0	0	1.1	50.4	3.6	.2	13.2	.1	2.1
0	0	.1	0	0	3.3	39	35.7	.4	43.8	.2	8.2
.1	0	.2	0	.1	6.5	131	33.5	.6	57.3	0.6	16.5
0	0	.1	0	0	.9	40.1	3.9	.3	13.4	.1	2.2
0	0	.1	0	0	.9	37.6	4	.3	17.4	.1	2.3
0	0	.2	0	0	.7	53.1	2.9	.2	4.2	.1	3.4
0	0	.4	0	0	8.5	71.1	7.1	.5	30.9	.3	11.9
0	0	.3	0	0	1.2	17.8	6.8	.4	16.6	.1	4.7
0	0	.3	0	0	1	40.3	12.5	.4	31.7	.1	4
0	0	.3	0	0	2.2	.2	1.9	.3	21.6	.1	7.2
0	0	.2	0	0	1	.1	.8	.1	4.5	0	3.3
0	0	.1	0	0	.7	1.3	4	.1	10.7	.1	3.4
0	0	.3	0	0	1	40.3	12.5	.4	31.7	.1	4
0	0	.3	0	0	1	40.3	12.5	.4	31.7	.1	4
.1	0	.2	0	0	10.5	42.9	8.8	.4	46.8	.2	13.1
0	0	.2	0	.1	4.3	9.9	5.7	.4	9.9	.2	2.1
0	0	.3	0	0	1.7	4.9	8.9	.4	30.1	.1	6.5
0	0	.2	0	0	2	39.5	6.2	.3	10.8	.1	1.4
0	0	.1	0	0	2.2	4.8	3.8	.1	64.8	.2	7.7
0	0	.2	0	0	4.5	37.6	3.8	.3	16.4	.2	6.3
0	0	.4	.1	0	1.8	57.9	7.6	.5	20.7	0	6.4
0	0	.2	0	0	1.3	20.1	13	.5	37.6	.2	8.3
0	0	.2	0	0	1.3	30.3	10.4	.2	15.4	.1	3.4
0	0	.2	0	0	1.6	21.1	2.7	.4	48.1	.1	3.6
0	0	.2	0	0	1.1	17.3	10.9	.3	24.2	.1	4.5
.1	0	.8	0	0	3	27.7	6.7	.4	28	.1	6.7
0	0	.7	0	0	3.7	56	6.2	.4	39.1	.2	7.4
0	0	.7	0	0	4.8	31.4	14.6	.5	56.7	.2	11.4
0	0	.2	0	0	1.5	24.9	12.9	.3	36.4	.1	4.1
0	0	.4	0	0	1.4	8.3	11.4	.6	43.5	0	4.8

	Calories (kcal)	Protein (gm)	Carbohydrates (gm)	Fat (gm)	Percent Saturated Fat	Cholesterol (mg)	Dietary Fiber (gm)	Vitamin A (RE)	Vitamin C (mg)
Raisin sandwich - 1 (30gm)	130	.9	22.6	4.4	25.4	6.8	.2	12.6	.1
Shortbread - 1 (15gm)	75	1.1	9.8	3.5	36.2	12.6	.1	3.6	0
Sugar - 1 (16gm)	71	.8	12.5	2.1	-	5.9	.1	2.3	0
Sugar, choc frosting - 1 medium (16gm)	66	.7	11.8	2.1	-	3.9	.3	5.1	0
Sugar, iced - 1 (16gm)	67	.5	12.2	1.9	28	6.3	0	8.4	0
Vanilla sandwich - 1 (11gm)	54	.5	7.6	2.5	24.6	0	.1	0	0
Whole wheat, dried fruit and nuts - 1 (14gm)	60	1	7.7	3.2	15.9	9.5	.7	24.4	.1

EGGS

	Calories (kcal)	Protein (gm)	Carbohydrates (gm)	Fat (gm)	Percent Saturated Fat	Cholesterol (mg)	Dietary Fiber (gm)	Vitamin A (RE)	Vitamin C (mg)
Chicken, raw - 1 (50gm)	79	6.1	.6	5.6	30	273.8	0	78	0
Chicken, yolk, raw - 1 (17gm)	63	2.8	0	5.6	30	272.4	0	93.8	0
Chicken, white, raw - 1 (33gm)	16	3.3	.4	0	0	0	0	0	0
Chicken, fried - 1 (46gm)	83	5.4	.5	6.4	37.5	245.8	0	82.8	0
Chicken, hard-boiled - 1 (50gm)	79	6.1	.6	5.6	30	273.8	0	78	0
Chicken, omelet - 1 (64gm)	94	6	1.4	7.1	39.9	248.4	0	89	.1
Chicken, poached - 1 (50gm)	79	6	.6	5.6	30	272.7	0	77.5	0
Chicken, scrambled - 1 (64gm)	94	6	1.4	7.1	39.9	248.4	0	89	.1
Duck, raw - 1 (70gm)	130	9	1	9.6	26.7	618.8	0	279.3	0
Goose, raw - 1 (144gm)	267	20	1.9	19.1	27.1	1226.7	0	553	0
Quail, raw - 1 (9gm)	14	1.2	0	1	-	76	0	8.1	0
Turkey, raw - 1 (79gm)	135	10.8	.9	9.4	30.6	737.1	0	131.1	0
Egg substitute, froz - ¼ c (60gm)	96	6.8	1.9	6.7	17.4	1.2	0	81	.3
Egg substitute, liquid - 1.5 fl oz (47gm)	39	5.6	.3	1.6	-	.5	0	101.5	0
Egg substitute, powder - .35 oz (9.9gm)	44	5.5	2.2	1.3	-	56.6	0	36.5	.1

FAST FOODS

(All portions are *one serving*)
Note: All fast food chains report vitamin A in IUs (International Units).

Arthur Treacher's

	Calories (kcal)	Protein (gm)	Carbohydrates (gm)	Fat (gm)	Percent Saturated Fat	Cholesterol (mg)	Dietary Fiber (gm)	IU	Vitamin C (mg)
Fish	355	19.2	25.4	19.8	-	55.7	-	111	1.5
Chicken	369	27.1	16.5	21.6	-	64.5	-	102	1.5
Shrimp	381	13.1	27.2	24.2	-	92.9	-	86	1.3

Thiamin (mg)	Riboflavin (mg)	Niacin (mg)	Vitamin B$_6$ (mg)	Vitamin B$_{12}$ (mcg)	Folacin (mcg)	Sodium (mg)	Calcium (mg)	Iron (mg)	Potassium (mg)	Zinc (mg)	Magnesium (mg)
0	0	.5	0	0	1.9	10.8	14.6	.7	56.2	.1	6.2
.1	0	.5	0	0	1.3	9	10.5	.4	9.9	.1	2.5
0	0	.3	0	0	1.2	40.8	14.7	.3	10.9	.1	1.7
0	0	.2	0	0	1	28.7	12.5	.2	18.7	.1	4.7
0	0	.2	0	0	.8	26.3	4.8	.2	8.1	0	1.2
0	0	.2	0	0	.7	53.1	2.9	.2	4.2	.1	3.4
0	0	.2	0	0	3.1	29.3	9.1	.4	54.6	.2	9.7

Source: USDA Food Consumption Survey

Thiamin (mg)	Riboflavin (mg)	Niacin (mg)	Vitamin B$_6$ (mg)	Vitamin B$_{12}$ (mcg)	Folacin (mcg)	Sodium (mg)	Calcium (mg)	Iron (mg)	Potassium (mg)	Zinc (mg)	Magnesium (mg)
0	.1	0	.1	.8	32.5	69.1	28.1	1	64.9	.7	6.1
0	.1	0	.1	.6	25.9	8.3	25.8	.9	15.3	.6	2.6
0	.1	0	0	0	5.2	50.3	3.6	0	45.3	0	2.9
0	.1	0	.1	.6	21.5	144	25.7	.9	57.9	.6	5.5
0	.1	0	.1	.7	24.5	69.1	28.1	1	64.9	.7	6.1
0	.2	0	.1	.6	22.2	155.2	47.1	.9	85	.7	7.9
0	.1	0	.1	.6	24.5	146.4	28.4	1	64.7	.7	6.1
0	.2	0	.1	.6	22.2	155.2	47.1	.9	85	.7	7.9
.1	.3	.1	.2	3.8	56	102.2	44.6	2.7	155.6	1	11.6
.2	.6	.3	.3	7.3	108.9	198.6	86.7	5.2	302.4	1.9	22.5
0	.1	0	0	.1	6	12.7	5.8	.3	11.9	.1	1.1
.1	.4	0	.1	1.3	56.2	119.5	78.2	3.2	112.3	1.2	10.6
.1	.2	.1	.1	.2	9.8	119.6	43.7	1.2	128	.6	9
.1	.1	.1	0	.1	7	83.2	24.9	1	155.1	.6	4.1
0	.2	.1	0	.3	12.4	79.2	32.3	.3	73.7	.2	6.4

Source: USDA Revised Handbook 8

Thiamin (mg)	Riboflavin (mg)	Niacin (mg)	Vitamin B$_6$ (mg)	Vitamin B$_{12}$ (mcg)	Folacin (mcg)	Sodium (mg)	Calcium (mg)	Iron (mg)	Potassium (mg)	Zinc (mg)	Magnesium (mg)
.1	.075	2.1	.178	1.56	-	450	14.9	.566	408.3	.573	27.7
.07	.148	11	.519	.61	-	495	11.2	.799	326.6	.623	26.8
.08	.051	1.7	.094	1.1	-	538	56.7	.638	99.1	.839	29

	Calories (kcal)	Protein (gm)	Carbohydrates (gm)	Fat (gm)	Percent Saturated Fat	Cholesterol (mg)	Dietary Fiber (gm)	Vitamin A (IU)	Vitamin C (mg)
Chips	276	4	34.9	13.2	-	.68	-	85	5.9
Krunch Pup	203	5.4	12	14.8	-	25	-	43	3.5
Cole slaw	123	1	11.1	8.2	-	6.59	-	170	59.1
Lemon Luvs	276	2.6	35.1	13.9	-	.42	-	64	.94
Chowder	112	4.6	11.2	5.4	-	8.96	-	340	1.7
Fish sandwich	440	16.4	39.4	24	-	41.6	-	117	1.6
Chicken sandwich	413	16.2	44	19.2	-	32	-	117	19.2

Burger Chef

	Calories (kcal)	Protein (gm)	Carbohydrates (gm)	Fat (gm)	Percent Saturated Fat	Cholesterol (mg)	Dietary Fiber (gm)	Vitamin A (IU)	Vitamin C (mg)
Hamburger	235	11	27	9	-	27	.2	113	1.2
Cheeseburger	278	14	28	12	-	37	.2	250	1.2
Double cheeseburger	402	23	28	22	-	74	.3	398	1.2
Big Shef	556	22	37	36	-	78	.5	293	1.6
Super Shef	604	27	35	39	-	99	.6	816	8.8
Top Shef	541	30	29	33	-	100	.3	304	-
Mushroom Burger	520	28	34	29	-	92	.6	339	2.9
Fun Meal	514	14	85	19	-	27	.9	113	9.4
French fries, regular	204	3	26	10	-	-	.6	-	7.2
French fries, large	285	4	36	14	-	-	.9	-	10.1
Apple turnover	237	2	38	9	-	-	.7	117	trace
Lettuce salad	11	1	3	.1	-	trace	.4	281	5.1
Vanilla shake	380	13	60	10	-	40	.2	387	trace
Chocolate shake	403	10	72	9	-	36	.9	292	trace
Hash Rounds	235	3	26	14	-	-	.8	-	3.6
Sunrise w/bacon	392	19	30	21	-	384	.1	560	-
Sunrise w/sausage	526	26	30	33	-	419	.1	560	1.1
Biscuit sandwich w/sausage	418	16	33	25	-	45	.1	37	1.1
Scrambled eggs and bacon platter	567	21	50	31	-	449	.6	546	-
Scrambled eggs and sausage platter	668	26	50	40	-	479	.6	546	4.2
Chicken club	521	36	33	25	-	-	-	498	8.9
Fisherman's Fillet	534	26	41	32	-	-	-	261	1

Hardee's

	Calories (kcal)	Protein (gm)	Carbohydrates (gm)	Fat (gm)	Percent Saturated Fat	Cholesterol (mg)	Dietary Fiber (gm)	Vitamin A (IU)	Vitamin C (mg)
Biscuit	275	5	35	13	-	82	-	44	1
Sausage biscuit	413	10	34	26	-	112	-	45	1
Sausage and egg biscuit	521	16	34	35	-	162	-	755	1
Steak biscuit	419	14	41	23	-	134	-	62	1
Steak and egg biscuit	527	20	41	31	-	162	-	772	1
Ham biscuit	349	12	37	17	-	108	-	127	1
Ham and egg biscuit	458	19	37	26	-	184	-	837	1
Bacon and egg biscuit	405	13	30	26	-	114	-	145	2
Biscuit w/jelly	324	5	47	13	-	100	-	46	1

Thiamin (mg)	Riboflavin (mg)	Niacin (mg)	Vitamin B$_6$ (mg)	Vitamin B$_{12}$ (mcg)	Folacin (mcg)	Sodium (mg)	Calcium (mg)	Iron (mg)	Potassium (mg)	Zinc (mg)	Magnesium (mg)
.17	.035	2.4	.308	.08	-	393	12.4	.473	598.8	.245	29
.05	.052	1.2	.050	.5	-	446	7.99	.601	70.3	.822	7.37
.026	.025	.43	.089	.06	-	266	24	.185	163.4	.0894	7.38
.18	.089	1.51	.027	.08	-	314	9.87	.851	432	.185	8.49
.07	.14	.39	.071	.48	-	835	61.4	.092	227.9	.202	12
.27	.215	4.1	.13	.94	-	836	88.9	1.49	247.9	.765	21.7
.17	.24	8.1	.327	.31	-	708	58.8	1.7	279.1	.633	27.3
.3	.2	3.6	.2	.4	20	480	75	2.2	144	1.8	17
.3	.3	3.6	.2	.5	21	641	145	2.3	162	2.1	19
.3	.4	5.2	.3	.9	23	835	218	2.9	244	3.9	26
.4	.4	5.9	.3	.8	37	840	178	3.6	267	3.8	26
.4	.5	6.8	.5	1.2	45	1088	241	3.8	424	5	36
.4	.5	7	.4	1.4	26	1007	226	3.5	303	5.1	28
.4	.6	7.9	.5	1.3	33	744	262	3.7	434	4.9	34
.4	.2	4.7	.2	.4	20	513	84	3	0	0	0
.1	trace	1.1	-	0	-	327	9	.8	469	.3	27
.2	trace	1.5	-	0	-	456	12	1	655	.4	37
trace	trace	.4	-	trace	-	-	24	1	-	-	-
.1	.1	.3	.1	trace	31	8	17	.4	149	.3	9
.1	.7	.5	.1	1.1	23	325	497	.3	622	1	40
.2	.8	.4	.1	1.1	17	378	449	.6	762	1	54
.1	trace	1.4	-	0	-	349	9	.9	434	.3	19
.4	.5	2.9	.1	1.1	54	978	186	3.3	209	2	23
.7	.6	4.7	.3	1.9	54	1412	201	3.8	350	3	30
.7	.4	4.4	.2	1	4	1313	155	2	326	1.8	25
.4	.5	3.5	.2	1.4	54	1108	146	3.9	574	2.2	39
.7	.6	4.9	.3	2	53	1411	160	4.2	688	3	45
.3	.4	15	-	-	-	-	77	3.6	-	-	-
.3	.3	4.1	-	-	-	-	146	2.7	-	-	-
1	1	1	-	-	-	650	149	2	117	-	-
1	1	3	-	-	-	864	134	3	217	-	-
1	1	3	-	-	-	1033	169	4	287	-	-
1	1	3	-	-	-	804	121	5	265	-	-
1	1	4	-	-	-	973	151	6	335	-	-
1	1	2	-	-	-	1415	181	3	235	-	-
1	1	2	-	-	-	1585	211	4	305	-	-
1	1	2	-	-	-	823	144	3	12	-	-
1	1	1	-	-	-	653	153	3	131	-	-

	Calories (kcal)	Protein (gm)	Carbohydrates (gm)	Fat (gm)	Percent Saturated Fat	Cholesterol (mg)	Dietary Fiber (gm)	Vitamin A (IU)	Vitamin C (mg)
Biscuit w/egg	383	11	35	22	-	158	-	754	1
One medium fried egg	108	6	1	7	-	50	-	710	-
Orange juice	81	2	20	1	-	-	-	360	75
Hash Rounds	200	2	20	13	-	10	-	-	4
Biscuit w/gravy	419	10	44	22	-	21	-	73	1
Cinnamon 'n' Raisin Biscuit	276	3	30	16	-	1	-	-	1
Hamburger	305	17	29	13	-	-	-	57	2
Cheeseburger	309	14	35	13	-	28	-	884	1
Big Deluxe	546	29	48	26	-	77	-	398	42
Bacon cheeseburger	686	35	42	42	-	295	-	832	3
Roast beef sandwich	377	20	36	17	-	57	-	542	3
Big Roast Beef	418	28	34	19	-	60	-	648	8
Mushroom 'n' Swiss	512	32	46	23	-	86	-	201	0
Hot Ham 'n' Cheese	376	23	37	15	-	59	-	178	1
Fisherman's Fillet	469	25	47	20	-	80	-	319	0
Turkey club	426	24	32	22	-	45	-	799	5
Chicken fillet	510	27	42	26	-	57	-	1098	13
Hot dog	346	11	26	22	-	42	-	trace	0
Chef salad	277	23	10	16	-	179	-	632	10
Shrimp salad	362	14	11	29	-	293	-	1690	20
Small french fries	239	3	28	13	-	4	-	trace	10
Large french fries	381	5	44	21	-	6	-	trace	16
Apple turnover	282	3	37	14	-	5	-	trace	0
Big Cookie	278	3	33	15	-	9	-	0	3
Milk shake	391	11	63	10	-	42	-	0	0

Jack in the Box

	Calories (kcal)	Protein (gm)	Carbohydrates (gm)	Fat (gm)	Percent Saturated Fat	Cholesterol (mg)	Dietary Fiber (gm)	Vitamin A (IU)	Vitamin C (mg)
Cheese nachos	571	14.5	49.4	35.1	-	37.1	-	511	2.89
Supreme nachos	718	22.9	66.1	40.2	-	55.1	-	1013	8.64
Swiss and bacon burger	643	32.9	30.6	43.2	-	99.4	-	378	2.7
Pita Pocket Supreme	284	22.4	29.7	8.4	-	42.7	-	247	4.45
Apple turnover	410	4	45	24	-	15	-	-	-
Jumbo Jack hamburger w/cheese	630	32	45	35	-	110	-	-	-
Pancake Breakfast	630	16	79	27	-	85	-	-	-
Scrambled Eggs Breakfast	720	26	55	44	-	260	-	-	-
Strawberry shake	380	10	63	10	-	35	-	-	-
Vanilla shake	340	10	54	9	-	35	-	-	-
Chocolate shake	360	10	59	10	-	35	-	-	-
Hamburger	276	12.7	30.1	11.7	-	29.4	-	49	1.37
Cheeseburger	323	15.7	31.9	14.7	-	41.8	-	305	1.36
Jumbo Jack	485	25.0	37.9	25.6	-	63.8	-	348	5.12
Bacon Cheeseburger Supreme	724	33.7	44.4	45.7	-	69.5	-	624	3.23

Thiamin (mg)	Riboflavin (mg)	Niacin (mg)	Vitamin B6 (mg)	Vitamin B12 (mcg)	Folacin (mcg)	Sodium (mg)	Calcium (mg)	Iron (mg)	Potassium (mg)	Zinc (mg)	Magnesium (mg)
1	1	1	-	-	-	819	179	4	187	-	-
1	1	1	-	-	-	169	30	2	70	-	-
1	1	1	-	-	-	2	17	1	335	-	-
1	-	2	-	-	-	310	-	1	300	-	-
1	1	2	-	-	-	1090	168	4	238	-	-
1	1	1	-	-	-	346	89	1	110	-	-
1	1	6	-	-	-	682	23	4	231	-	-
1	1	5	-	-	-	825	123	1	197	-	-
1	1	11	-	-	-	1083	98	7	594	-	-
1	1	6	-	-	-	1074	152	6	33	-	-
1	1	4	-	-	-	1030	56	6	205	-	-
1	1	5	-	-	-	1770	74	8	470	-	-
1	1	6	-	-	-	1051	111	4	437	-	-
1	1	3	-	-	-	1067	207	4	317	-	-
1	1	3	-	-	-	1013	139	2	465	-	-
1	1	9	-	-	-	1185	39	2	444	-	-
1	1	9	-	-	-	360	83	5	334	-	-
1	1	4	-	-	-	744	43	3	120	-	-
1	1	6	-	-	-	517	212	2	414	-	-
1	1	1	-	-	-	941	104	3	696	-	-
1	1	1	-	-	-	121	13	1	433	-	-
1	1	2	-	-	-	192	21	1	689	-	-
1	1	1	-	-	-	-	19	1	17	-	-
1	1	1	-	-	-	258	16	1	64	-	-
1	1	1	-	-	-	-	450	1	652	-	-

Thiamin (mg)	Riboflavin (mg)	Niacin (mg)	Vitamin B6 (mg)	Vitamin B12 (mcg)	Folacin (mcg)	Sodium (mg)	Calcium (mg)	Iron (mg)	Potassium (mg)	Zinc (mg)	Magnesium (mg)
.102	.187	1.02	.272	.17	-	1154	367	1.45	225	2.4	72.8
.149	.253	3.28	.506	.596	-	1782	414	3.21	611	4.51	103
.45	.414	6.84	.234	2.88	-	1354	226	4.65	418	5.11	43.3
.775	.330	7.75	.28	.660	-	953	83.5	2.44	398	2	33.6
-	-	-	-	-	-	350	-	-	-	-	-
-	-	-	-	-	-	1665	-	-	-	-	-
-	-	-	-	-	-	1670	-	-	-	-	-
-	-	-	-	-	-	1110	-	-	-	-	-
-	-	-	-	-	-	270	-	-	-	-	-
-	-	-	-	-	-	265	-	-	-	-	-
-	-	-	-	-	-	295	-	-	-	-	-
.353	.243	3.26	.113	1.27	-	521	68.8	2.62	-	1.7	20.4
.35	.266	3.31	.123	1.58	-	749	157	2.7	-	1.99	23.3
.512	.213	7.03	.264	2.46	-	905	96.8	6.93	-	4.14	42.9
.554	.513	8.87	.259	2.31	-	1307	314	4.85	-	4.64	44.5

	Calories (kcal)	Protein (gm)	Carbohydrates (gm)	Fat (gm)	Percent Saturated Fat	Cholesterol (mg)	Dietary Fiber (gm)	Vitamin A (IU)	Vitamin C (mg)
Regular taco	191	7.5	15.6	10.9	-	20.5	-	397	-
Super Taco	288	12	21.1	17.3	-	37	-	580	1.62
Chicken Supreme	601	30.6	39.2	35.8	-	60.2	-	456	4.33
Moby Jack	444	16.4	38.8	24.8	-	47	-	274	-
Taco salad	377	30.8	10.4	23.6	-	102	-	1146	6.8
Croissant Supreme	547	20.3	27.4	39.6	-	178	-	526	-
Sausage croissant	584	22	27.8	42.7	-	187	-	530	-
Bacon croissant	480	17.6	27.1	33.5	-	194	-	538	-
Ham croissant	447	18.3	24.5	30.7	-	166	-	432	-
Breakfast Jack	307	18.8	29.6	12.6	-	203	-	-	-
Chicken Strips Dinner	689	39.8	65.2	29.9	-	99.8	-	417	11.9
Shrimp Dinner	731	22	77.4	37	-	157	-	421	11.7
Sirloin Steak Dinner	699	38.1	75.1	27.4	-	75.1	-	167	8.02
French fries	221	2.4	27	11.5	-	8.16	-	0	2.86
Onion rings	382	5	39.1	22.9	-	26.7	-	0	2.81

Kentucky Fried Chicken

	Calories (kcal)	Protein (gm)	Carbohydrates (gm)	Fat (gm)	Percent Saturated Fat	Cholesterol (mg)	Dietary Fiber (gm)	Vitamin A (IU)	Vitamin C (mg)
Chicken wing, Original Recipe	136	9.6	4.2	9	-	54.6	.2	8	.85
Chicken drumstick, Original Recipe	117	12.1	2.6	6.5	-	63	.1	9	1
Chicken side breast, Original Recipe	199	16.2	7.1	11.7	-	69.8	.1	14	1.4
Chicken thigh, Original Recipe	257	18.4	6.5	17.5	-	109	.1	17	1.8
Chicken keel, Original Recipe	236	23.9	7.4	12.3	-	86.7	.1	19	1.9
Chicken wing, Extra Crispy	201	11.2	8.7	13.5	-	58.7	.1	11	1.1
Chicken drumstick, Extra Crispy	155	13.3	5.1	9	-	65.5	.1	12	1.2
Chicken side breast, Extra Crispy	286	17.2	14.1	17.8	-	65.1	.2	17	1.7
Chicken thigh, Extra Crispy	343	20.4	12.6	23.4	-	109	.2	22	2.2
Chicken keel, Extra Crispy	297	23.6	13.6	16.4	-	78.8	.1	21	2.1
Mashed potatoes	63.9	1.5	12.2	.9	-	.2	.2	18	4.9
Gravy	22.7	.4	1.3	1.8	-	.44	.1	3	.15
Roll	60.6	1.8	10.9	1.1	-	.64	.1	5	.25
Corn	169	4.6	31.2	2.8	-	.14	.7	162	2.6
Cole slaw	121	.9	12.7	7.5	-	7.18	.5	255	31.7
Kentucky fries	184	3.2	27.7	6.7	-	-	.792	20	14.4
2-Piece Colonel's Special Dinner [includes mashed potatoes, gravy, cole slaw, roll] Dark—drumstick and thigh, Original Recipe	643	35.1	46.2	35.2	-	180	.8	255	36.6
2-Piece Colonel's Special Dinner [includes mashed potatoes, gravy, cole slaw, roll] Combination—wing and thigh, Original Recipe	661	32.6	47.8	37.8	-	172	1	255	36.6

Thiamin (mg)	Riboflavin (mg)	Niacin (mg)	Vitamin B$_6$ (mg)	Vitamin B$_{12}$ (mcg)	Folacin (mcg)	Sodium (mg)	Calcium (mg)	Iron (mg)	Potassium (mg)	Zinc (mg)	Magnesium (mg)
.0729	.176	1.09	.13	.356	-	406	97.4	1.13	-	1.07	35.2
.121	.0821	1.48	.221	.634	-	765	151	1.59	-	1.67	48.3
.524	.374	10.5	.467	.684	-	1582	235	2.96	-	1.78	56
.397	.251	2.86	.112	1.14	-	820	159	2.18	-	1.04	29.7
.179	.53	6.09	.291	1.86	-	1436	283	4.37	-	5.18	52.7
.642	.539	4.19	.175	1.02	-	1053	147	2.66	-	1.99	26.8
.593	.512	4.66	.159	1.87	-	1012	169	2.89	-	2.25	28.3
.487	.476	3.42	.107	.862	-	935	147	2.34	-	1.62	23.3
.537	.507	3.88	.155	.93	-	848	143	2.71	-	1.83	25.2
.466	.413	3.04	.155	1.11	-	871	168	3.01	-	1.78	24.9
.449	.295	18.6	1.09	.321	-	1213	114	3.98	-	1.8	82.5
.391	.175	6.92	.632	.451	-	1510	374	4.88	918	1.93	80.1
.668	.501	12.4	.935	1.5	-	969	216	9.59	1216	4.94	75.1
.0748	.0252	1.21	.216	.0224	-	164	9.71	.53	-	.184	20.5
.205	.125	1.81	.0611	.105	-	407	28.5	1.36	-	.324	17.6
.03	.04	2.28	.097	-	-	302	21.6	.68	86.3	.58	9.77
.04	.09	2.38	.085	-	-	207	12.1	.8	122	1.29	12.6
.06	.08	5.66	.2	-	-	558	50.1	.98	176	.774	19.1
.08	.16	4.03	.167	-	-	566	34.2	1.45	217	1.65	21.6
.08	.11	7.57	.313	-	-	631	29.8	1.17	267	.72	27.7
.06	.09	2.94	.112	-	-	312	15.5	.65	99.9	.673	11.6
.07	.11	3.07	.157	-	-	263	11	.95	147	1.32	14
.12	.13	5.37	.237	-	-	564	56.8	1.12	188	.879	21.1
.12	.19	5.35	.171	-	-	549	49	1.49	228	1.73	24.1
.11	.11	7.89	.302	-	-	584	62.2	1.29	244	.77	29.3
.01	.02	.76	.11	-	-	268	15.6	.46	232	.17	14.9
.003	.01	.11	.002	-	-	57.1	1.69	.13	8.29	.014	.851
.10	.04	.98	.014	-	-	118	21.3	.53	28.6	.2	5.89
.12	.07	1.2	.207	-	-	11.1	6.14	.76	305	.931	50.9
.03	.02	.19	.081	-	-	225	31.8	.53	132	.146	10.6
-	-	-	-	-	-	-	-	-	-	-	-
.25	.32	8.46	.459	-	-	1441	116	3.9	720	3.47	66.4
.24	.27	8.36	.471	-	-	1536	126	3.78	684	2.76	63.6

	Calories (kcal)	Protein (gm)	Carbohydrates (gm)	Fat (gm)	Percent Saturated Fat	Cholesterol (mg)	Dietary Fiber (gm)	Vitamin A (IU)	Vitamin C (mg)
2 Piece Colonel's Special Dinner [includes mashed potatoes, gravy, cole slaw, roll] White—wing and side breast, Original Recipe	604	30.4	48.3	32.1	-	133	1	255	36.6
2-Piece Colonel's Special Dinner [includes mashed potatoes, gravy, cole slaw, roll] White—wing and side breast, Extra Crispy	755	33	59.9	42.6	-	132	1	255	36.6
2-Piece Colonel's Special Dinner [includes mashed potatoes, gravy, cole slaw, roll] Dark—drumstick and thigh, Extra Crispy	765	38.3	54.7	53.7	-	183	1	255	36.6
2-Piece Colonel's Special Dinner [includes mashed potatoes, gravy, cole slaw, roll] Combination—wing and thigh, Extra Crispy	902	36.2	58.4	48.2	-	176	1	255	36.6
Chicken breast fillet sandwich	436	24.8	33.8	22.5	-	-	.471	47	3.61

McDonald's

English muffin w/butter	186	5	29.5	5.3	-	15.4	-	164	1
Hash brown potatoes	125	1.5	14	7	-	7.15	-	13	4.14
Biscuit, plain	330	4.9	36.6	18.2	-	9.2	-	179	.85
Biscuit w/sausage	467	12.1	35.3	30.9	-	48	-	61	1.2
Biscuit w/sausage and egg	585	19.8	36.4	39.9	-	285.3	-	420	1.75
Biscuit w/bacon, egg, and cheese	483	16.5	33.2	31.6	-	262.5	-	653	1.6
Sausage McMuffin	427	17.6	30	26.3	-	59	-	380	1.27
Sausage McMuffin w/egg	517	22.9	32.2	32.9	-	287	-	660	1.65
Hamburger	263	12.4	28.3	11.3	-	29.1	-	100	1.79
Cheeseburger	318	15	28.5	16	-	40.6	-	353	2.05
Quarter Pounder	427	24.6	29.3	23.5	-	81	-	128	2.56
Quarter Pounder w/cheese	525	29.6	30.5	31.6	-	107	-	614	2.79
Big Mac	570	24.6	39.2	35	-	83	-	380	3
Filet O' Fish	435	14.7	35.9	25.7	-	45.2	-	186	2.15
Regular fries	220	3	26.1	11.5	-	8.57	-	17	12.53
Chicken McNuggets	323	19.1	13.7	21.3	-	72.8	-	109	2.07
Hot mustard sauce	63	.6	10.5	2.1	-	2.7	-	9	.3
Barbeque sauce	60	.4	13.7	.4	-	.3	-	45	.64
Sweet & sour sauce	64	.2	15	.3	-	.1	-	200	.3
Honey	50	.04	12.4	.04	-	.1	-	14	.15
Vanilla shake	352	9.3	59.6	8.4	-	30.6	-	349	3.2
Chocolate shake	383	9.9	65.5	9	-	29.7	-	349	2.91
Strawberry shake	362	9	62.1	8.7	-	32.2	-	377	4.06

Thiamin (mg)	Riboflavin (mg)	Niacin (mg)	Vitamin B$_6$ (mg)	Vitamin B$_{12}$ (mcg)	Folacin (mcg)	Sodium (mg)	Calcium (mg)	Iron (mg)	Potassium (mg)	Zinc (mg)	Magnesium (mg)
.22	.19	10	.504	-	-	1528	142	3.31	643	1.88	61.1
.31	.29	10.4	.556	-	-	1544	143	6.03	689	2.08	65
.32	.38	10.4	.535	-	-	1480	130	4.09	776	3.58	70.3
.31	.35	10.3	.49	-	-	1529	135	6.4	729	2.93	67.9
-	-	-	-	-	-	-	-	-	-	-	-
.28	.49	2.61	.04	-	-	310	117	1.5	-	.5	13
.06	.01	.82	.13	.01	-	325	5	.4	-	.2	13
.21	.15	1.7	.03	.11	-	786	74	1.3	-	.33	10.2
.56	.22	3.39	.12	.52	-	1147	82	2.05	-	1.3	17.2
.53	.49	3.85	.19	1.33	-	1301	119	3.43	-	2.1	23.9
.3	.43	2.32	.11	1.06	-	1269	2	2.57	-	1.6	19.8
.7	.25	4.14	.15	.08	-	942	168	2.25	-	1.68	23.8
.84	.5	4.46	.2	1.37	-	1044	196	3.47	-	2.36	29.8
.31	.22	4.08	.15	.83	-	506	84	2.85	-	1.85	19.9
.30	.24	4.33	.14	1	-	743	169	2.84	-	2.22	22.8
.35	.32	7.2	.32	1.92	-	718	98	4.3	-	4	33
.37	.41	7.07	.3	2.23	-	1220	255	4.84	-	4.74	39.9
.48	.38	7.2	.28	1.7	-	979	203	4.9	-	4	37.7
.36	.23	3	.13	.69	-	799	133	2.47	-	.84	25.8
.12	.02	2.26	.22	.03	-	109	9	.61	-	.32	26.7
.16	.14	7.52	.38	.36	-	512	11	1.25	-	.89	26.3
.01	.003	.08	.01	.02	-	259	8	.17	-	.09	6.22
.01	.01	.08	.02	.13	-	309	4	.12	-	.05	4.99
.01	.01	.07	.01	.01	-	186	2	.08	-	.02	2
.002	.003	.03	.001	.01	-	2	1	.02	-	.01	.24
.12	.7	.35	.12	1.19	-	201	329	.18	-	1.16	30.8
.12	.44	.5	.13	1.16	-	300	320	.84	-	1.4	48.9
.12	.44	.35	.14	1.16	-	207	322	.17	-	1.16	30.7

	Calories (kcal)	Protein (gm)	Carbohydrates (gm)	Fat (gm)	Percent Saturated Fat	Cholesterol (mg)	Dietary Fiber (gm)	Vitamin A (IU)	Vitamin C (mg)
Strawberry sundae	320	6	54	8.7	-	24.6	-	230	2.79
Hot fudge sundae	357	7	58	10.8	-	26.6	-	230	2.46
Caramel sundae	361	7.2	608	10	-	31.4	-	279	3.61
Cone	185	4.3	30.2	5.2	-	23.5	-	218	1.15
Apple pie	253	1.87	29.3	14.3	-	12.4	-	34	.85
Cherry pie	260	2	32.1	13.6	-	13.4	-	114	.88
McDonaldland cookies	308	4.2	48.7	10.8	-	10.2	-	27	.94
Chocolaty chip cookies	342	4.2	44.8	16.3	-	17.7	-	76	1.04
Egg McMuffin	340	18.5	31	15.8	-	259	-	591	1.38
Hotcakes w/butter and syrup	500	7.9	93.9	10.3	-	47.1	-	257	4.71
Scrambled eggs	180	13.2	2.5	13	-	514.2	-	652	1.18
Sausage	210	9.8	.6	18.6	-	38.8	-	32	.53

Ponderosa

	Calories (kcal)	Protein (gm)	Carbohydrates (gm)	Fat (gm)	Percent Saturated Fat	Cholesterol (mg)	Dietary Fiber (gm)	Vitamin A (IU)	Vitamin C (mg)
King prime rib	409	47.9	0	22.7	-	118.1	-	40	-
Baked potato	145	4	32.8	.2	-	-	-	trace	31
Kaiser roll	184	5	33	3.4	-	-	-	trace	trace
Prime rib	286	33.5	73.6	15.9	-	82.6	-	28	-
T-Bone	240	37.4	0	8.8	-	84.2	-	12	-
New York Strip	362	44.3	-	19.2	-	122	-	-	-
Super sirloin	383	59.1	0	14.2	-	128	-	25	-
Sirloin	197	30.4	0	7.3	-	65.8	-	13	-
Sirloin tips	192.4	34.8	-	4.7	-	73.5	-	-	-
Filet Mignon	152	17.8	.15	8.3	-	70	-	-	-
Ribeye	197	23	0	10.9	-	56.4	-	19	-
Shrimp	139	12.5	6.2	6.7	-	77	-	32	0
Ribeye	197	23	0	10.9	-	56.4	-	19	-
Chicken strips	282	26.9	15.8	11.7	-	60	-	423	-
Shrimp dinner	220	19.9	9.8	10.6	-	122.5	-	51	0
Baked fish	268	25	11.6	13.5	-	97.8	-	255	-
Filet of sole dinner	125	14.9	4.4	4.9	-	59	-	-	-
Filet of sole sandwich	315	20.9	39.4	7.9	-	59	-	trace	trace
French fries	230	3.6	30.2	11.1	-	-	-	trace	16.8
Chopped beef	209	26.2	0	10.8	-	66.9	-	19	-
Big chopped beef	295	36.9	0	15.2	-	94.3	-	27	-
Double Deluxe	552	51.4	35	21.8	-	115.8	-	33	trace
Steakhouse Deluxe	371	28.7	35	12.4	-	57.9	-	17	trace
Ham 'n Cheese	450	23	36.88	23.3	-	54	-	183	trace
Child's chicken strips	141	13.4	7.9	5.8	-	30	-	211	-
Gelatin	97	1.7	23.5	trace	-	-	-	-	1
Pudding, vanilla	195	2.4	27.5	8.8	-	16	-	129	1
Pudding, chocolate	213	2.7	27.1	10.6	-	15.4	-	-	-
Pudding, butterscotch	200	2.6	27.4	8.8	-	2.6	-	129	-

Thiamin (mg)	Riboflavin (mg)	Niacin (mg)	Vitamin B_6 (mg)	Vitamin B_{12} (mcg)	Folacin (mcg)	Sodium (mg)	Calcium (mg)	Iron (mg)	Potassium (mg)	Zinc (mg)	Magnesium (mg)
.07	.3	1.03	.05	.61	-	90	174	.38	-	.8	28.2
.07	.31	1.12	.13	.67	-	170	215	.61	-	.98	35.1
.07	.31	1.01	.05	.64	-	145	200	.23	-	.87	29.5
.06	.36	.44	.06	.03	-	109	183	.12	⌐	.64	17.1
.02	.02	.19	.02	.03	-	398	14	.62	-	.16	6.35
.03	.02	.25	.02	.04	-	427	12	.59	-	.15	6.51
.23	.23	2.85	.03	.03	-	358	12	1.47	-	.34	10.8
.12	.21	1.7	.03	.08	-	313	29	1.56	-	.5	28.7
.47	.44	3.77	.21	.75	-	885	226	2.93	-	1.92	25.8
.26	.36	2.27	.12	.19	-	1070	103	2.23	-	.69	28.2
.08	.47	.2	.2	.93	-	205	61	2.53	-	1.66	13.1
.27	.11	2.07	.18	.53	-	423	16	.82	-	1.47	9.17

Thiamin (mg)	Riboflavin (mg)	Niacin (mg)	Vitamin B_6 (mg)	Vitamin B_{12} (mcg)	Folacin (mcg)	Sodium (mg)	Calcium (mg)	Iron (mg)	Potassium (mg)	Zinc (mg)	Magnesium (mg)
.11	.36	8.7	.73	3	-	100.6	20	6.2	536.5	-	38
.15	.07	2.7	.47	0	-	6	14	1.1	782	-	-
.18	.11	1.3	-	-	-	311	45.4	1.1	58	-	23
.08	.25	6.1	.51	2.1	-	70.6	14	4.3	375.2	-	26.6
.10	.29	7.2	.52	2.2	-	545	14.5	4.5	518	-	24.6
173.8	799.3	5.7	.75	trace	-	79.2	25	6.7	757.6	-	36
.18	.47	11.7	.79	3.3	-	695.2	23.6	7.1	663.8	-	38.2
.1	.24	6	.41	1.69	-	372	12.1	3.6	342	-	19.9
124.8	686.4	3.4	.48	2	-	374.6	18.2	5.2	517	-	2.6
61.6	337	1.85	.46	1.9	-	82	9.4	2.7	483	-	14.3
.06	.17	4.2	.35	1.45	-	271	9.6	2.4	258	-	25.8
.06	.19	1.01	.06	.55	-	114.4	84.9	.4	140.8	-	31.4
.06	.17	4.2	.35	1.45	-	271	9.6	2.4	258	-	25.8
.1	.14	10	.68	.45	-	420	38.9	1.8	26.8	-	6
.09	.31	1.6	.098	.88	-	182	135	.63	224	-	50
.12	.15	4.2	.25	1.8	-	363	43.5	1.4	579	-	-
.03	.05	2.3	-	-	-	46.4	17.5	.05	231	-	18.2
.23	.18	4.1	.03	trace	-	380.4	65.9	1.8	292.6	-	42.4
.12	.07	2.6	.15	0	-	4.8	12.6	1.2	717.6	-	-
.09	.22	5.8	-	-	-	57.5	11.5	3.3	297.5	-	20
.12	.31	8.1	-	-	-	81	16.2	4.7	419	-	28.2
.34	.51	11.72	.75	3	-	433.1	68.2	7.1	985.6	-	59.4
.27	.32	6.76	.39	1.5	-	383.8	58.3	4.2	523.6	-	41.8
.64	.31	4.2	.35	.61	-	1368.6	230.7	1.58	278	-	30.6
.05	.07	5	.34	.22	-	210	19.4	.9	13.4	-	3
.01	.01	.2	-	-	-	55	2	.1	81	-	-
.03	.12	-	-	-	-	127	38	.3	38	-	8
.03	.12	.07	-	-	-	177	76	1	17.6	-	19
.03	.13	-	-	-	•	192	38	.3	128	-	7

	Calories (kcal)	Protein (gm)	Carbohydrates (gm)	Fat (gm)	Percent Saturated Fat	Cholesterol (mg)	Dietary Fiber (gm)	Vitamin A (IU)	Vitamin C (mg)
Child's hot dog	248	7.7	20.9	14.8	-	50	-	-	0
Child's Square Shooter	215	15.5	21	6.8	-	31.4	-	9	trace

Wendy's

	Calories (kcal)	Protein (gm)	Carbohydrates (gm)	Fat (gm)	Percent Saturated Fat	Cholesterol (mg)	Dietary Fiber (gm)	Vitamin A (IU)	Vitamin C (mg)
Single hamburger on multi-grain wheat bun*	340	25	20	17	-	67	-	-	-
Single hamburger on white bun	350	21	27	18	-	65	-	-	-
Double hamburger on white bun	560	41	24	34	-	125	-	-	-
Bacon cheeseburger on white bun	460	29	23	28	-	65	-	412	-
Chicken sandwich on white bun	366	25.5	39.2	11.9	-	56.2	-	-	-
Chicken sandwich on multi-grain wheat bun	320	25	31	10	-	59	-	-	-
Kid's Meal hamburger	220	13	11	8	-	20	-	-	-
Chili	260	21	26	8	-	30	-	-	5.89
French fries, salted (regular size)	280	4	35	14	-	15	-	-	11.3
Taco salad	390	23	36	18	-	40	-	-	-
Pick-up window side salad*	110	8	5	6	-	15	-	-	-
Frosty dairy dessert	400	8	59	14	-	50	-	535	trace
White bun	160	5	28	3	-	trace	-	-	-
Multigrain wheat bun*	135	5	23	3	-	2	-	-	.771
Hot stfd bkd potato, plain *	250	6	52	2	-	trace	-	-	6.5
Hot stfd bkd potato, sour crm and chives	460	6	53	24	-	15	-	-	-
Hot stfd bkd potato, cheese	590	17	55	34	-	22	-	-	-
Hot stfd bkd potato, chili and cheese	510	22	63	20	-	22	-	-	-
Hot stfd bkd potato, bacon and cheese	570	19	57	30	-	22	-	-	-
Hot stfd bkd potato, broccoli and cheese	500	13	54	25	-	22	-	-	-
Hot stfd bkd potato, stroganoff and sour crm	490	14	60	21	-	43	-	-	-
Hot stfd bkd potato, chicken a la king	350	15	59	6	-	20	-	-	-
Omelet #1—ham and cheese	250	18	6	17	-	450	-	1038	-
Omelet #2—ham, cheese, mushroom	290	18	7	21	-	355	-	1015	-
Omelet #3—ham, cheese, onion, grn pepper	280	19	7	19	-	525	-	960	5.5
Omelet #4—mushroom, onion, grn pepper	210	14	7	15	-	460	-	741	6.5
Breakfast sandwich	370	17	33	19	-	200	-	929	-

Thiamin (mg)	Riboflavin (mg)	Niacin (mg)	Vitamin B$_6$ (mg)	Vitamin B$_{12}$ (mcg)	Folacin (mcg)	Sodium (mg)	Calcium (mg)	Iron (mg)	Potassium (mg)	Zinc (mg)	Magnesium (mg)
.18	.15	2.8	.22	-	-	805	30	.47	108	-	9
.15	.18	3.8	.2	.81	-	223.9	55.4	2.5	286.5	-	24.1

Thiamin (mg)	Riboflavin (mg)	Niacin (mg)	Vitamin B$_6$ (mg)	Vitamin B$_{12}$ (mcg)	Folacin (mcg)	Sodium (mg)	Calcium (mg)	Iron (mg)	Potassium (mg)	Zinc (mg)	Magnesium (mg)
-	-	-	-	-	-	290	-	-	310	-	-
.2	.2	.5	-	-	-	410	39	4	275	4.01	25
-	-	-	-	-	-	575	-	-	485	-	-
.265	.279	5.73	-	-	-	860	136	3.54	330	5.14	33.4
.251	.251	10.8	-	-	-	545	40.9	1.72	314	.977	38.4
-	-	-	-	-	-	500	-	-	320	-	-
-	-	-	-	-	-	265	-	-	150	-	-
.102	.179	3.33	-	-	-	1070	72.3	4.4	584	3.79	48.3
.137	.0343	2.74	-	-	-	96.7	12.2	.951	635	.47	41.7
-	-	-	-	-	-	1100	-	-	790	-	-
-	-	-	-	-	-	540	-	-	320	-	-
.121	.510	.345	-	-	-	220	289	.972	585	1.04	48.9
-	-	-	-	-	-	266	-	-	48	-	-
.193	.053	1.301	-	-	-	220	19.4	.738	80	.656	23.8
.275	.112	3.82	-	-	-	60	34.1	2.82	1360	.65	66.5
-	-	-	-	-	-	230	-	-	1420	-	-
-	-	-	-	-	-	450	-	-	1380	-	-
-	-	-	-	-	-	610	-	-	1590	-	-
-	-	-	-	-	-	1180	-	-	1380	-	-
-	-	-	-	-	-	430	-	-	1550	-	-
-	-	-	-	-	-	910	-	-	1920	-	-
-	-	-	-	-	-	820	-	-	1550	-	-
.189	.566	1.03	-	-	-	405	120	3	180	2.27	19.6
.148	.559	.866	-	-	-	570	103	2.79	190	2.17	17.4
.166	.563	.666	-	-	-	485	130	3.15	200	2.48	21.1
.0798	.524	.244	-	-	-	200	65.3	2.87	190	1.8	16.5
.477	.464	3.22	-	-	-	770	1.59	3.73	155	1.72	26.7

	Calories (kcal)	Protein (gm)	Carbohydrates (gm)	Fat (gm)	Percent Saturated Fat	Cholesterol (mg)	Dietary Fiber (gm)	Vitamin A (IU)	Vitamin C (mg)
Scrambled eggs	190	14	7	12	-	450	-	837	-
French toast	400	11	45	19	-	115	-	513	-
Home fries	360	4	37	22	-	20	-	-	4.22
Sausage	200	9	1	18	-	30	-	-	-

*Part of Light Menu

FATS AND OILS

Fat   RE

	Calories (kcal)	Protein (gm)	Carbohydrates (gm)	Fat (gm)	Percent Saturated Fat	Cholesterol (mg)	Dietary Fiber (gm)	Vitamin A (IU)	Vitamin C (mg)
Butter, salted - 1 tbsp (14gm)	100	0	0	11	62.2	31	0	106	0
Butter, salted - ½ c (1 stick) (113gm)	810	1	0	92	62.3	247	0	852	0
Fat, beef tallow - 1 tbsp (12.8gm)	115	0	0	12.8	50	14	0	0	0
Fat, chicken - 1 tbsp (12.8gm)	115	0	0	12.8	29.7	11	0	0	0
Fat, duck - 1 tbsp (12.8gm)	115	0	0	12.8	33.6	13	0	0	0
Fat, goose - 1 tbsp (12.8gm)	115	0	0	12.8	27.3	13	0	0	0
Fat, mutton tallow - 1 tbsp (12.8gm)	115	0	0	12.8	47.7	13	0	0	0
Fat, turkey - 1 tbsp (12. 8gm)	115	0	0	12.8	29.7	13	0	0	0
Lard - 1 tbsp (12. 8gm)	115	0	0	12.8	39.1	12	0	0	0
Lard - 1 c (205gm)	1849	.1	.1	205	39.1	195	0	.1	.1
Oil, almond - 1 tbsp (13.6gm)	120	0	0	13.6	8.1	0	0	0	0
Oil, apricot kernel - 1 tbsp (13.6gm)	120	0	0	13.6	6.6	0	0	0	0
Oil, cocoa butter - 1 tbsp (13.6gm)	120	0	0	13.6	59.6	0	0	0	0
Oil, coconut - 1 tbsp (13.6gm)	120	0	0	13.6	86.8	0	0	0	0
Oil, corn - 1 tbsp (13.6gm)	120	0	0	13.6	12.5	0	0	0	0
Oil, corn - 1 c (218 g)	1927	.1	.1	218	12.5	.1	0	.1	.1
Oil, cottonseed - 1 tbsp (13.6gm)	120	0	0	13.6	25.7	0	0	0	0
Oil, hazelnut - 1 tbsp (13.6gm)	120	0	0	13.6	7.4	0	0	0	0
Oil, linseed - 1 tbsp (13.6gm)	120	0	0	13.6	9.6	0	0	0	0
Oil, olive - 1 tbsp (13.5gm)	119	0	0	13.5	13.3	0	0	0	0
Oil, olive - 1 c (216gm)	1909	.1	.1	216	13.3	.1	0	.1	.1
Oil, palm - 1 tbsp (13.6gm)	120	0	0	13.6	49.3	0	0	0	0
Oil, palm kernel - 1 tbsp (13.6gm)	120	0	0	13.6	81.6	0	0	0	0
Oil, peanut - 1 tbsp (13.5gm)	119	0	0	13.5	17	0	0	0	0
Oil, safflower - 1 tbsp (13.6gm)	120	0	0	13.6	8.8	0	0	0	0
Oil, safflower - 1 c (218gm)	1927	.1	.1	218	-	.1	0	.1	.1
Oil, sesame - 1 tbsp (13.6gm)	120	0	0	13.6	14	0	0	0	0

Thiamin (mg)	Riboflavin (mg)	Niacin (mg)	Vitamin B$_6$ (mg)	Vitamin B$_{12}$ (mcg)	Folacin (mcg)	Sodium (mg)	Calcium (mg)	Iron (mg)	Potassium (mg)	Zinc (mg)	Magnesium (mg)
.0637	.491	.0855	-	-	-	160	59.8	2.48	130	1.59	13.5
.58	.499	3.91	-	-	-	850	89	1.66	175	.621	21
.124	.035	2.78	-	-	-	745	21.5	.855	615	.484	35
-	-	-	-	-	-	410	-	-	125	-	-

Source: Fast Food Companies

Thiamin (mg)	Riboflavin (mg)	Niacin (mg)	Vitamin B$_6$ (mg)	Vitamin B$_{12}$ (mcg)	Folacin (mcg)	Sodium (mg)	Calcium (mg)	Iron (mg)	Potassium (mg)	Zinc (mg)	Magnesium (mg)
0	0	0	0	0	.3	116	3.6	0	4	0	.3
0	0	0	0	0	.8	933	27	0	29	0	.8
0	0	0	0	0	0	0	0	0	0	0	0
0	0	0	0	0	0	0	0	0	0	0	0
0	0	0	0	0	0	0	0	0	0	0	0
0	0	0	0	0	0	0	0	0	0	0	0
0	0	0	0	0	0	0	0	0	0	0	0
0	0	0	0	0	0	0	0	0	0	0	0
0	0	0	0	0	0	0	0	0	0	0	0
.1	.1	.1	.1	.1	.1	.1	.2	.1	.1	.3	.1
0	0	0	0	0	0	0	0	0	0	0	0
0	0	0	0	0	0	0	0	0	0	0	0
0	0	0	0	0	0	0	0	0	0	0	0
0	0	0	0	0	0	0	0	0	0	0	0
0	0	0	0	0	0	0	0	0	0	0	0
.1	.1	.1	.1	.1	.1	.1	.1	.1	.1	.1	.1
0	-	0	0	0	0	0	0	0	0	0	0
0	0	0	0	0	0	0	0	0	0	0	0
0	0	0	0	0	0	0	0	0	0	0	0
0	0	0	0	0	0	0	0	.1	0	0	0
.1	.1	.1	.1	.1	.1	.1	.4	.9	.1	.2	.1
.0	0	0	0	0	0	0	0	0	0	-	0
0	0	0	0	0	0	0	0	0	0	0	0
0	0	0	0	0	0	0	0	0	0	0	0
0	0	0	0	0	0	0	0	0	0	0	0
.1	.1	.1	.1	.1	.1	.1	.1	.1	.1	.1	.1
0	0	0	0	0	0	0	0	0	0	0	0

	Calories (kcal)	Protein (gm)	Carbohydrates (gm)	Fat (gm)	Percent Saturated Fat	Cholesterol (mg)	Dietary Fiber (gm)	Vitamin A (RE)	Vitamin C (mg)
Oil, soybean - 1 tbsp (13.6 gm)	120	0	0	13.6	14.7	0	0	0	0
Oil, soybean - 1 c (218gm)	1927	.1	.1	218	-	.1	0	.1	.1
Oil, sunflower - 1 tbsp (13.6gm)	120	0	0	13.6	10.3	0	0	0	0
Oil, walnut - 1 tbsp (13.6gm)	120	0	0	13.6	8.8	0	0	0	0
Oil, wheat germ - 1 tbsp (13.6gm)	120	0	0	13.6	19.1	0	0	0	0
Margarine, hard, coconut, sflwr and palm - 1 tsp (4.7gm)	34	0	0	3.8	71.1	0	0	47	0
Margarine, hard, coconut, sflwr and palm - 1 stick (113.4gm)	815	1	1	91.3	71.1	.1	0	1126	.2
Margarine, hard, corn - 1 tsp (4.7gm)	34	0	0	3.8	18.4	0	0	47	0
Margarine, hard, corn - 1 stick (113.4gm)	815	1	1	91.3	18.4	.1	0	1126	.2
Margarine, hard, soybean - 1 tsp (4.7gm)	34	0	0	3.8	15.8	0	0	47	0
Margarine, soft, corn - 1 tsp (4.7gm)	34	0	0	3.8	18.4	0	0	47	0
Margarine, soft, corn - 1 c (227gm)	1626	1.7	1.2	182.6	18.4	.1	0	2254	.4
Margarine, soft, soybean and cttnsd - 1 tsp (4.7gm)	34	0	0	3.8	21.1	0	0	47	0
Margarine, liquid, soybean and cttnsd - 1 tsp (4.7gm)	34	.1	0	3.8	15.8	0	0	47	0
Margarine, imitation corn - 1 tsp (4.8gm)	17	0	0	1.9	15.8	0	0	48	0
Shortening, lard and veg oil - 1 c (205gm)	1845	.1	.1	205	40.6	115	0	.1	.1
Shortening, soybean and palm - 1 c (205gm)	1812	.1	.1	205	30.5	.1	0	.1	.1
Shortening, soybean and cttnsd - 1 c (205gm)	1812	.1	.1	205	25	.1	0	.1	.1
Shortening, lard and veg oil - 1 tbsp (12.8gm)	115	0	0	12.8	40.6	7	0	0	0
Shortening, soybean and palm - 1 tbsp (12. 8gm)	113	0	0	12.8	30.5	0	0	0	0
Shortening, soybean and cttnsd - 1 tbsp (12.8gm)	113	0	0	12.8	25	0	0	0	0

Salad Dressing

Blue or roquefort cheese - 1 tbsp (15.3gm)	77	.7	1.1	8	18.8	3	0	10	.3
French - 1 tbsp (15.6gm)	67	.1	2.7	6.4	23.4	9	0	3	0
French, diet, lowfat - 1 tbsp (16.3gm)	22	0	3.5	.9	-	1	0	0	0

Thiamin (mg)	Riboflavin (mg)	Niacin (mg)	Vitamin B₆ (mg)	Vitamin B₁₂ (mcg)	Folacin (mcg)	Sodium (mg)	Calcium (mg)	Iron (mg)	Potassium (mg)	Zinc (mg)	Magnesium (mg)
0	0	0	0	0	0	0	0	0	0	0	0
.1	.1	.1	.1	.1	.1	.1	.1	.1	.1	.1	.1
0	0	0	0	0	0	0	0	0	0	0	0
0	0	0	0	0	0	0	0	0	0	0	0
0	0	0	0	0	0	0	0	0	0	0	0
0	0	0	0	0	.1	44.3	1.4	0	2	-	.1
.1	.1	.1	.1	.2	1.4	1069.9	34	.1	48.1	-	3
0	0	0	0	0	.1	44.3	1.4	0	2	0	.1
.1	.1	.1	.1	.2	1.4	1069.9	34	.1	48.1	.1	3
0	0	0	0	0	.1	44.3	1.4	0	2	-	.1
0	0	0	0	0	.1	50.7	1.3	0	1.8	0	.1
.1	.1	.1	.1	.2	2.4	2448.6	60.2	.1	85.6	.1	5.3
0	0	0	0	0	.1	50.7	1.3	0	1.8	0	.1
0	0	0	0	0	.1	36.7	3.1	0	4.4	0	.3
0	0	0	0	0	0	46.1	.9	0	1.2	0	.1
.1	.1	.1	.1	.1	.1	.1	.1	.1	.1	.1	.1
.1	.1	.1	.1	.1	.1	.1	.1	.1	.1	.1	.1
.1	.1	.1	.1	.1	.1	.1	.1	.1	.1	.1	.1
0	0	0	0	0	0	0	0	0	0	0	0
0	0	0	0	0	0	0	0	0	0	0	0
0	0	0	0	0	0	0	0	0	0	0	0
0	0	0	0	0	1.2	167.4	12.4	0	5.7	0	0
0	0	0	0	0	.6	213.7	1.7	.1	12.3	0	0
0	0	0	0	0	0	128.3	1.8	.1	12.9	0	0

	Calories (kcal)	Protein (gm)	Carbohydrates (gm)	Fat (gm)	Percent Saturated Fat	Cholesterol (mg)	Dietary Fiber (gm)	Vitamin A (RE)	Vitamin C (mg)
French, home recipe - 1 tbsp (14gm)	88	0	.5	9.8	18.4	0	0	22	.1
Italian, diet - 1 tbsp (15gm)	16	0	.7	1.5	-	1	0	0	0
Italian - 1 tbsp (14.7gm)	69	.1	1.5	7.1	14.1	0	0	4	0
Mayonnaise type - 1 tbsp (14.7gm)	57	.1	3.5	4.9	14.3	4	0	12	0
Mayonnaise, imitn, milk cream - 1 tbsp (15gm)	14	.3	1.7	.8	-	6	0	0	.1
Mayonnaise, imitn, soybean - 1 tbsp (15gm)	35	0	2.4	2.9	17.2	4	0	0	0
Mayonnaise - 1 tbsp (13.8 gm)	99	.2	.4	11	10.9	8	0	12	0
Russian, low-cal - 1 tbsp (16.3gm)	23	.1	4.5	.7	-	1	0	3	1
Russian - 1 tbsp (15.3gm)	76	.2	1.6	7.8	14.1	3	0	32	.9
Sesame seed - 1 tbsp (15.3gm)	68	.5	1.3	6.9	13	0	0	32	0
Thousand island - 1 tbsp (15.6gm)	59	.1	2.4	5.6	16.1	4	0	15	0
Thousand island, diet - 1 tbsp (15.3gm)	24	.1	2.5	1.6	-	2	0	15	0

FRUIT

	Calories (kcal)	Protein (gm)	Carbohydrates (gm)	Fat (gm)	Percent Saturated Fat	Cholesterol (mg)	Dietary Fiber (gm)	Vitamin A (RE)	Vitamin C (mg)
Acerola (cherry), raw - 1 (4.8gm)	2	.1	.4	.1	-	.1	-	4	80.5
Apples, raw w/skin 1 (3 per lb) (138gm)	81	.3	21.1	.5	-	.1	2.8	7	7.8
Apples, raw, wo/skin - 1 (3 per lb) (128gm)	72	.2	19	.4	-	.1	-	6	5.1
Apples, peeled, cooked - ½ c slices (86gm)	46	.3	11.8	.4	-	.1	1.7	1	.2
Apples, canned, swtnd - ½ c slices (102gm)	68	.2	17.1	.5	-	.1	1.9	5	.4
Apples, dried - 10 rings (64gm)	155	.6	42.2	.2	-	.1	-	.1	2.5
Apples, dried, stewed, w/sgr - ½ c (140gm)	116	.3	29.1	.1	-	.1	-	2	1.3
Apples, dried, stewed, wo/sgr - ½ c (128gm)	72	.3	19.7	.1	-	.1	-	2	1.3
Apples, froz - ½ c slices (103gm)	48	.3	12.4	.4	-	.1	2	2	.4
Applesauce, canned, swtnd, w/salt - ½ c (128gm)	97	.3	25.5	.3	-	.1	1.5	1	2.2
Applesauce, canned, swtnd - ½ c (128gm)	97	.3	25.5	.3	-	.1	1.5	1	2.2
Applesauce, canned, unswtnd w/vit C - ½ c (122gm)	53	.2	13.8	.1	-	.1	1	3	25.9

Thiamin (mg)	Riboflavin (mg)	Niacin (mg)	Vitamin B_6 (mg)	Vitamin B_{12} (mcg)	Folacin (mcg)	Sodium (mg)	Calcium (mg)	Iron (mg)	Potassium (mg)	Zinc (mg)	Magnesium (mg)
0	0	0	0	0	0	92.1	.8	0	3.3	0	0
0	0	0	0	0	0	118.1	.3	0	2.3	0	0
0	0	0	0	0	.7	115.7	1.5	0	2.2	0	.1
0	0	0	0	0	.9	104.5	2.1	0	1.3	0	.3
0	0	0	0	0	.4	75.6	10.8	.1	14.6	0	1.1
0	0	0	0	0	0	74.6	0	0	1.5	0	0
0	0	0	.1	0	1.1	78.4	2.5	.1	4.7	0	.1
0	0	0	0	0	.6	141.5	3.1	.1	25.6	0	.1
0	0	.1	0	0	1.6	132.8	2.9	.1	24	.1	.2
0	0	0	0	0	0	153	2.9	.1	24	0	0
0	0	0	0	0	1	109.2	1.7	.1	17.6	0	.3
0	0	0	0	0	.9	153	1.7	.1	17.3	0	.1

Source: USDA Revised *Handbook 8*

Thiamin (mg)	Riboflavin (mg)	Niacin (mg)	Vitamin B_6 (mg)	Vitamin B_{12} (mcg)	Folacin (mcg)	Sodium (mg)	Calcium (mg)	Iron (mg)	Potassium (mg)	Zinc (mg)	Magnesium (mg)
.1	.1	.1	.1	.1	-	.1	1	.1	7	-	1
.1	.1	.2	.1	.1	3.9	1	10	.3	159	.1	6
.1	.1	.2	.1	.1	.5	.1	5	.1	144	.1	4
.1	.1	.1	.1	.1	.5	1	4	.2	76	.1	3
.1	.1	.1	.1	.1	.3	3	4	.3	69	.1	2
.1	.2	.6	.1	.1	.1	56	9	.9	288	.2	10
.1	.1	.2	.1	.1	.1	27	4	.5	137	.1	5
.1	.1	.2	.1	.1	.1	26	4	.5	134	.1	5
.1	.1	.1	.1	.1	.6	3	5	.2	78	.1	3
.1	.1	.3	.1	.1	.7	35	5	.5	78	.1	4
.1	.1	.3	.1	.1	.7	4	5	.5	78	.1	4
.1	.1	.3	.1	.1	.7	2	4	.2	91	.1	4

	Calories (kcal)	Protein (gm)	Carbohydrates (gm)	Fat (gm)	Percent Saturated Fat	Cholesterol (mg)	Dietary Fiber (gm)	Vitamin A (RE)	Vitamin C (mg)
Applesauce, canned - ½ c (122gm)	53	.2	13.8	.1	-	.1	1	3	1.5
Apricots, raw - 3 (12 per lb) (106gm)	51	1.5	11.8	.5	-	.1	1.4	277	10.6
Apricots, canned, hvy syrup - 3 hlvs, 1¾ tbsp lq (85gm)	70	.5	18.3	.1	-	.1	-	105	2.6
Apricots, canned, x-hvy syrup - 2 fruits, 2 tbsp lq (90gm)	87	.5	22.4	.1	-	.1	-	132	2.2
Apricots, canned, juice - 3 hlvs, 1¾ tbsp lq (84gm)	40	.6	10.4	.1	-	.1	.4	142	4.1
Apricots, canned, lt syrup - 3 hlvs, 1¾ tbsp lq (85gm)	54	.5	14.1	.1	-	.1	-	112	2.3
Apricots, canned, water - 3 hlvs, 1¾ tbsp lq (84gm)	22	.6	5.4	.2	-	.1	-	109	2.9
Apricots, dried - 10 halves (35gm)	83	1.3	21.7	.2	-	.1	-	253	.8
Apricots, dried, stewed, w/sgr - ½ c hlvs (135gm)	153	1.6	39.5	.2	-	.1	-	289	1.9
Apricots, dried, stewed - ½ c hlvs (125gm)	106	1.7	27.4	.2	-	.1	-	295	2
Avocado, California - 1 (173gm)	306	3.7	12	30	15	.1	-	106	13.7
Avocado, Florida - 1 (304gm)	339	4.9	27.1	27	20	.1	-	186	24
Banana, raw - 1 (114gm)	105	1.2	26.8	.6	-	.1	1.6	9	10.3
Blackberries, raw - ½ c (72 gm)	37	.6	9.2	.3	-	.1	3.3	12	15.1
Blackberries, canned, hvy syrup - ½ c (128gm)	118	1.7	29.6	.2	-	.1	5.8	28	3.6
Blackberries, froz - 1 c (151gm)	97	1.8	23.7	.7	-	.1	6.7	17	4.7
Blueberries, raw - 1 c (145gm)	82	1	20.5	.6	-	.1	-	15	18.9
Blueberries, canned, hvy syrup - ½ c (128gm)	112	.9	28.3	.5	-	.1	2.2	8	1.4
Blueberries, froz, swtnd - 1 c thawed (230gm)	187	1	50.5	.4	-	.1	-	10	2.3
Blueberries, froz - 1 c, (155gm)	78	.7	18.9	1	-	.1	3.3	13	3.8
Boysenberries, canned, hvy syrup - ½ c (128gm)	113	1.3	28.6	.2	-	.1	4.9	5	7.9
Boysenberries, froz - 1 c (132gm)	66	1.5	16.1	.4	-	.1	4.8	9	4.1
Breadfruit, raw - ¼ small (96gm)	99	1.1	26.1	.3	-	.1	-	4	27.8
Carambola (starfruit), raw - 1 (127gm)	42	.7	10	.5	-	.1	1.5	63	26.9
Carissa (natal-plum), raw - 1 (20gm)	12	.1	2.8	.3	-	.1	-	1	7.6
Cherimoya, raw - 1 (547gm)	515	7.2	131.3	2.2	-	.1	-	5	49.2

Thiamin (mg)	Riboflavin (mg)	Niacin (mg)	Vitamin B_6 (mg)	Vitamin B_{12} (mcg)	Folacin (mcg)	Sodium (mg)	Calcium (mg)	Iron (mg)	Potassium (mg)	Zinc (mg)	Magnesium (mg)
.1	.1	.3	.1	.1	.7	2	4	.2	91	.1	4
.1	.1	.7	.1	.1	9.1	1	15	.6	313	.3	8
.1	.1	.4	.1	.1	1.4	3	7	.3	119	.1	6
.1	.1	.4	.1	.1	1.5	12	7	.6	113	.1	7
.1	.1	.3	.1	.1	1.4	3	10	.3	139	.1	8
.1	.1	.3	.1	.1	1.4	3	10	.4	117	.1	7
.1	.1	.4	.1	.1	1.5	2	7	.3	161	.1	6
.1	.1	1.1	.1	.1	3.6	3	16	1.7	482	.3	16
.1	.1	1.2	.2	.1	.1	4	20	2.1	598	.4	20
.1	.1	1.2	.2	.1	.1	4	20	2.1	611	.4	21
.2	.3	3.4	.5	.1	113.3	21	19	2.1	1097	.8	70
.4	.4	5.9	.9	.1	161.9	14	33	1.6	1484	1.3	104
.1	.2	.7	.7	.1	21.8	1	7	.4	451	.2	33
.1	.1	.3	.1	.1	24.5	.1	23	.5	141	.2	14
.1	.1	.4	.1	.1	33.9	3	27	.9	127	.3	22
.1	.1	1.9	.1	.1	51.3	2	44	1.3	211	.4	33
.1	.1	.6	.1	.1	9.3	9	9	.3	129	.2	7
.1	.1	.2	.1	.1	2.1	4	7	.5	51	.1	4
.1	.2	.6	.2	.1	15.5	3	13	.9	137	.2	6
.1	.1	.9	.1	.1	10.4	1	12	.3	83	.2	8
.1	.1	.3	.1	.1	44.1	4	23	.6	115	.3	14
.1	.1	1.1	.1	.1	83.6	2	36	1.2	183	.3	21
.2	.1	.9	-	.1	-	2	17	.6	470	.2	24
.1	.1	.6	-	.1	-	2	6	.4	207	.2	12
.1	.1	.1	-	.1	-	1	2	.3	52	-	3
.6	.7	7.2	-	.1	-	-	126	2.8	-	-	-

	Calories (kcal)	Protein (gm)	Carbohydrates (gm)	Fat (gm)	Percent Saturated Fat	Cholesterol (mg)	Dietary Fiber (gm)	Vitamin A (RE)	Vitamin C (mg)
Cherries, sour, red, raw - 1 c w/pits (103gm)	51	1.1	12.6	.4	-	.1	-	132	10.3
Cherries, sour, red, cnd, hvy syrup - ½ c (128gm)	116	1	29.8	.2	-	.1		91	2.5
Cherries, sour, red, cnd, x-hvy syrup - ½ c (130gm)	148	1	38	.2	-	.1	-	90	2.5
Cherries, sour, red, cnd, lt syrup - ½ c (126gm)	94	1	24.4	.2	-	.1	-	91	2.5
Cherries, sour, red, cnd, water - ½ c (122gm)	43	1	11	.2	-	.1	-	92	2.5
Cherries, sour, red, froz - 1 c (155gm)	72	1.5	17.1	.7	-	.1	1.3	135	2.6
Cherries, sweet, raw - 10 (68gm)	49	.9	11.3	.7	-	.1	1.1	15	4.8
Cherries, sweet, cnd, hvy syrup - ½ c pitted (129gm)	107	.8	27.5	.2	-	.1	-	20	4.7
Cherries, sweet, cnd, x-hvy syrup - ½ c pitted (130gm)	133	.8	34.1	.2	-	.1	-	20	4.6
Cherries, sweet, cnd, juice - ½ c pitted (125gm)	68	1.2	17.3	.1	-	.1	.4	16	3.1
Cherries, sweet, cnd, lt syrup - ½ c, pitted (126gm)	85	.8	21.8	.2	-	.1	-	20	4.7
Cherries, sweet, cnd, water - ½ c pitted (124gm)	57	1	14.6	.2	-	.1	-	20	2.7
Cherries, sweet, froz, swtnd - 1 c (259gm)	232	3	57.9	.4	-	.1	-	49	2.6
Crabapples, raw - 1 c slices, w/skin (130gm)	83	.5	22	.4	-	.1	-	4	8.8
Cranberries, raw - 1 c whole (95gm)	46	.4	12.1	.2	-	.1	-	4	12.8
Cranberry sauce, cnd, swtnd - ½ c (138gm)	209	.3	53.7	.3	-	.1	-	3	2.8
Cranberry-orange relish, cnd - ½ c (138gm)	246	.5	63.8	.2	-	.1	-	10	24.8
Currants, black, raw - ½ c (56gm)	36	.8	8.7	.3	-	.1	3.1	13	101.4
Currants, red and white, raw - ½ c (56gm)	31	.8	7.8	.2	-	.1	-	7	23
Currants, Zante, dried - ½ c (72gm)	204	3	53.4	.2	-	.1	-	5	3.4
Dates - 10 (83gm)	228	1.7	61.1	.4	-	.1	-	4	.1
Elderberries, raw - 1 c (145gm)	105	1	26.7	.8	-	.1	-	87	52.2
Figs, raw - 1 med (50gm)	37	.4	9.6	.2	-	.1	-	7	1
Figs, cnd, hvy syrup - 3 (85gm)	75	.4	19.5	.1	-	.1	-	3	.9
Figs, cnd, x-hvy syrup - 3 (85gm)	91	.4	23.7	.1	-	.1	-	3	.8
Figs, cnd, lt syrup - 3 (85gm)	58	.4	15.3	.1	-	.1	-	3	.9

Thiamin (mg)	Riboflavin (mg)	Niacin (mg)	Vitamin B$_6$ (mg)	Vitamin B$_{12}$ (mcg)	Folacin (mcg)	Sodium (mg)	Calcium (mg)	Iron (mg)	Potassium (mg)	Zinc (mg)	Magnesium (mg)
.1	.1	.5	.1	.1	7.7	3	16	.4	178	.1	9
.1	.1	.3	.1	.1	9.7	9	13	1.7	119	.1	7
.1	.1	.3	.1	.1	9.6	9	13	1.7	118	.1	7
.1	.1	.3	.1	.1	9.7	9	13	1.7	119	.1	7
.1	.1	.3	.1	.1	9.8	9	13	1.7	120	.1	7
.1	.1	.3	.2	.1	7	1	20	.9	192	.2	13
.1	.1	.3	.1	.1	2.8	.1	10	.3	152	.1	8
.1	.1	.6	.1	.1	5.4	3	12	.5	187	.2	11
.1	.1	.6	.1	.1	5.4	3	11	.5	185	.2	11
.1	.1	.6	.1	.1	5.2	3	17	.8	163	.2	16
.1	.1	.6	.1	.1	5.3	3	12	.5	186	.2	11
.1	.1	.6	.1	.1	5.2	2	13	.5	162	.1	11
.1	.2	.5	.1	.1	10.9	3	31	.9	514	.1	26
.1	.1	.2	-	.1	-	1	20	.4	213	-	7
.1	.1	.1	.1	.1	1.6	1	7	.2	67	.2	5
.1	.1	.2	.1	.1	-	40	5	.3	35	.1	4
.1	.1	.2	-	.1	-	44	15	.3	53	-	6
.1	.1	.2	.1	.1	-	1	31	.9	180	.2	14
.1	.1	.1	.1	.1	-	1	18	.6	154	.2	7
.2	.2	1.2	.3	.1	7.3	6	62	2.4	642	.5	30
.1	.1	1.9	.2	.1	10.4	2	27	1	541	.3	29
.2	.1	.8	.4	.1	-	-	55	2.4	406	-	-
.1	.1	.2	.1	.1	-	1	18	.2	116	.1	8
.1	.1	.4	-	.1	-	1	23	.3	85	.1	8
.1	.1	.4	-	.1	-	1	22	.3	83	.1	8
.1	.1	.4	-	.1	-	1	23	.3	86	.1	9

	Calories (kcal)	Protein (gm)	Carbohydrates (gm)	Fat (gm)	Percent Saturated Fat	Cholesterol (mg)	Dietary Fiber (gm)	Vitamin A (RE)	Vitamin C (mg)
Figs, cnd, water - 3 (80gm)	42	.4	11.2	.1	-	.1	-	3	.8
Figs, dried - 10 (187gm)	477	5.7	122.2	2.2	-	.1	-	25	1.6
Figs, dried, stewed - ½ c (130gm)	140	1.7	35.9	.7	-	.1	-	21	5.8
Fruit cktl, cnd, hvy syrup - ½ c (128gm)	93	.5	24.3	.1	-	.1	-	26	2.4
Fruit cktl, cnd, x-hvy syrup - ½ c (130gm)	115	.5	29.8	.1	-	.1	-	26	2.4
Fruit cktl, cnd, lt syrup - ½ c (126gm)	72	.5	18.9	.1	-	.1	-	26	2.4
Fruit cktl, cnd, water - ½ c (122gm)	40	.6	10.4	.1	-	.1	-	30	2.5
Fruit cktl, cnd, juice - ½ c (124gm)	56	.6	14.8	.1	-	.1	.8	38	3.4
Fruit salad, cnd, hvy syrup - ½ c (128gm)	94	.5	24.5	.1	-	.1	-	65	3
Fruit salad, cnd, x-hvy syrup - ½ c (130gm)	114	.5	29.6	.1	-	.1	-	83	2.7
Fruit salad, cnd, juice - ½ c (124gm)	62	.7	16.2	.1	-	.1	.9	74	4.1
Fruit salad, cnd, lt syrup - ½ c (126gm)	73	.5	19.1	.1	-	.1	-	54	3.1
Fruit salad, cnd, water - ½ c (122gm)	37	.5	9.6	.1	-	.1	-	54	2.3
Fruit salad, tropical, cnd, - ½ c (128gm)	110	.6	28.7	.2	-	.1	-	16	22.4
Gooseberries, raw - 1 c (150gm)	67	1.4	15.3	.9	-	.1	-	44	41.6
Gooseberries, canned - ½ c (126gm)	93	.9	23.7	.3	-	.1	2.7	17	12.6
Grapefruit, raw - ½ (120gm)	38	.8	9.7	.2	-	.1	-	15	41.3
Grapefruit, sections, cnd, juice - ½ c (124gm)	46	.9	11.5	.2	-	.1	.3	.1	42
Grapefruit, sections, cnd, lt syrup - ½ c (127gm)	76	.8	19.6	.2	-	.1	-	.1	27
Grapefruit, sections, cnd, water - ½ c (122gm)	44	.8	11.2	.2	-	.1	-	.1	26.6
Grapes, American type (slip skin), raw - 10 (24gm)	15	.2	4.2	.1	-	.1	-	2	1
Grapes, cnd, Thompson sdls, hvy syrup - ½ c (128gm)	94	.7	25.2	.2	-	.1	-	8	1.3
Grapes, cnd, Thompson sdls, water - ½ c (122gm)	48	.7	12.6	.2	-	.1	-	8	1.3
Grapes, European type (adherent skin), raw - 10 (50gm)	36	.4	8.9	.3	-	.1	.9	4	5.4
Groundcherries, raw - ½ c (70gm)	37	1.4	7.9	.5	-	.1	-	50	7.7
Guava, raw - 1 (90gm)	45	.8	10.7	.6	-	.1	-	71	165.1

Thiamin (mg)	Riboflavin (mg)	Niacin (mg)	Vitamin B$_6$ (mg)	Vitamin B$_{12}$ (mcg)	Folacin (mcg)	Sodium (mg)	Calcium (mg)	Iron (mg)	Potassium (mg)	Zinc (mg)	Magnesium (mg)
.1	.1	.4	-	.1	-	1	22	.3	83	.1	8
.2	.2	1.3	.5	.1	14.1	20	269	4.2	1332	1	111
.1	.2	.9	.2	.1	1.3	6	79	1.3	391	.3	33
.1	.1	.5	.1	.1	3.4	7	8	.4	112	.2	7
.1	.1	.5	.1	.1	3.4	7	8	.4	112	.2	7
.1	.1	.5	.1	.1	3.4	7	8	.4	112	.2	7
.1	.1	.5	.1	.1	3.3	5	6	.4	115	.2	8
.1	.1	.5	.1	.1	3.1	4	10	.3	118	.2	9
.1	.1	.5	.1	.1	3.3	7	8	.4	103	.1	7
.1	.1	.5	.1	.1	3.2	7	8	.4	104	.1	7
.1	.1	.5	.1	.1	3.3	7	14	.4	144	.2	10
.1	.1	.5	.1	.1	3.3	7	8	.4	104	.1	7
.1	.1	.5	.1	.1	3.2	4	8	.4	95	.1	7
.1	.1	.8	-	.1	-	3	17	.7	168	.2	17
.1	.1	.5	.2	.1	-	1	38	.5	297	.2	15
.1	.1	.2	.1	.1	4	3	20	.5	97	.2	8
.1	.1	.3	.1	.1	12.2	.1	14	.1	167	.1	10
.1	.1	.4	.1	.1	10.9	9	19	.3	209	.1	13
.1	.1	.4	.1	.1	10.8	2	18	.6	164	.2	13
.1	.1	.4	.1	.1	10.7	2	18	.5	161	.2	12
.1	.1	.1	.1	.1	.9	.1	3	.1	46	.1	1
.1	.1	.2	.1	.1	3.3	7	13	1.2	132	.1	8
.1	.1	.2	.1	.1	3.1	7	13	1.2	131	.1	8
.1	.1	.2	.1	.1	2	1	5	.2	93	.1	3
.1	.1	2	-	.1	-	-	6	.7	-	-	-
.1	.1	1.1	.2	.1	-	2	18	.3	256	.3	9

	Calories (kcal)	Protein (gm)	Carbohydrates (gm)	Fat (gm)	Percent Saturated Fat	Cholesterol (mg)	Dietary Fiber (gm)	Vitamin A (RE)	Vitamin C (mg)
Guava sauce, cooked - ½ c (119gm)	43	.4	11.3	.2	-	.1	-	34	174.2
Kiwifruit, raw - 1 (76gm)	46	.8	11.4	.4	-	.1	-	13	74.5
Kumquat, raw - 1 (19gm)	12	.2	3.2	.1	-	.1	-	6	7.1
Lemon, raw, w/peel - 1 (108gm)	22	1.3	11.6	.4	-	.1	-	3	83.2
Lemon, raw, wo/peel - 1 (58gm)	17	.7	5.5	.2	-	.1	-	2	30.7
Lemon peel, raw - 1 tsp (2gm)	-	.1	.4	.1	-	.1	-	.1	2.6
Lime, raw - 1 (67gm)	20	.5	7.1	.2	-	.1	-	1	19.5
Litchi, raw - 1 (9.6gm)	6	.1	1.6	.1	-	.1	-	.1	6.9
Loganberries, froz - 1 c (167gm)	80	2.3	19.2	.5	-	.1	6.5	5	22.5
Loquat, raw - 1 (9.9gm)	5	.1	1.2	.1	-	.1	-	15	.1
Mammy-apple, raw - 1 (846gm)	431	4.3	105.8	4.3	-	.1	-	195	118.4
Mango, raw - 1 (207gm)	135	1.1	35.2	.6	-	.1	2.3	806	57.3
Melon, cantaloupe, raw - ½ (267gm)	94	2.4	22.4	.8	-	.1	.9	861	112.7
Melon, casaba, raw - 1/10 (164gm)	43	1.5	10.2	.2	-	.1	-	5	26.2
Melon, honeydew, raw - 1/10 (129gm)	46	.6	11.9	.2	-	.1	-	5	32
Melon balls, froz - 1 c (173gm)	58	1.5	13.8	.5	-	.1	1.3	307	10.7
Mixed, cnd, hvy syrp, - ½ c (128gm)	92	.5	24.1	.2	-	.1	-	25	88.3
Mixed , dried - 1 oz (28.4gm)	.1	.1	.1	.1	-	.1	-	.1	.1
Mixed, froz, swtnd - 1 c (250gm)	245	3.6	60.6	.5	-	.1	-	81	187.6
Mulberries, raw - 10 (15gm)	7	.3	1.5	.1	-	.1	-	.1	5.5
Nectarine, raw - 1 (136gm)	67	1.3	16.1	.7	-	.1	-	100	7.3
Orange, raw - 1 (131gm)	62	1.3	15.4	.2	-	.1	-	27	69.7
Orange peel, raw - 1 tsp (2gm)	-	.1	.5	.1	-	.1	-	1	2.7
Papaya, raw - 1 (304gm)	117	1.9	29.9	.5	-	.1	2.8	612	187.8
Passion fruit, purple, raw - 1 (18gm)	18	.4	4.3	.2	-	.1	-	13	5.4
Peach, raw - 1 (4 per lb) (87gm)	37	.7	9.7	.1	-	.1	.6	47	5.7
Peaches, cnd, hvy syrup - 1 half (81gm)	60	.4	16.2	.1	-	.1	-	27	2.2
Peaches, cnd, x-hvy syrup - 1 half (81gm)	77	.4	21.2	.1	-	.1	-	11	1
Peaches, cnd, juice - 1 half (77gm)	34	.5	9	.1	-	.1	.4	29	2.7

Thiamin (mg)	Riboflavin (mg)	Niacin (mg)	Vitamin B$_6$ (mg)	Vitamin B$_{12}$ (mcg)	Folacin (mcg)	Sodium (mg)	Calcium (mg)	Iron (mg)	Potassium (mg)	Zinc (mg)	Magnesium (mg)
.1	.1	.5	-	.1	-	4	8	.3	268	.2	8
.1	.1	.4	-	.1	-	4	20	.4	252	-	23
.1	.1	.1	-	.1	-	1	8	.1	37	.1	2
.1	.1	.3	.2	.1	-	3	66	.8	157	.2	13
.1	.1	.1	.1	.1	6.2	1	15	.4	80	.1	5
.1	.1	.1	.1	.1	-	.1	3	.1	3	-	.1
.1	.1	.2	.1	.1	5.5	1	22	.4	68	.1	4
.1	.1	.1	-	.1	-	.1	.1	.1	16	.1	1
.1	.1	1.3	.1	.1	37.8	1	38	1	213	.5	32
.1	.1	.1	-	.1	-	.1	2	.1	26	.1	1
.2	.4	3.4	-	.1	-	127	93	6	398	-	-
.2	.2	1.3	.3	.1	-	4	21	.3	322	.1	18
.1	.1	1.6	.4	.1	45.5	23	28	.6	825	.5	28
.1	.1	.7	-	.1	-	20	8	.7	344	-	13
.1	.1	.8	.1	.1	-	13	8	.1	350	-	9
.3	.1	1.2	.2	.1	44.5	53	17	.5	484	.3	24
.1	.1	.8	.1	.1	3.8	5	1	.5	108	.1	6
.1	.1	.1	.1	.1	.1	.1	.1	.1	.1	.1	.1
.1	.1	1	.1	.1	19	8	18	.7	327	.2	14
.1	.1	.1	-	.1	-	2	6	.3	29	-	3
.1	.1	1.4	.1	.1	5.1	.1	6	.3	288	.2	11
.2	.1	.4	.1	.1	39.7	.1	52	.2	237	.1	13
.1	.1	.1	.1	.1	-	.1	3	.1	4.	-	.1
.1	.1	1.1	.1	.1	-	8	72	.3	780	.3	31
.1	.1	.3	-	.1	-	5	2	.3	63	-	5
.1	.1	.9	.1	.1	3	.1	5	.1	171	.2	6
.1	.1	.5	.1	.1	2.6	5	2	.3	74	.1	4
.1	.1	.5	.1	.1	2.5	6	3	.3	67	.1	4
.1	.1	.5	.1	.1	2.6	3	5	.3	98	.1	6

	Calories (kcal)	Protein (gm)	Carbohydrates (gm)	Fat (gm)	Percent Saturated Fat	Cholesterol (mg)	Dietary Fiber (gm)	Vitamin A (RE)	Vitamin C (mg)
Peaches; cnd, lt syrup - 1 half 1¾ tbsp lg (81gm)	44	.4	11.8	.1	-	.1	-	29	1.9
Peaches, cnd, water - 1 half (77gm)	18	.4	4.7	.1	-	.1	-	41	2.2
Peaches, dried, sulfured, unckd - 10 hlvs (130gm)	311	4.7	79.8	1	-	.1	-	281	6.3
Peaches, dried, stewed, w/sgr - ½ c hlvs (135gm)	139	1.5	36	.3	-	.1	-	24	4.6
Peaches, dried, stewed - ½ c hlvs (129gm)	99	1.5	25.5	.4	-	.1	-	25	4.8
Peaches, froz, swtnd - 1 c slices unthawed (250gm)	235	1.6	60	.4	-	.1	-	71	235.4
Peaches, spiced, cnd - 1 (88gm)	66	.4	17.7	.1	-	.1	-	28	4.6
Pear, raw - 1 (2½ per lb) (166gm)	98	.7	25.1	.7	-	.1	4.1	3	6.6
Pears, cnd, hvy syrup - 1 half (79gm)	58	0.2	15.2	.1	-	.1	-	.1	.9
Pears, cnd, x-hvy syrup - 1 half (79gm)	77	.2	20	.1	-	.1	-	.1	.9
Pears, cnd, juice - 1 half (77gm)	38	.3	10	.1	-	.1	.7	.1	1.2
Pears, cnd, lt syrup - 1 half (79gm)	45	.2	12	.1	-	.1	-	.1	.6
Pears, cnd, water - 1 half (77gm)	22	.2	6.1	.1	-	.1	-	.1	.8
Pears, dried - 10 hlvs (175gm)	459	3.3	122	1.1	-	.1	-	1	12.3
Pears, dried, stewed, w/sgr - ½ c hlvs (140gm)	196	1.3	52	.5	-	.1	-	6	5.3
Pears, dried, stewed - ½ c hlvs (128gm)	163	1.2	43.3	.4	-	.1	-	5	5.1
Persimmon, Japanese, raw - 1 (168gm)	118	1	31.3	.4	-	.1	-	364	12.6
Persimmon, native, raw - 1 (25gm)	32	.2	8.4	.1	-	.1	-	-	16.5
Persimmon, Japanese, dried - 1 (34gm)	93	.5	25	.2	-	.1	-	19	.1
Pineapple, raw - 1 slice (84gm)	42	.4	10.5	.4	-	.1	1.3	2	13
Pineapple, cnd, hvy syrup - 1 slice (58gm)	45	.2	11.8	.1	-	.1	-	1	4.3
Pineapple, cnd, juice - 1 slice (28gm)	35	.3	9.1	.1	-	.1	.5	2	5.5
Pineapple, cnd, lt syrup - 1 slice (58gm)	30	.3	7.8	.1	-	.1	-	1	4.4
Pineapple, cnd, water - 1 slice (58gm)	19	.3	4.9	.1	-	.1	-	1	4.5
Pineapple, froz, swtnd - ½ c chunks (122gm)	104	.5	27.1	.2	-	.1	-	4	9.8

Thiamin (mg)	Riboflavin (mg)	Niacin (mg)	Vitamin B$_6$ (mg)	Vitamin B$_{12}$ (mcg)	Folacin (mcg)	Sodium (mg)	Calcium (mg)	Iron (mg)	Potassium (mg)	Zinc (mg)	Magnesium (mg)
.1	.1	.5	.1	.1	2.6	4	3	.3	79	.1	4
.1	.1	.5	.1	.1	2.6	3	2	.3	76	.1	4
.1	.3	5.7	.1	.1	.4	9	37	5.3	1295	.8	54
.1	.1	1.9	.1	.1	.1	3	11	1.7	395	.3	16
.1	.1	2	.1	.1	.1	3	12	1.7	413	.3	17
.1	.1	1.7	.1	.1	8	16	6	1	325	.2	12
.1	.1	.5	.1	.1	2.8	3	5	.3	75	.1	6
.1	.1	.2	.1	.1	12.1	1	19	.5	208	.2	9
.1	.1	.2	.1	.1	.9	4	4	.2	51	.1	3
.1	.1	.2	.1	.1	.9	4	4	.2	50	.1	3
.1	.1	.2	.1	.1	1	3	7	.3	74	.1	5
.1	.1	.2	.1	.1	1	4	4	.3	52	.1	3
.1	.1	.1	.1	.1	1	2	3	.2	41	.1	3
.1	.3	2.5	.2	.1	.1	10	59	3.7	932	.7	58
.1	.1	.5	.1	.1	.1	4	22	1.4	344	.3	21
.1	.1	.5	.1	.1	.1	4	21	1.3	331	.3	21
.1	.1	.2	-	.1	12.6	3	13	.3	270	.2	15
-	-	-	-	.1	-	.1	7	.7	78	-	-
-	.1	.1	-	.1	-	1	8	.3	273	.2	11
.1	.1	.4	.1	.1	8.9	1	6	.4	95	.1	11
.1	.1	.2	.1	.1	2.7	1	8	.3	60	.1	9
.1	.1	.2	.1	.1	2.8	1	8	.2	70	.1	8
.1	.1	.2	.1	.1	2.7	1	8	.3	61	.1	9
.1	.1	.2	.1	.1	2.8	1	9	.3	74	.1	10
.2	.1	.4	.1	.1	12.9	2	11	.5	122	.2	12

	Calories (kcal)	Protein (gm)	Carbohydrates (gm)	Fat (gm)	Percent Saturated Fat	Cholesterol (mg)	Dietary Fiber (gm)	Vitamin A (RE)	Vitamin C (mg)
Plantain, raw - 1 (17gm)	218	2.4	57.1	.7	-	.1	-	202	32.9
Plantain, cooked - ½ c slices (77gm)	89	.7	24	.2	-	.1	-	70	8.4
Plum, raw - 1 (66gm)	36	.6	8.6	.5	-	.1	-	21	6.3
Plums, cnd, hvy syrup - 3 (133gm)	119	.5	31	.2	-	.1	-	34	.6
Plum, cnd, x-hvy syrup - 3 (133gm)	135	.5	35	.2	-	.1	-	34	.5
Plum, cnd, lt syrup - 3 (133gm)	83	.5	21.7	.2	-	.1	-	35	.6
Plum, cnd, water - 3 (95gm)	39	.4	10.5	.1	-	.1	-	87	2.6
Plums, cnd, juice - 3 (95gm)	55	.5	14.4	.1	-	.1	.4	96	2.6
Pomegranate, raw - 1 (154gm)	104	1.5	26.5	.5	-	.1	-	.1	9.4
Pricklypear, raw - 1 (103gm)	42	.8	9.9	.6	-	.1	-	5	14.4
Prunes, cnd, hvy syrup - 5 (86gm)	90	.8	24	.2	-	.1	-	69	2.4
Prunes, dried, 10 pitted (84gm)	201	2.2	52.7	.5	-	.1	-	167	2.8
Prunes, dried, stewed, w/sgr - ½ c pitted (119gm)	147	1.3	39.2	.3	-	.1	-	34	3.2
Prunes, dried, stewed - ½ c pitted (106gm)	113	1.3	29.8	.3	-	.1	-	32	3.1
Quince, raw - 1 (92gm)	53	.4	14.1	.1	-	.1	-	4	13.8
Raisins, seeded - 1 c (145gm)	428	3.7	113.8	.8	-	.1	-	.1	7.9
Raisins, seedless - 1 c (145gm)	434	4.7	114.8	.7	-	.1	-	1	4.8
Raspberries, raw - 1 c (123gm)	61	1.2	14.3	.7	-	.1	5.8	16	30.8
Raspberries, cnd, red, hvy syrup - ½ c (128gm)	117	1.1	29.9	.2	-	.1	3.6	4	11.2
Raspberries, froz, red, swtnd, unthawed - 1 c (250gm)	256	1.8	65.4	.4	-	.1	-	15	41.3
Rhubarb, raw - ½ c diced (61gm)	13	.6	2.8	.2	-	.1	-	6	4.9
Rhubarb, froz, ckd, w/sgr - ½ c (120gm)	139	.5	37.5	.1	-	.1	1.2	8	3.9
Rhubarb, froz, unthawed - 1 c diced (137gm)	14	.4	3.5	.1	-	.1	.9	7	3.3
Strawberries, raw - 1 c (149gm)	45	1	10.5	.6	-	.1	2.9	4	84.5
Strawberries, cnd, hvy syrup - ½ c (127gm)	117	.8	29.9	.4	-	.1	1.6	3	40.2
Strawberries, froz, swtnd, sl, unthawed - 1 c (265gm)	245	1.4	66.1	.4	-	.1	-	6	105.6
Strawberries, froz, swtnd, whole, unthawed - 1 c (255gm)	200	1.4	53.6	.4	-	.1	-	7	100.7

Thiamin (mg)	Riboflavin (mg)	Niacin (mg)	Vitamin B$_6$ (mg)	Vitamin B$_{12}$ (mcg)	Folacin (mcg)	Sodium (mg)	Calcium (mg)	Iron (mg)	Potassium (mg)	Zinc (mg)	Magnesium (mg)
.1	.1	1.3	.6	.1	39.4	7	5	1.1	893	.3	66
.1	.1	.6	.2	.1	20	4	2	.5	358	.1	25
.1	.1	.4	.1	.1	1.4	.1	2	.1	113	.1	4
.1	.1	.4	.1	.1	3.3	26	12	1.2	121	.1	7
.1	.1	.4	.1	.1	3.3	25	12	1.1	118	.1	7
.1	.1	.4	.1	.1	3.4	26	13	1.2	123	.1	7
.1	.1	.4	.1	.1	2.5	1	6	.2	120	.1	5
.1	.1	.5	.1	.1	2.5	1	9	.4	147	.1	8
.1	.1	.5	.2	.1	-	5	5	.5	399	-	5
.1	.1	.5	-	.1	-	6	58	.4	226	-	88
.1	.2	.8	.2	.1	.1	2	15	.4	194	.2	13
.1	.2	1.7	.3	.1	3.1	3	43	2.1	626	.5	38
.1	.2	.9	.3	.1	.1	2	25	1.3	371	.3	22
.1	.2	.8	.3	.1	.1	2	24	1.2	354	.3	21
.1	.1	.2	.1	.1	-	4	10	.7	181	-	7
.2	.3	1.7	.3	.1	4.8	41	41	3.8	1197	.3	43
.3	.2	1.2	.4	.1	4.8	17	71	3.1	1089	.4	48
.1	.2	1.2	.1	.1	32	.1	27	.7	187	.6	22
.1	.1	.6	.1	.1	13.4	4	14	.6	120	.2	16
.1	.2	.6	.1	.1	65	1	38	1.7	285	.5	32
.1	.1	.2	.1	.1	4.3	2	52	.2	175	.1	7
.1	.1	.3	.1	.1	6.4	2	174	.3	115	.1	15
.1	.1	.2	.1	.1	5.6	1	132	.2	73	.1	12
.1	.1	.4	.1	.1	26.4	2	21	.6	247	.2	16
.1	.1	.1	.1	.1	35.6	5	16	.7	109	.2	11
.1	.2	1.1	.1	.1	37.9	8	28	1.5	249	.2	18
.1	.2	.8	.1	.1	9.7	3	29	1.3	249	.2	16

	Calories (kcal)	Protein (gm)	Carbohydrates (gm)	Fat (gm)	Percent Saturated Fat	Cholesterol (mg)	Dietary Fiber (gm)	Vitamin A (RE)	Vitamin C (mg)
Strawberries, froz, unthawed - 1 c (149gm)	52	.7	13.6	.2	-	.1	-	7	61.4
Tangerine, raw - 1 (84gm)	37	.6	9.4	.2	-	.1	-	77	25.9
Tangerines, cnd, juice - ½ c (124gm)	46	.8	11.9	.1	-	.1	-	106	42.5
Tangerines, cnd, lt syrup - ½ c (126gm)	76	.6	20.4	.2	-	.1	-	106	25
Watermelon, raw - 1/16 (10" dia) (482gm)	152	3	34.7	2.1	-	.1	1	176	46.5

FRUIT JUICES

All juices are unsweetened unless noted.

	Calories (kcal)	Protein (gm)	Carbohydrates (gm)	Fat (gm)	Percent Saturated Fat	Cholesterol (mg)	Dietary Fiber (gm)	Vitamin A (RE)	Vitamin C (mg)
Apple, cnd/btld, w/vit C - 1 fl oz (31gm)	15	.1	3.7	.1	-	.1	-	.1	12.9
Apple, cnd/btld - 1 fl oz (31gm)	15	.1	3.7	.1	-	.1	-	.1	.3
Apple, froz rcnstd - 1 fl oz (29.9gm)	14	.1	3.5	.1	-	.1	-	.1	.2
Apple, froz, rcnstd w/vit C - 1 fl oz (29.9gm)	14	.1	-	.1	-	.1	-	.1	7.5
Apple, froz, conc, w/vit C - 6 fl oz (211gm)	349	1.1	86.6	.8	-	.1	-	.1	187.7
Apple, froz, conc, - 6 fl oz (211gm)	349	1.1	86.6	.8	-	.1	-	.1	4.4
Apricot nectar, cnd, w/vit C - 1 fl oz (31.4gm)	18	.2	4.6	.1	-	.1	.1	41	17.1
Apricot nectar, cnd - 1 fl oz (31.4gm)	18	.2	4.6	.1	-	.1	.1	41	.2
Cranberry cktl, btld - 1 fl oz (31.6gm)	18	.1	4.7	.1	-	.1	-	.1	13.5
Grape, cnd/btld - 1 fl oz (31.6gm)	19	.2	4.8	.1	-	.1	-	.1	.1
Grape, froz, conc, swtnd, rcnstd - 1 fl oz (31.2gm)	16	.1	4	.1	-	.1	.1	.1	7.5
Grape, froz, swtnd - 6 fl oz (216gm)	386	1.4	95.9	.7	-	.1	.2	6	179.5
Grapefruit, pink, raw - juice 1 fruit (196gm)	76	1	18.1	.2	-	.1	-	86	74.5
Grapefruit, white, raw - juice 1 fruit (196gm)	76	1	18.1	.2	-	.1	-	2	74.5
Grapefruit, cnd, swtnd - 1 fl oz (31.2gm)	14	.2	3.5	.1	-	.1	-	.1	8.4
Grapefruit, cnd - 1 fl oz (30.9gm)	12	.2	2.8	.1	-	.1	-	.1	9
Grapefruit, froz, rcnstd - 1 fl oz (30.9gm)	13	.2	3.1	.1	-	.1	-	.1	10.4

Thiamin (mg)	Riboflavin (mg)	Niacin (mg)	Vitamin B6 (mg)	Vitamin B12 (mcg)	Folacin (mcg)	Sodium (mg)	Calcium (mg)	Iron (mg)	Potassium (mg)	Zinc (mg)	Magnesium (mg)
.1	.1	.7	.1	.1	25	3	23	1.2	220	.2	16
.1	.1	.2	.1	.1	17.1	1	12	.1	132	.2	10
.2	.1	.6	.1	.1	5.7	7	14	.4	165	.7	14
.1	.1	.6	.1	.1	5.8	8	9	.5	99	.3	10
.4	.1	1	.7	.1	10.4	10	38	.9	560	.4	52

Source: USDA Revised *Handbook 8*

Thiamin (mg)	Riboflavin (mg)	Niacin (mg)	Vitamin B6 (mg)	Vitamin B12 (mcg)	Folacin (mcg)	Sodium (mg)	Calcium (mg)	Iron (mg)	Potassium (mg)	Zinc (mg)	Magnesium (mg)
.1	.1	-	.1	.1	.1	1	2	.2	37	.1	1
.1	.1	.1	.1	.1	.1	1	2	.2	37	.1	1
.1	.1	.1	.1	.1	.1	2	2	.1	38	.1	1
.1	.1	.1	.1	.1	.1	2	2	.1	38	.1	1
.1	.2	.3	.3	.1	2.1	54	43	2	945	.3	37
.1	.2	.3	.3	.1	2.1	54	43	2	945	.3	37
.1	.1	.1	.1	.1	.4	1	2	.2	36	.1	2
.1	.1	.1	.1	.1	.4	1	2	.2	36	.1	2
.1	.1	.1	-	.1	.1	1	1	.1	8	.1	1
.1	.1	.1	.1	.1	.8	1	3	.1	42	.1	3
.1	.1	.1	.1	.1	.4	1	1	.1	7	.1	1
.2	.2	1	.4	.1	9.4	15	28	.8	159	.3	32
.1	.1	.4	.1	.1	20	2	18	.4	318	.1	24
.1	.1	.4	.1	.1	20	2	18	.4	318	.1	24
.1	.1	.1	.1	.1	3.2	.1	2	.2	51	.1	3
.1	.1	.1	.1	.1	3.2	.1	2	.1	47	.1	3
.1	.1	.1	.1	.1	1.1	.1	2	.1	42	.1	3

	Calories (kcal)	Protein (gm)	Carbohydrates (gm)	Fat (gm)	Percent Saturated Fat	Cholesterol (mg)	Dietary Fiber (gm)	Vitamin A (RE)	Vitamin C (mg)
Grapefruit, froz, conc - 6 fl oz (207gm)	302	4.1	71.6	1	-	.1	-	6	248.1
Lemon, raw - 1 tbsp (15.2gm)	4	.1	1.4	.1	-	.1	-	.1	7
Lemon, cnd/btld - 1 tbsp (15.2gm)	3	.1	1	.1	-	.1	-	.1	3.8
Lemon, froz - 1 tbsp (15.2gm)	3	.1	1	.1	-	.1	.1	.1	4.8
Lime, raw - 1 tbsp (15.4gm)	4	.1	1.4	.1	-	.1	-	.1	4.5
Lime, cnd/btld - 1 tbsp (15.4gm)	3	.1	1.1	.1	-	.1	-	.1	1
Orange, raw - juice 1 fruit (86gm)	39	.6	9	.2	-	.1	-	17	43
Orange - 1 fl oz (31gm)	14	.3	3.2	.1	-	.1	.1	5	13.3
Orange, cnd, - 1 fl oz (31.1gm)	13	.2	3.1	.1	-	.1	-	5	10.7
Orange, froz, recnstd - 1 fl oz (31.1gm)	14	.3	3.4	.1	-	.1	-	2	12.1
Orange, froz - 6 fl oz (213gm)	339	5.1	81.3	.5	-	.1	-	59	293.6
Orange-grapefruit, cnd - 1 fl oz (31gm)	13	.2	3.2	.1	-	.1	-	4	9
Papaya nectar, cnd - 1 fl oz (31gm)	18	.1	4.6	.1	-	.1	.1	3	.9
Passionfruit, purple, raw - 1 fl oz (31gm)	16	.2	4.2	.1	-	.1	-	22	9.2
Passionfruit, yellow, raw - 1 fl oz (31gm)	19	.3	4.5	.1	-	.1	-	74	5.6
Peach nectar, cnd, w/vit C - 1 fl oz (31.1gm)	17	.1	4.4	.1	-	.1	.1	8	8.3
Peach nectar, cnd - 1 fl oz (31.1 oz)	17	.1	4.4	.1	-	.1	.1	8	1.6
Pear nectar, cnd, w/vit C - 1 fl oz (31.2gm)	19	.1	5	.1	-	.1	.2	.1	8.4
Pear nectar, cnd - 1 fl oz (31.2gm)	19	.1	5	.1	-	.1	.2	.1	.3
Pineapple, cnd, - 1 fl oz (31.3gm)	17	.1	4.4	.1	-	.1	-	.1	3.3
Pineapple, cnd, w/vit C - 1 fl oz (31.3gm)	17	.1	4.4	.1	-	.1	-	.1	12.1
Pineapple, froz, rcnstd - 1 fl oz (31.2gm)	16	.2	4	.1	-	.1	-	.1	3.7
Pineapple, froz, conc - 6 fl oz (216gm)	387	2.9	95.7	.3	-	.1	-	11	90.7
Prune, cnd - 1 fl oz (32gm)	23	.2	5.6	.1	-	.1	-	.1	1.3
Tangerine, raw - 1 fl oz (30.9gm)	13	.2	3.2	.1	-	.1	-	13	9.6
Tangerine, cnd, swtnd - 1 fl oz (31.1gm)	16	.2	3.8	.1	-	.1	-	13	6.8
Tangerine, froz swt, reconstituted - 1 fl oz (30.1gm)	14	.2	3.4	.1	-	.1	.1	17	7.3

Thiamin (mg)	Riboflavin (mg)	Niacin (mg)	Vitamin B$_6$ (mg)	Vitamin B$_{12}$ (mcg)	Folacin (mcg)	Sodium (mg)	Calcium (mg)	Iron (mg)	Potassium (mg)	Zinc (mg)	Magnesium (mg)
.3	.2	1.6	.4	.1	26.4	6	56	1.1	1002	.4	78
.1	.1	.1	.1	.1	2	.1	1	.1	19	.1	1
.1	.1	.1	.1	.1	1.5	3	2	.1	15	.1	1
.1	.1	.1	.1	.1	1.4	.1	1	.1	14	.1	1
.1	.1	.1	.1	.1	1.3	.1	1	.1	17	.1	1
.1	.1	.1	.1	.1	1.2	2	2	.1	12	.1	1
.1	.1	.4	.1	.1	26.1	1	9	.2	172	.1	9
.1	.1	.1	.1	.1	9	.1	3	.1	59	.1	3
.1	.1	.1	.1	.1	5.6	1	3	.2	54	.1	3
.1	.1	.1	.1	.1	13.6	.1	3	.1	59	.1	3
.6	.2	1.6	.4	.1	330.7	7	67	.8	1435	.4	73
.1	.1	.2	.1	.1	4.4	1	3	.2	49	.1	3
.1	.1	.1	.1	.1	.6	2	3	.2	10	.1	1
.1	.1	.5	-	.1	-	2	1	.1	86	-	5
.1	.1	.7	-	.1	-	2	1	.2	86	-	5
.1	.1	.1	.1	.1	.4	2	2	.1	13	.1	1
.1	.1	.1	.1	.1	.4	2	2	.1	13	.1	1
.1	.1	.1	.1	.1	.4	1	1	.1	4	.1	1
.1	.1	.1	.1	.1	.4	1	1	.1	4	.1	1
.1	.1	.1	.1	.1	7.2	.1	5	.1	42	.1	4
.1	.1	.1	.1	.1	7.2	.1	5	.1	42	.1	4
.1	.1	.1	.1	.1	3.3	.1	3	.1	42	.1	3
.5	.2	2	.6	.1	79.5	6	84	2	1020	.9	76
.1	.1	.3	.1	.1	.1	1	4	.4	88	.1	4
.1	.1	.1	.1	.1	1.4	.1	6	.1	55	.1	2
.1	.1	.1	.1	.1	1.4	.1	6	.1	55	.1	2
.1	.1	.1	.1	.1	1.4	.1	2	.1	34	.1	2

	Calories (kcal)	Protein (gm)	Carbohydrates (gm)	Fat (gm)	Percent Saturated Fat	Cholesterol (mg)	Dietary Fiber (gm)	Vitamin A (RE)	Vitamin C (mg)
Tangerine, froz, conc, swt - 6 fl oz (214gm)	344	3.2	83.2	.9	-	.1	.5	431	182.1

GRAINS (Flour, Pasta, Rice, Pancakes and Waffles, Tortillas)

Note: Cooked rice and pasta have high sodium figures because "ordinary amounts of salt" were added during cooking. Without added salt, raw rice has 9 to 17 mg of sodium per cup. Cooked unsalted pasta has 1 mg of sodium per cup.

Grains

	Calories (kcal)	Protein (gm)	Carbohydrates (gm)	Fat (gm)	Percent Saturated Fat	Cholesterol (mg)	Dietary Fiber (gm)	Vitamin A (RE)	Vitamin C (mg)
Barley, pearled, light - 1 c dry (200gm)	698	16.4	157.6	2	0	0	-	0	0
Barley, pearled, pot or scotch - 1 c dry (200gm)	696	19.2	154.4	2.2	0	0	-	0	0
Bulgur, parboiled - 1 c dry (175gm)	628	15.2	139.1	2.4	0	0	-	0	0
Bulgur, cnd - ⅔ c ckd (90gm)	151	5.6	31.5	.6	12.9	0	4	0	0
Rice, brown - ⅔ c ckd (131gm)	156	3.3	33.4	.8	26.7	0	1.4	0	0
Rice, brown and wild - ⅔ c ckd (101gm)	151	4.5	32.3	.6	23.5	0	1.1	0	0
Rice, white, regular - ⅔ c ckd (137gm)	149	2.7	33.2	.1	30	0	.3	0	0
Rice, white converted - ⅔ c ckd (117gm)	124	2.5	27.3	.1	30	0	.2	0	0
Rice, white, instant - ⅔ c ckd (111gm)	121	2.4	26.9	0	0	0	.2	0	0
Rice, white and wild - ⅔ c ckd (101gm)	107	3	23.4	.2	17.6	0	.3	0	0
Rice, wild - ⅔ c ckd (87gm)	78	3.1	16.7	.2	12.9	0	.4	0	0

Flour and Meal

	Calories (kcal)	Protein (gm)	Carbohydrates (gm)	Fat (gm)	Percent Saturated Fat	Cholesterol (mg)	Dietary Fiber (gm)	Vitamin A (RE)	Vitamin C (mg)
Buckwheat, dark - 1 c (98gm)	326	11.5	70.6	2.4	0	0	-	0	0
Buckwheat, light - 1 c (98gm)	340	6.3	77.9	1.2	0	0	-	0	0
Buckwheat, whl grn - 1 c (100gm)	335	11.7	72.9	2.4	0	0	-	0	0
Carob - 1 c (140gm)	252	6.3	113	2	0	0	-	0	0
Corn, white - 1 c (117gm)	431	9.1	89.9	3	11.1	0	-	0	0
Corn, yellow - 1 c (117gm)	431	9.1	89.9	3	11.1	0	-	40	0
Cornmeal, yellow, enr - 1 c dry (138gm)	502	10.9	108.2	1.7	0	0	-	61	0
Cornmeal, yellow, unenr - 1 c dry (138gm)	502	10.9	108.2	1.7	0	0	-	61	0
Cornmeal, yellow, whl grn - 1 c (122gm)	442	11	90.9	4.1	10.9	0	-	58	0
Cornmeal, white, whl grn - 1 c (122gm)	442	11.0	90.9	4.1	10.9	0	-	0	0
Cornmeal, white, enr - 1 c (138gm)	502	10.9	108.2	1.7	0	0	-	0	0

Thiamin (mg)	Riboflavin (mg)	Niacin (mg)	Vitamin B$_6$ (mg)	Vitamin B$_{12}$ (mcg)	Folacin (mcg)	Sodium (mg)	Calcium (mg)	Iron (mg)	Potassium (mg)	Zinc (mg)	Magnesium (mg)
.4	.2	.8	.4	.1	34.6	7	57	.8	850	.2	60

Source: USDA Revised *Handbook 8*

Thiamin (mg)	Riboflavin (mg)	Niacin (mg)	Vitamin B$_6$ (mg)	Vitamin B$_{12}$ (mcg)	Folacin (mcg)	Sodium (mg)	Calcium (mg)	Iron (mg)	Potassium (mg)	Zinc (mg)	Magnesium (mg)
.2	.1	6.2	-	-	-	6	32	4	320	-	-
.4	.1	7.4	-	-	-	8	68	5.4	592	-	-
.5	.2	7.4	-	-	-	7	52.5	8.2	458.5	-	-
0	0	2.2	.3	0	158.4	539.1	18	5	78.3	1.9	146.7
.1	0	1.8	.1	0	6.5	369.4	15.7	.8	91.7	.7	48.5
.1	.1	2.3	.1	0	4.9	266.2	14	1.2	87.1	1.3	51.6
.2	0	1.4	.1	0	2.7	512.4	13.7	1.9	38.4	.6	15.1
.1	0	1.4	.1	0	2.3	418.9	22.2	2.9	50.3	.5	11.7
.1	0	1.1	0	0	34.4	303	3.3	1.6	0	.4	11.1
.1	.1	1.4	.1	0	2.8	321	10.2	1.3	43	.9	24.9
.1	.1	1.4	.1	0	2.6	319	7.8	.9	46.3	1	30.1

Thiamin (mg)	Riboflavin (mg)	Niacin (mg)	Vitamin B$_6$ (mg)	Vitamin B$_{12}$ (mcg)	Folacin (mcg)	Sodium (mg)	Calcium (mg)	Iron (mg)	Potassium (mg)	Zinc (mg)	Magnesium (mg)
.6	.1	2.8	-	-	-	2	32.3	2.7	376.3	-	-
.1	0	.4	-	-	-	2	10.8	1	313.6	-	-
.6	.1	4.4	-	-	-	2	114	3.1	448	-	-
0	0	0	-	-	-	0	492.8	0	0	-	-
.2	.1	1.6	-	-	-	1.2	7	2.1	270.3	-	-
.2	.1	1.6	-	-	-	1.2	7	2.1	270.3	-	-
.6	.4	4.8	-	-	-	1.4	8.3	4	165.6	-	-
.2	.1	1.4	-	-	-	1.4	8.3	1.5	165.6	-	-
.4	.1	2.3	-	-	-	1.2	20.7	2.2	302.6	-	-
.4	.1	2.3	-	-	-	1.2	20.7	2.2	302.6	-	-
.6	.4	4.8	-	-	-	1.4	8.3	4	165.6		

	Calories (kcal)	Protein (gm)	Carbohydrates (gm)	Fat (gm)	Percent Saturated Fat	Cholesterol (mg)	Dietary Fiber (gm)	Vitamin A (RE)	Vitamin C (mg)
Cornmeal, white, unenr - 1 c (138gm)	502	10.9	108.2	1.7	0	0	-	0	0
Rye, whl grn - 1 c (100gm)	334	12.1	73.4	1.7	0	0	-	0	0
Soybean, full fat - 1 c not stirred (85gm)	358	31.2	25.8	17.3	15	0	-	9	0
White - 1 c (125gm)	455	13.1	95.1	1.3	16	0	2.9	0	0
Whole wheat - 1 c (120gm)	400	16	85.2	2.4	14	0	15.1	0	0

Pasta

	Calories (kcal)	Protein (gm)	Carbohydrates (gm)	Fat (gm)	Percent Saturated Fat	Cholesterol (mg)	Dietary Fiber (gm)	Vitamin A (RE)	Vitamin C (mg)
Macaroni - 1 c ckd (140gm)	154	4.7	32	.6	15.1	0	1.1	0	0
Noodles, egg - 1 c ckd (160gm)	199	6.5	37.1	2.4	22	49.3	1.1	4.8	0
Noodles, spinach - 1 c ckd (160gm)	190	6.4	38.6	.8	13.8	0	.5	4.4	0
Noodles, whole wheat - 1 c ckd (160gm)	174	7	37.4	1	15	0	4.6	0	0
Noodles, chow mein - 1 c (45gm)	220	5.9	26.1	10.6	19.5	5.4	1.3	0	0
Spaghetti - 1 c ckd (140gm)	154	4.7	32	.6	15.1	0	1.1	0	0
Spaghetti, hi protein - 1 c ckd (140gm)	153	9.5	27.4	.6	15	0	1.1	0	0

Pancakes

	Calories (kcal)	Protein (gm)	Carbohydrates (gm)	Fat (gm)	Percent Saturated Fat	Cholesterol (mg)	Dietary Fiber (gm)	Vitamin A (RE)	Vitamin C (mg)
Pancake, plain - 1 (73gm)	162	5.1	22.5	5.7	35.5	60.4	.4	30.2	.4
Pancake, buckwheat - 1 (73gm)	135	4.9	18.2	5.1	35.9	54	1.6	27	.3
Pancake, cornmeal - 1 (73gm)	148	3.6	22.8	4.6	25.9	38.4	1	62.8	.1
Pancake, whole wheat - 1 (73gm)	173	5.6	20.9	8.1	24.3	57.7	2.8	28.9	.4
Pancake w/fruit - 1 (73gm)	153	4.7	22.1	5.2	35.3	54.6	.7	28.5	1.9
Tortilla, corn - 1 (15gm)	32	.8	6.4	.5	-	0	.4	2.5	0
Tortilla, flour - 1 (40gm)	118	2.9	21.8	3	24.7	0	.9	0	0
Waffles - 2 (74gm)	204	6.2	32.4	5.5	37.8	47.7	.6	29.6	.5

GRAVY

	Calories (kcal)	Protein (gm)	Carbohydrates (gm)	Fat (gm)	Percent Saturated Fat	Cholesterol (mg)	Dietary Fiber (gm)	Vitamin A (RE)	Vitamin C (mg)
Au jus, cnd - 1 c (238gm)	38	2.9	6	.5	-	1	-	0	2.4
Au jus, mix, prep - 1 c (8 fl oz) (246gm)	19	.7	2.4	.8	-	1	-	0	.5
Beef, cnd - 1 c (232.8gm)	124	8.7	11.2	5.5	50.1	7	-	0	0
Brown, mix, dry - 1 c (23gm)	80	2.6	14	1.9	-	2	-	0	1.6
Brown, mix, prep - 1 c (8 fl oz) (260gm)	9	.3	1.5	.2	-	0	-	0	0
Chicken, cnd - 1 c (238gm)	189	4.6	12.9	13.6	24.7	5	-	265	0

Thiamin (mg)	Riboflavin (mg)	Niacin (mg)	Vitamin B$_6$ (mg)	Vitamin B$_{12}$ (mcg)	Folacin (mcg)	Sodium (mg)	Calcium (mg)	Iron (mg)	Potassium (mg)	Zinc (mg)	Magnesium (mg)
.2	.1	1.4	-	-	-	1.4	8.3	1.5	165.6	-	-
.4	.2	1.6	-	-	-	1	38	3.7	467	-	-
.7	.3	1.8	-	-	-	.9	169.1	7.1	1411	-	-
.8	.5	6.6	0	0	20	2.5	20	5.5	118.7	.8	26.3
.7	.1	5.2	.4	0	57.6	3.6	49.2	5.2	444	3	168
.2	.1	1.5	.1	0	8.3	325	13.2	1.7	84.9	.5	16.3
.2	.1	1.9	.1	0	9.5	373	18.3	2.4	70	.8	21.8
.3	.1	2	.1	0	26.4	284.5	35.2	2.3	21.2	1.2	18.6
.1	0	1.4	.1	0	25.6	1.6	22.4	1.8	195.2	1.3	59.2
0	0	.6	0	0	3.1	450	14.4	1.6	32.8	.5	31
.2	.1	1.5	.1	0	8.3	325	13.2	1.7	84.9	.5	17.7
.3	.1	1.9	.1	0	8.4	0	11.2	1.3	36.4	.5	70
.1	.2	.7	.1	.3	8.5	417.7	182.3	1.1	128.5	.5	13.8
.1	.1	.6	.1	.2	9.6	338.3	162.8	.9	185.3	.7	31.1
.1	.1	1	0	.1	8.1	427.6	87.4	1.3	65.2	.4	12
.1	.1	.9	.1	.3	14.1	347.3	132.9	1.2	173	.9	39.5
.1	.2	.7	.1	.2	8.5	378.7	165.8	1	127.5	.5	13.1
0	0	.2	0	0	2.8	2.8	29.7	.2	21.3	.2	9
.1	.1	1.4	0	0	17.6	151.2	24	.6	39.6	.3	14.4
.2	.2	1.1	.1	.3	8.5	599.4	250.4	1.4	162	.6	17.8

Source: USDA Food Consumption Survey and "nonupdated" database

Thiamin (mg)	Riboflavin (mg)	Niacin (mg)	Vitamin B$_6$ (mg)	Vitamin B$_{12}$ (mcg)	Folacin (mcg)	Sodium (mg)	Calcium (mg)	Iron (mg)	Potassium (mg)	Zinc (mg)	Magnesium (mg)
0	.1	2.1	0	.2	4.8	119	10	1.4	193	2.4	5
0	0	.2	0	.1	.7	579	11	.7	32	0	2
.1	.1	1.5	0	.2	4.7	117	14	1.6	189	2.3	5
0	.1	.9	0	.2	3.3	1145	66	.2	61	.3	8
0	0	.1	0	0	.3	125	7	0	7	0	1
0	.1	1.1	0	.2	4.8	1375	48	1.1	260	1.9	5

	Calories (kcal)	Protein (gm)	Carbohydrates (gm)	Fat (gm)	Percent Saturated Fat	Cholesterol (mg)	Dietary Fiber (gm)	Vitamin A (RE)	Vitamin C (mg)
Chicken, mix, prep - 1 c (8 fl oz) (259gm)	83	2.6	14.3	1.9	-	3	-	0	2.6
Mushroom, cnd - 1 c (238.4gm)	120	3	13	6.5	14.9	0	-	0	0
Mushroom, mix, dry - 1 c (21.3gm)	70	2.1	13.8	.9	-	1	-	0	1.5
Mushroom, mix, prep - 1 c (8 fl oz) (257.9gm)	70	2.1	13.8	.9	-	1	-	0	1.5
Onion, mix, dry - 1 c (24gm)	77	2.2	16.2	.7	-	0	-	0	1.7
Onion, mix, prep - 1 c (8 fl oz) (261.4gm)	80	2.2	16.8	.7	-	1	-	0	1.8
Pork, mix, dry - 1 c (21.3gm)	76	1.9	13.4	1.9	-	2	-	0	1.5
Pork, mix, prep - 1 c (8 fl oz) (257.9gm)	76	1.9	13.4	1.9	-	3	-	0	1.5
Turkey, cnd - 1 c (238.4gm)	122	6.2	12.2	5	29.5	5	-	0	0
Turkey, mix, dry - 1 c (24.8gm)	87	2.9	15.1	1.9	-	2	-	0	1.7
Turkey, mix, prep - 1 c (8 fl oz) (261.4gm)	87	2.9	15	1.9	-	3	-	0	1.8

LEGUMES

Note: unsalted, cooked dried beans have from 3 to 13 mg of sodium per cup, lentils about 26 mg per cup.

	Calories (kcal)	Protein (gm)	Carbohydrates (gm)	Fat (gm)	Percent Saturated Fat	Cholesterol (mg)	Dietary Fiber (gm)	Vitamin A (RE)	Vitamin C (mg)
Baked beans/tomato sauce -½ c (128gm)	156	7.8	31.4	.7	-	0	5.6	57	16.2
Baked beans w/pork and sweet sauce - ½ c (127gm)	190	7.9	26.8	6	-	19	8.6	16.5	2.5
Black, brown, boyo beans, dry, ckd ½ cup (86gm)	98	6.4	17.7	.4	-	0	4.4	.3	0
Boston baked beans - ½ c (127gm)	193	7.4	26.9	6.7	34	6.4	4.9	0	1.4
Chickpeas (garbanzo) - ½ c ckd (82gm)	146	8.3	24.7	1.9	-	0	6.2	2.8	0
Cowpeas, dry - ½ c ckd (87gm)	66	4.4	11.9	.3	-	0	4.7	.9	0
Lentils, dry - ½ c ckd (96gm)	101	7.4	18.4	0	0	0	2.7	1	0
Lima beans, dry - ½ c ckd (94gm)	129	7.7	23.9	.6	-	0	4.9	0	0
Pinto, calico, Mex beans, dry - ½ c ckd (88gm)	102	6.7	18.5	.3	-	0	4.4	0	0
Pork and beans - ½ c (127gm)	155	7.7	24.1	3.3	31.9	19	8.6	21.6	2.5
Red kidney beans, dry - ½ c ckd (88gm)	103	6.8	18.7	.4	-	0	4.6	.9	0
Refried beans - ½ c (127gm)	208	9	25.1	8.5	12.7	0	6	0	0
Soybeans, dried - 1 c ckd (180gm)	234	19.8	19.4	10.3	15.1	0	-	5	0

Thiamin (mg)	Riboflavin (mg)	Niacin (mg)	Vitamin B$_6$ (mg)	Vitamin B$_{12}$ (mcg)	Folacin (mcg)	Sodium (mg)	Calcium (mg)	Iron (mg)	Potassium (mg)	Zinc (mg)	Magnesium (mg)
.1	.1	.8	0	.2	2.6	1133	39	.3	62	.3	10
.1	.1	1.6	0	0	28.6	1359	17	1.6	253	1.7	5
0	.1	.8	0	.1	3	1402	49	.2	56	.3	7
.1	.1	.8	0	.1	2.6	1402	49	.3	57	.3	8
0	.1	.9	0	.2	3.4	1005	67	.2	63	.2	8
.1	.1	1	0	.2	2.6	1036	69	.3	65	.2	8
0	.1	.8	0	.1	3	1235	32	.2	56	.3	10
.1	.1	.8	0	.1	3.1	1235	32	.3	57	.3	10
0	.2	3.1	0	.2	4.8	1376	10	1.7	260	1.9	5
.1	.1	.9	0	.2	3.5	1500	50	.3	65	.3	11
.1	.1	1	0	.3	3.4	1498	50	.3	65	.3	10

Source: USDA Revised *Handbook 8*

Thiamin (mg)	Riboflavin (mg)	Niacin (mg)	Vitamin B$_6$ (mg)	Vitamin B$_{12}$ (mcg)	Folacin (mcg)	Sodium (mg)	Calcium (mg)	Iron (mg)	Potassium (mg)	Zinc (mg)	Magnesium (mg)
.2	.1	1.3	.2	0	67.5	441.1	77.9	2.7	613	1	72
.1	.1	.6	0	.1	34.3	482.6	80	2.8	266.7	2	47
.1	0	.4	.1	0	64.2	188.3	39.6	1.2	270.2	1.1	51.6
.2	.1	.7	.1	0	63.9	537.4	71.9	2.3	431.3	.9	61.9
.1	0	.5	.1	0	70.1	198.6	59.9	1.9	274.7	1.1	52.4
.1	0	.3	.1	0	179.9	208	16	1.9	198.1	1.3	56
.1	.1	.6	.2	0	172.7	234.3	25.3	2.3	237.6	1.4	42.7
.1	.1	.7	.1	0	78.5	219.2	28.5	1.6	571.9	1	48.3
.2	0	.4	.1	0	78.5	188.6	39.9	1.3	257.9	.6	47.3
.1	0	.8	.1	0	30.5	588	68.6	1.7	266.7	1.1	25.4
.1	.1	.6	.1	0	113.7	206	34.6	2	297.4	1	42.6
.2	.1	.6	.1	0	106	280.2	54.1	1.8	348.5	.8	64
.4	.2	1.1	-	-	-	3.6	131.4	4.9	972	-	-

	Calories (kcal)	Protein (gm)	Carbohydrates (gm)	Fat (gm)	Percent Saturated Fat	Cholesterol (mg)	Dietary Fiber (gm)	Vitamin A (RE)	Vitamin C (mg)
Split peas, grn/yellow, dry - ½ c ckd -(101gm)	116	8.1	21	.3	-	0	5.5	4	0
Bean curd (tofu) - ½ c (92gm)	66	7.2	2.2	3.9	14.5	0	.4	0	0
White beans, dry - ½ c ckd (88gm)	103	6.8	18.5	.5	-	0	4.6	0	0

LUNCHEON MEATS AND SAUSAGE

	Calories (kcal)	Protein (gm)	Carbohydrates (gm)	Fat (gm)	Percent Saturated Fat	Cholesterol (mg)	Dietary Fiber (gm)	Vitamin A (RE)	Vitamin C (mg)
Barbeque loaf - 1 oz (28.4gm)	49	4.5	1.8	2.5	35.7	11	0	2	5
Beerwurst (beer salami), beef - 1 slice (23gm)	75	2.8	.4	6.8	40.8	13	0	0	3
Beerwurst (beer salami), pork - 1 slice (23gm)	55	3.3	.5	4.3	33.3	13	0	0	7
Berliner sausage - 1 oz (28.4gm)	65	4.3	.7	4.9	35.2	13	0	0	2
Blood sausage or blood pudding - 1 oz (28.4gm)	107	4.1	.4	9.8	38.8	34	0	0	0
Bockwurst - 1 link (65gm)	200	8.7	.4	18	-	38	0	4	.1
Bologna, beef - 1 slice (28.4gm)	89	3.3	.6	8	41.2	16	0	0	5
Bologna, beef and pork - 1 slice (28.4gm)	89	3.3	.8	8	37.8	16	0	0	6
Bologna, pork - 1 slice (23gm)	57	3.6	.2	4.6	-	14	0	.1	8
Bologna, turkey - 1 oz (28.4gm)	57	3.9	.3	4.4	-	28	0	.1	.1
Bratwurst - 1 link (85gm)	256	12	1.8	22	-	51	0	.1	1
Braunschweiger - 1 oz (28.4gm)	102	3.8	.9	9.1	34	44	0	1196	3
Brotwurst - 1 link (70gm)	226	10	2.1	19.5	-	44	0	.1	20
Cheesefurter, cheese smokie - 1 (43gm)	141	6.1	.7	12.5	-	29	0	16	8
Chicken roll, light meat - 2 slices (56.8gm)	90	11.1	1.4	4.2	-	28	0	14	.1
Chicken spread, cnd - 1 tbsp (13gm)	25	2	.7	1.6	-	7	0	3	.1
Chorizo sausage - 1 link (60gm)	273	14.5	1.2	23	-	53	0	.1	.1
Corned beef loaf, jellied - 1 slice (28.4gm)	46	6.7	0	1.9	39.4	12	0	0	2
Dutch brand loaf - 1 slice (28.4gm)	68	3.8	1.6	5.1	35.6	13	0	0	5
Frankfurter, raw, beef - 1 (45gm)	145	5.1	1.1	13.2	40.6	22	0	0	11
Frankfurter, raw, beef and pork - 1 (45gm)	144	5.1	1.1	13.1	36.9	23	0	0	12
Frankfurter, raw, chicken - 1 (45gm)	116	5.8	3.1	8.8	28.4	45	0	17	0

Thiamin (mg)	Riboflavin (mg)	Niacin (mg)	Vitamin B_6 (mg)	Vitamin B_{12} (mcg)	Folacin (mcg)	Sodium (mg)	Calcium (mg)	Iron (mg)	Potassium (mg)	Zinc (mg)	Magnesium (mg)
.2	.1	.9	.2	0	103	13.1	11.1	1.6	299	1.2	43.4
.1	0	.1	0	0	9.2	6.4	117.8	1.3	38.6	.7	93.8
.1	.1	.6	.1	0	119.8	209.5	45.1	2.4	363.9	.9	60.1

Source: USDA Food Consumption Survey and "nonupdated" database

Thiamin (mg)	Riboflavin (mg)	Niacin (mg)	Vitamin B_6 (mg)	Vitamin B_{12} (mcg)	Folacin (mcg)	Sodium (mg)	Calcium (mg)	Iron (mg)	Potassium (mg)	Zinc (mg)	Magnesium (mg)
.1	.1	.6	.1	.5	3	378	15	.3	93	.7	5
0	0	.7	.1	.5	1	214	2	.3	42	.6	3
.1	0	.7	.1	.2	1	285	2	.2	58	.4	3
.1	.1	.9	.1	.8	1	368	3	.3	80	.7	4
0	0	.3	0	.3	1	193	2	1.8	11	.4	2
.3	.2	2.7	.2	.6	4	718	10	.5	176	1.1	12
0	0	.7	.1	.4	1	284	3	.4	44	.6	3
0	0	.7	.1	.4	1	289	3	.4	51	.6	3
.2	.1	.9	.1	.3	1	272	3	.2	65	.5	3
.1	.1	1	.1	.1	2	249	24	.5	56	.5	4
.5	.2	2.8	.2	.9	2	473	38	1.1	180	2	12
.1	.4	2.4	.1	5.7	12	324	2	2.6	57	.8	3
.2	.2	2.4	.1	1.5	4	778	34	.8	197	1.5	11
.2	.1	1.3	.1	.8	1	465	25	.5	89	1	5
.1	.1	3	.2	.1	1	331	24	.6	129	.5	10
.1	.1	.4	.1	.1	.1	50	16	.3	14	.2	2
.4	.2	3.1	.4	1.2	1	741	5	1	239	2.1	11
0	0	.5	0	.3	1	294	3	.6	25	1.1	3
.1	.1	.7	.1	.4	1	354	24	.4	107	.5	6
0	0	1.1	.1	.7	2	461	6	.6	71	.9	4
.1	.1	1.2	.1	.6	2	504	5	.5	75	.8	5
0	.1	1.4	.1	.1	2	617	43	.9	38	.5	5

	Calories (kcal)	Protein (gm)	Carbohydrates (gm)	Fat (gm)	Percent Saturated Fat	Cholesterol (mg)	Dietary Fiber (gm)	Vitamin A (RE)	Vitamin C (mg)
Frankfurter, raw, turkey - 1 (45gm)	102	6.4	.7	8	33.3	48	0	0	0
Ham, chopped - 1 slice (28.4gm)	65	4.9	0	4.9	33.1	15	0	0	6
Ham, chopped, spiced, cnd - 1 oz (28.4gm)	68	4.6	.1	5.3	33.3	14	0	0	0
Ham, minced - 1 oz (28.4gm)	75	4.6	.5	5.9	34.6	20	0	0	8
Ham, extra lean, approx 5% fat - 1 slice (28.4gm)	37	5.5	.3	1.5	-	13	0	.1	7
Ham, approx 11% fat - 1 slice (28.4gm)	52	5	.9	3	-	16	0	.1	8
Ham and cheese loaf/roll - 1 slice (28.4gm)	73	4.7	.4	5.7	37.2	16	0	6	7
Ham and cheese spread - 1 tbsp (15gm)	37	2.5	.4	2.8	-	9	0	14	1
Ham salad spread - 1 tbsp (15gm)	32	1.3	1.6	2.4	-	6	0	.1	1
Headcheese - 1 slice (28.4gm)	60	4.5	.1	4.5	31.3	23	0	0	6
Honey loaf - 1 slice (28.4gm)	36	4.5	1.5	1.3	32.3	10	0	0	6
Honey roll sausage - 1 oz (28.4gm)	52	5.3	.6	3	38.9	14	0	0	5
Italian sausage, ckd - 1 link (83gm)	268	16.6	1.3	21.3	35.3	65	0	0	1
Kielbasa - 1 oz (28.4gm)	88	3.8	.6	7.7	36.5	19	0	0	6
Knockwurst - 1 link (68gm)	209	8.1	1.2	18.9	-	39	0	.1	18
Lebanon bologna - 1 oz (28gm)	64	5.6	.6	4.2	41.6	19	0	0	10
Liver cheese - 1 oz (28gm)	86	4.3	.6	7.3	35	49	0	1489	1
Liverwurst, fresh - 1 oz (28.4gm)	93	4	.6	8.1	37.1	45	0	2353	0
Luncheon meat, beef, loaf - 1 slice (28.4gm)	87	4.1	.8	7.4	42.7	18	0	0	4
Luncheon meat, beef, thin sliced - 1 oz (28.4gm)	35	6.2	.1	.9	41.6	12	0	0	4
Luncheon meat, pork and beef chopped - 1 slice (28.4gm)	100	3.6	.7	9.1	36.1	15	0	0	4
Luncheon meat, pork, cnd - 1 oz (28.4gm)	95	3.5	.6	8.6	35.7	18	0	0	0
Luncheon type sausage - 1 oz (28.4gm)	74	4.4	.4	5.9	36.4	18	0	0	5
Luxury loaf - 1 slice (28.4gm)	40	5.2	1.4	1.4	32.8	10	0	0	6
Mortadella - 1 oz (28.4gm)	88	4.6	.9	7.2	37.5	16	0	0	7
Mother's loaf - 1 oz (28.4gm)	80	3.4	2.1	6.3	35.6	13	0	0	0
New England brand sausage - 1 oz (28.4gm)	46	4.9	1.4	2.1	33.5	14	0	0	6
Olive loaf - 1 slice (28.4gm)	67	3.4	2.6	4.7	35.5	11	0	6	2

Thiamin (mg)	Riboflavin (mg)	Niacin (mg)	Vitamin B_6 (mg)	Vitamin B_{12} (mcg)	Folacin (mcg)	Sodium (mg)	Calcium (mg)	Iron (mg)	Potassium (mg)	Zinc (mg)	Magnesium (mg)
0	.1	1.9	.1	.1	4	642	48	.8	80	1.4	6
.2	.1	1.1	.1	.3	0	389	2	.2	91	.6	4
.2	0	.9	.1	.2	0	387	2	.3	81	.5	4
.2	.1	1.2	.1	.3	0	353	3 .	.2	88	.5	5
.3	.1	1.4	.2	.3	1	405	2	.3	99	.6	5
.3	.1	1.5	.1	.3	1	373	2	.3	94	.7	5
.2	.1	1	.1	.2	1	381	16	.3	83	.6	5
.1	.1	.4	.1	.2	.1	179	33	.2	24	.4	3
.1	.1	.4	.1	.2	.1	137	1	.1	22	.2	1
0	.1	.3	.1	.3	1	356	4	.3	9	.4	3
.1	.1	.9	.1	.3	2	374	5	.4	97	.7	5
0	.1	1.2	.1	.7	1	375	3	.6	83	.9	4
.5	.2	3.5	.3	1.1	4	765	20	1.2	253	2	15
.1	.1	.8	.1	.5	1	305	12	.4	77	.6	5
.3	.1	1.9	.2	.8	1	687	7	.7	136	1.2	8
0	.1	1.3	.1	.8	1	359	4	.7	87	1.1	4
.1	.6	3.3	.1	7	29	347	2	3.1	64	1.1	3
.1	.3	1.2	.1	3.8	8	244	7	1.8	48	.6	3
0	.1	1	.1	1.1	2	377	3	.7	59	.7	4
0	.1	1.5	.1	.7	3	470	1	.6	116	1.1	5
.1	0	.8	.1	.4	2	367	3	.2	57	.5	4
.1	.1	.9	.1	.3	2	365	2	.2	61	.4	3
.1	.1	1	.1	.6	1	335	4	.4	70	.7	4
.2	.1	1·	.1	.4	1	347	10	.3	107	.9	6
0	0	.8	0	.4	1	353	5	.4	46	.6	3
.2	0	.9	.1	.3	2	320	12	.4	64	.4	4
.2	.1	1	.1	.4	2	346	2	.3	91	.8	4
.1	.1	.5	.1	.4	1	421	31	.1	84	.4	5

	Calories (kcal)	Protein (gm)	Carbohydrates (gm)	Fat (gm)	Percent Saturated Fat	Cholesterol (mg)	Dietary Fiber (gm)	Vitamin A (RE)	Vitamin C (mg)
Pastrami, turkey - 2 slices - (56.8gm)	80	10.5	1	3.6	-	31	0	.1	.1
Pâté - 1 oz (28.4gm)	90	4	.4	7.9	34.1	72	0	283	0
Peppered loaf - 1 slice (28.4gm)	42	4.9	1.3	1.8	35.9	13	0	0	7
Pepperoni - 1 slice (5.5gm)	27	1.1	.2	2.4	36.8	4	0	0	0
Pickle and pimiento loaf - 1 slice (28.4gm)	74	3.3	1.7	6	37.2	10	0	2	4
Picnic loaf - 1 slice (28.4gm)	66	4.2	1.4	4.7	36.4	11	0	0	5
Polish sausage - 1 oz (28.4gm)	92	4	.5	8.1	36	20	0	0	0
Pork and beef sausage, fresh, ckd - 1 link (13gm)	52	1.8	.4	4.7	35.7	9	0	0	0
Pork sausage, links or bulk, ckd - 1 link (13gm)	48	2.6	.1	4.1	34.6	11	0	0	0
Salami, beef - 1 oz (28.4gm)	72	4.2	.7	5.7	41.9	17	0	0	4
Salami, beef, and pork - 1 oz (28.4gm)	71	3.9	.6	5.7	40.2	18	0	0	3
Salami, beef and pork, dry - 1 slice (10gm)	42	2.3	.3	3.5	-	8	0	.1	3
Salami, pork, dry or hard - 1 slice (10gm)	41	2.3	.2	3.4	-	8	0	.1	.1
Smoked link sausage, pork - 1 link (16gm)	62	3.6	.3	5.1	35.6	11	0	0	0
Smoked link sausage, pork and beef - 1 link (16gm)	54	2.1	.2	4.9	35.1	11	0	0	3
Thuringer - 1 oz (28.4gm)	98	4.6	.6	8.5	40.2	19	0	0	7
Turkey-ham luncheon meat - 2 slices (56.8gm)	73	10.8	.3	2.9	-	32	0	.1	.1
Turkey loaf - 2 slices (42.6gm)	47	9.6	.1	.7	-	17	0	.1	.1
Vienna sausage, cnd - 1 (16gm)	45	1.7	.4	4.1	-	8	0	.1	.1

MEAT AND GAME

Note: All meat is cooked; weight applies to *cooked* portions unless noted.
Lean means the portions after all separable fat has been trimmed. Lean/fat means both lean and fat as trimmed at time of purchase.

Beef

	Calories (kcal)	Protein (gm)	Carbohydrates (gm)	Fat (gm)	Percent Saturated Fat	Cholesterol (mg)	Dietary Fiber (gm)	Vitamin A (RE)	Vitamin C (mg)
Brisket, whole, lean/fat, braised - 3 oz (85gm)	332	19.5	0	27.6	40.6	79	0	-	0
Brisket, whole, lean, braised - 3 oz (85gm)	205	25	0	10	39.1	79	0	-	0
Chuck, arm pot roast, lean/fat, choice, braised - 3 oz (85gm)	301	22.9	0	22.5	41	84	0	-	0
Chuck, arm pot roast, lean/fat, good, braised - 3 oz (85 gm)	287	23.3	0	20.8	41.1	84	0	-	0

Thiamin (mg)	Riboflavin (mg)	Niacin (mg)	Vitamin B$_6$ (mg)	Vitamin B$_{12}$ (mcg)	Folacin (mcg)	Sodium (mg)	Calcium (mg)	Iron (mg)	Potassium (mg)	Zinc (mg)	Magnesium (mg)
.1	.2	2	.2	.2	3	593	5	1	147	1.3	8
0	.2	.9	0	.9	17	198	20	1.6	39	.8	4
.1	.1	.9	.1	.6	1	432	15	.3	112	.9	6
0	0	.3	0	.1	0	112	1	.1	19	.1	1
.1	.1	.6	.1	.3	1	394	27	.3	96	.4	5
.1	.1	.7	.1	.4	1	330	13	.3	76	.6	4
.1	0	1	.1	.3	1	248	3	.4	67	.6	4
0	0	.4	0	.1	0	105	1	.1	25	.2	1
.1	0	.6	0	.2	0	168	4	.2	47	.3	2
0	.1	1	.1	1.4	1	328	2	.6	64	.6	4
.1	.1	1	.1	1	1	302	4	.8	56	.6	4
.1	.1	.5	.1	.2	.1	186	1	.2	38	.4	2
.1	.1	.6	.1	.3	.1	226	1	.2	38	.5	2
.1	0	.7	.1	.3	1	240	5	.2	54	.4	3
0	0	.5	0	.2	0	151	2	.2	30	.3	2
0	.1	1.2	.1	1.3	1	412	2	.6	65	.6	3
.1	.2	2	.2	.2	3	565	5	1.6	184	1.7	9
.1	.1	3.6	.2	.9	2	608	3	.2	118	.5	9
.1	.1	.3	.1	.2	1	152	2	.2	16	.3	1

Source: USDA Revised *Handbook 8*

0	.1	2.6	.2	1.9	5	52	7	1.9	195	4.3	15
.1	.2	3.2	.3	2.2	7	61	5	2.4	244	5.9	20
.1	.2	2.7	.2	2.5	7	50	9	2.6	207	5.7	16
.1	.2	2.7	.2	2.5	8	51	9	2.6	209	5.8	17

	Calories (kcal)	Protein (gm)	Carbohydrates (gm)	Fat (gm)	Percent Saturated Fat	Cholesterol (mg)	Dietary Fiber (gm)	Vitamin A (RE)	Vitamin C (mg)
Chuck, arm pot roast, lean, choice, braised - 3 oz (85gm)	199	28.1	0	8.8	38	85	0	-	0
Chuck, arm pot roast, lean, good, braised - 3 oz (85gm)	189	28.1	0	7.6	37.9	85	0	-	0
Flank, lean/fat, choice, braised - 3 oz (85gm)	218	23.4	0	13.1	42.8	61	0	-	0
Flank, lean/fat, choice, broiled - 3 oz (85gm)	216	21.3	0	13.9	42.7	60	0	-	0
Flank, lean, choice, braised - 3 oz (85gm)	208	23.8	0	11.8	42.9	60	0	-	0
Flank, lean, choice, broiled - 3 oz (85gm)	207	21.6	0	12.7	42.7	60	0	-	0
Ground, ext lean, raw - 4 oz (113gm)	265	21.1	0	19.3	40	78	0	-	0
Ground, ext lean, broiled, medium - 3 oz (85gm)	217	21.6	0	13.9	39.3	71	0	-	0
Ground, ext lean, broiled, well done - 3 oz (85gm)	225	24.3	0	13.4	39.3	84	0	-	0
Ground, ext lean, fried, medium - 3 oz (85gm)	216	21.2	0	14	39.3	69	0	-	0
Ground, ext lean, fried, well done - 3 oz (85gm)	224	23.8	0	13.6	39.3	79	0	-	0
Ground, lean, broiled, medium - 3 oz (85gm)	231	21	0	15.7	39.3	74	0	-	0
Ground, lean, broiled, well done - 3 oz (85gm)	238	24	0	15	39.3	86	0	-	0
Ground, lean, fried, medium - 3 oz (85gm)	234	20.6	0	16.2	39.3	71	0	-	0
Ground, lean, fried, well done - 3 oz (85gm)	235	23.4	0	15	39.3	81	0	-	0
Ground, reg, raw - 4 oz (113gm)	351	18.8	0	30	40.6	96	0	-	0
Ground, reg, broiled, medium - 3 oz (85gm)	246	20.5	0	17.6	39.3	76	0	-	0
Ground, reg, broiled, well done - 3 oz (85gm)	248	23.1	0	16.5	39.3	86	0	-	0
Ground, reg, fried, medium - 3 oz (85gm)	260	20.3	0	19.2	39.3	75	0	-	0
Ground, reg, fried, well done - 3 oz (85gm)	243	22.9	0	16.1	39.3	83	0	-	0
Rib, whole, lean/fat, choice, broiled - 3 oz (85gm)	313	18.2	0	26.1	42.2	73	0	-	0
Rib, whole, lean/fat, choice, roasted - 3 oz (85gm)	328	18.6	0	27.6	42.4	72	0	-	0
Rib, whole lean/fat, good, broiled - 3 oz (85gm)	313	18.2	0	26.1	42.2	73	0	-	0
Rib, whole, lean/fat, good, roasted - 3 oz (85gm)	306	19	0	24.9	42.4	72	0	-	0
Rib, whole, lean, choice, roasted - 3 oz (85gm)	209	23.1	0	12.2	42.6	68	0	-	0

Thiamin (mg)	Riboflavin (mg)	Niacin (mg)	Vitamin B$_6$ (mg)	Vitamin B$_{12}$ (mcg)	Folacin (mcg)	Sodium (mg)	Calcium (mg)	Iron (mg)	Potassium (mg)	Zinc (mg)	Magnesium (mg)
.1	.2	3.2	.3	2.9	9	56	7	3.2	246	7.4	21
.1	.2	3.2	.3	2.9	9	56	7	3.2	246	7.4	21
.1	.2	3.8	.3	2.9	7	61	6	2.9	293	5	20
.1	.2	4.1	.4	2.6	7	70	5	2.1	338	4	21
.1	.2	3.9	.3	2.9	7	61	6	2.9	298	5.1	20
.1	.2	4.2	.4	2.6	7	70	5	2.1	344	4.1	21
.1	.3	5.1	.3	2.3	9	75	7	2.2	321	4.7	22
.1	.2	4.2	.2	1.8	8	59	6	2	266	4.6	18
.1	.3	5	.3	2.2	9	70	7	2.4	314	5.5	21
.1	.2	4	.2	1.7	7	59	6	2	265	4.6	18
.1	.3	4.6	.3	2	9	69	7	2.3	306	5.3	21
0	.2	4.4	.2	2	8	65	9	1.8	256	4.6	18
.1	.2	5.1	.3	2.3	9	76	10	2.1	296	5.3	20
0	.2	4.1	.2	1.9	8	65	8	1.9	254	4.4	17
.1	.2	4.6	.3	2.2	9	74	9	2.1	289	5	20
0	.2	5.1	.3	3	8	77	10	2	258	4	18
0	.2	4.9	.2	2.5	8	70	9	2.1	248	4.4	17
0	.2	5.5	.3	2.8	9	79	10	2.3	278	4.9	19
0	.2	5	.2	2.3	8	71	10	2.1	255	4.3	17
0	.2	5.5	.2	2.6	8	79	11	2.3	283	4.8	19
.1	0	2.6	.3	2.4	5	52	10	1.8	256	4.3	17
.1	.1	2.8	.2	2.1	6	54	10	1.8	249	4.4	16
.1	0	2.7	.3	2.4	5	52	9	1.8	262	4.4	17
.1	.1	2.9	.2	2.1	6	54	10	1.8	255	4.5	16
.1	.2	3.5	.3	2.5	7	63	9	2.2	320	5.9	21

	Calories (kcal)	Protein (gm)	Carbohydrates (gm)	Fat (gm)	Percent Saturated Fat	Cholesterol (mg)	Dietary Fiber (gm)	Vitamin A (RE)	Vitamin C (mg)
Rib, whole, lean, choice, broiled - 3 oz (85gm)	198	22.1	0	11.5	42	69	0	-	0
Rib eye, lean/fat, choice, broiled - 3 oz (85gm)	250	21.6	0	17.5	42.3	70	0	-	0
Rib eye, lean, choice, broiled - 3 oz (85gm)	191	23.8	0	9.9	42.3	68	0	-	0
Ribs, short, lean/fat, choice, braised - 3 oz (85gm)	400	18.3	0	35.7	42.4	80	0	-	0
Ribs, short, lean, choice, braised -3 oz (85gm)	251	26.1	0	15.4	42.7	79	0	-	0
Round, lean/fat, choice, broiled - 3 oz (85gm)	233	21.7	0	15.5	40	71	0	-	0
Round, lean/fat, good, broiled - 3 oz (85gm)	222	21.8	0	14.3	40.1	71	0	-	0
Round, lean, choice, broiled - 3 oz (85gm)	165	24.2	0	6.8	36.2	70	0	-	0
Round, lean, good, broiled - 3 oz (85gm)	157	24.2	0	5.9	36	70	0	-	0
Shank crosscuts, lean, choice, simmered - 3 oz (85gm)	171	28.6	0	5.4	35.9	66	0	-	0
Steak, porterhouse, lean/fat, choice, broiled - 3 oz (85gm)	254	21.3	0	18	41.4	70	0	-	0
Steak, porterhouse, lean, choice, broiled - 3 oz (85gm)	185	23.9	0	9.2	40.1	68	0	-	0
Steak, T-bone, lean/fat, choice, broiled - 3 oz (85gm)	276	20.4	0	20.9	41.6	71	0	-	0
Steak, T-bone, lean, choice, broiled - 3 oz (85gm)	182	23.9	0	8.8	40	68	0	-	0
Tenderloin, lean/fat, choice, broiled - 3 oz (85gm)	230	22	0	15.1	40.7	73	0	-	0
Tenderloin, lean/fat, choice, roasted -3 oz (85gm)	262	20.7	0	19.2	40.9	74	0	-	0
Tenderloin, lean/fat, good, broiled - 3 oz (85gm)	216	22.2	0	13.4	40.8	73	0	-	0
Tenderloin, lean/fat, good, roasted - 3 oz (85gm)	245	21	0	17.3	41	74	0	-	0
Tenderloin, lean/fat, prime, broiled - 3 oz (85gm)	270	21.1	0	19.9	40.9	73	0	-	0
Tenderloin, lean, prime, broiled - 3 oz (85gm)	197	24	0	10.5	39.1	72	0	-	0
Tenderloin, lean, choice, broiled - 3 oz (85gm)	176	24	0	8.1	39	72	0	-	0
Tenderloin, lean, choice, roasted - 3 oz (85gm)	189	23.4	0	9.9	39.1	73	0	-	0
Tenderloin, lean, good, broiled - 3 oz (85gm)	167	24	0	7.1	39	72	0	-	0
Tenderloin, lean, good, roasted - 3 oz (85gm)	177	23.4	0	8.6	39.1	73	0	-	0

Thiamin (mg)	Riboflavin (mg)	Niacin (mg)	Vitamin B$_6$ (mg)	Vitamin B$_{12}$ (mcg)	Folacin (mcg)	Sodium (mg)	Calcium (mg)	Iron (mg)	Potassium (mg)	Zinc (mg)	Magnesium (mg)
.1	.2	3.2	.3	2.8	6	59	9	2.1	323	5.6	21
.1	.2	3.7	.3	2.6	6	55	11	2	299	5.2	20
.1	.2	4.1	.3	2.8	7	58	11	2.2	335	5.9	23
0	.1	2.1	.2	2.2	4	43	10	2	191	4.1	13
.1	.2	2.7	.2	2.9	6	50	9	2.9	266	6.6	19
.1	.2	3.2	.4	2.3	8	51	6	2.1	311	3.5	21
.1	.2	3.2	.4	2.4	8	51	6	2.1	313	3.5	21
.1	.2	3.5	.4	2.5	9	54	5	2.3	352	4	24
.1	.2	3.5	.4	2.5	9	54	5	2.3	352	4	24
.2	.2	5	.3	3.2	8	54	27	3.3	380	8.9	26
.1	.2	3.5	.3	1.8	6	52	7	2.3	303	4	21
.1	.2	3.9	.3	1.9	7	56	6	2.6	346	4.6	25
.1	.2	3.3	.3	1.8	6	51	8	2.2	288	3.8	20
.1	.2	.9	.3	1.9	7	56	6	2.6	346	4.6	25
.1	.2	3.1	.3	2.1	6	51	6	2.8	322	4.2	23
.1	.2	2.6	.3	2.2	6	47	7	2.7	290	3.8	20
.1	.2	3.1	.3	2.1	6	52	6	2.8	326	4.3	23
.1	.2	2.6	.3	2.2	6	48	7	2.7	294	3.9	20
.1	.2	2.9	.3	2	6	50	7	2.6	307	4.1	22
.1	.3	3.3	.4	2.2	6	54	6	3.1	356	4.8	26
.1	.3	3.3	.4	2.2	6	54	6	3.1	356	4.8	26
.1	.3	2.9	.3	2.4	7	50	6	3.1	334	4.4	23
.1	.3	3.3	.4	2.2	6	54	6	3.1	356	4.8	26
.1	.3	2.9	.3	2.4	7	50	6	3.1	334	4.4	23

	Calories (kcal)	Protein (gm)	Carbohydrates (gm)	Fat (gm)	Percent Saturated Fat	Cholesterol (mg)	Dietary Fiber (gm)	Vitamin A (RE)	Vitamin C (mg)
Top loin, lean/fat, choice, broiled - 3 oz (85gm)	243	21.8	0	16.6	41.3	68	0	-	0
Top loin, lean/fat, good, broiled - 3 oz (85gm)	223	22.1	0	14.3	41.1	67	0	-	0
Top loin, lean/fat, prime, broiled - 3 oz (85gm)	288	21	0	22	41.4	68	0	-	0
Top loin, lean, choice, broiled - 3 oz (85gm)	176	24.3	0	8	40.1	65	0	-	0
Top loin, lean, good, broiled - 3 oz (85gm)	162	24.3	0	6.4	39.9	65	0	-	0
Top loin, lean, prime, broiled - 3 oz (85gm)	208	24.3	0	11.6	40.1	65	0	-	0
Brains, fried - 3 oz (85gm)	167	10.7	0	13.5	23.6	1696	0	0	2.8
Brains, simmered - 3 oz (85gm)	136	9.4	0	10.6	23.3	1746	0	0	.8
Heart, braised - 3 oz (85gm)	148	24	.3	4.8	80	164	0	0	1.2
Kidneys, simmered - 3 oz (85gm)	122	21.7	.8	2.9	31.8	329	0	317	.7
Liver, braised - 3 oz (85gm)	137	20.7	2.9	4.2	38.9	331	0	9011	19.2
Liver, fried - 3 oz (85gm)	184	22.7	6.7	6.8	35.3	410	0	9119	19.4
Tongue, simmered - 3 oz (85gm)	241	18.8	.3	17.6	43.1	91	0	-	.4

Beef, cured

	Calories (kcal)	Protein (gm)	Carbohydrates (gm)	Fat (gm)	Percent Saturated Fat	Cholesterol (mg)	Dietary Fiber (gm)	Vitamin A (RE)	Vitamin C (mg)
Corned brisket, ckd - 3 oz (85gm)	213	15.4	.4	16.1	33.4	83	0	-	13.6
Corned beef, canned -1 oz (28gm)	71	7.7	0	4.2	41.4	24	0	0	.4
Dried- 1 oz (28gm)	47	8.3	.4	1.1	40.5	-	0	-	-
Pastrami - 1 oz (28gm)	99	4.9	.9	8.3	35.7	26	0	-	.9

Lamb

	Calories (kcal)	Protein (gm)	Carbohydrates (gm)	Fat (gm)	Percent Saturated Fat	Cholesterol (mg)	Dietary Fiber (gm)	Vitamin A (RE)	Vitamin C (mg)
Chop, loin, lean - 1 med (5 oz, w/bone raw) (62gm)	116	17.4	0	4.6	41.1	57.9	0	0	0
Chop, loin, lean/fat - 1 med (5 oz, w/bone, raw) (89gm)	318	19.5	0	26	45.5	85.8	0	0	0
Chop, shldr, lean - 1 med (7 oz, w/bone, raw) (91gm)	185	24.2	0	9	42.9	83.2	0	0	0
Chop, shldr, lean/fat - 1 med (7 oz, w/bone, raw) (127gm)	427	27.4	0	34.3	46.8	121.2	0	0	0
Ground - 2.7 oz ckd, 4 oz raw (76.7gm)	275	16.8	0	22.5	45.5	74.2	0	0	0
Hocks - 4 oz w/bone* (85gm)	236	21.4	0	16	44	77.7	0	0	0
Leg, roast, lean* - 3 oz, bnls (63gm)	117	18.1	0	4.4	42	56.1	0	0	0
Leg roast, lean/fat - 3 oz (85.2gm)	237	21.5	0	16.1	44	78.2	0	0	0

Thiamin (mg)	Riboflavin (mg)	Niacin (mg)	Vitamin B₆ (mg)	Vitamin B₁₂ (mcg)	Folacin (mcg)	Sodium (mg)	Calcium (mg)	Iron (mg)	Potassium (mg)	Zinc (mg)	Magnesium (mg)
.1	.2	4	.3	1.6	6	54	8	1.9	297	3.9	20
.1	.2	4.1	.3	1.6	6	54	7	1.9	302	4	21
.1	.1	3.8	.3	1.6	6	53	8	1.8	285	3.7	19
.1	.2	4.5	.4	1.7	7	57	7	2.1	336	4.4	23
.1	.2	4.5	.4	1.7	7	57	7	2.1	336	4.4	23
.1	.2	4.5	.4	1.7	7	57	7	2.1	336	4.4	23
.1	.2	3.2	.3	12.9	5	134	8	1.9	301	1.1	12
.1	.1	1.9	.2	7.3	6	102	8	1.9	204	1.1	12
.1	1.3	3.4	.2	12	2	54	5	6.4	198	2.3	22
.2	3.5	5.1	.4	43.6	83	114	15	6.2	152	3.6	15
.2	3.5	9.1	.8	60.4	185	60	6	5.8	200	5.2	17
.2	3.5	12.3	1.2	95	187	90	9	5.3	309	4.6	20
0	.3	1.8	.1	5	4	51	6	2.9	153	4.1	14

Thiamin (mg)	Riboflavin (mg)	Niacin (mg)	Vitamin B₆ (mg)	Vitamin B₁₂ (mcg)	Folacin (mcg)	Sodium (mg)	Calcium (mg)	Iron (mg)	Potassium (mg)	Zinc (mg)	Magnesium (mg)
0	.1	2.6	.2	1.4	-	964	7	1.6	123	3.9	11
0	0	89	0	.5	-	285	-	.6	39	1	4
-	-	-	-	-	-	984	2	1.3	126	1.5	9
0	0	1.4	.1	.5	-	348	2	.5	65	1.2	5

Source: USDA Revised *Handbook 8*

Thiamin (mg)	Riboflavin (mg)	Niacin (mg)	Vitamin B₆ (mg)	Vitamin B₁₂ (mcg)	Folacin (mcg)	Sodium (mg)	Calcium (mg)	Iron (mg)	Potassium (mg)	Zinc (mg)	Magnesium (mg)
.1	.2	3.8	.1	1.6	14.8	185.9	8.3	1.2	194.6	2.5	17.7
.1	.2	4.4	.1	2.2	17.7	253.4	9.3	1.6	218	3.2	23.6
.1	.3	5.2	.1	2.5	19.9	269.8	12.2	1.6	271.6	5.9	24.2
.2	.3	5.9	.2	3.5	22.7	360.7	14.5	2.1	306.8	7.3	31.2
.1	.2	3.8	.1	1.9	15.3	219.2	8.1	1.4	188.6	2.8	20.4
.1	.2	4.6	.1	2.2	16.9	248.9	10.6	1.7	239.5	3.8	20.9
.1	.2	3.9	.1	1.7	14.5	44.3	8.2	1.3	202.5	3.1	16.4
.1	.2	4.7	.1	2.2	17	52.7	9.3	1.7	240.9	3.8	20.4

	Calories (kcal)	Protein (gm)	Carbohydrates (gm)	Fat (gm)	Percent Saturated Fat	Cholesterol (mg)	Dietary Fiber (gm)	Vitamin A (RE)	Vitamin C (mg)
Liver, brld - 1.6 oz slice (45gm)	117	14.5	1.3	5.6	24.2	197	-	10160	16.2
Ribs - 6 oz w/bone, ckd, 3 oz meat (85gm)	178	23	0	8.9	43.8	74.4	0	0	0
Shoulder, lean - 3 oz, bnls* (63gm)	128	16.8	0	6.3	42.9	57.6	0	0	0
Shoulder, lean/fat - 3 oz, bnls (85.2gm)	286	18.3	0	23	46.8	81.1	0	0	0

*3 ounces includes fat, which is trimmed and not eaten.

Veal

	Calories (kcal)	Protein (gm)	Carbohydrates (gm)	Fat (gm)	Percent Saturated Fat	Cholesterol (mg)	Dietary Fiber (gm)	Vitamin A (RE)	Vitamin C (mg)
Chop, lean - 1 med (6.5 oz, w/bone, raw) (85gm)	177	27.7	0	6.6	41.8	143.6	0	0	0
Chop, fried, lean/fat - 1 med (6.5 oz, w/bone, raw) (107gm)	282	26.7	0	18.6	37.8	102.3	0	0	0
Cutlet/steak, lean - 3 oz, bnls* (78gm)	140	25.6	0	3.5	41.6	106.2	0	0	0
Cutlet/steak, lean/fat - 3 oz, bnls (85.2gm)	182	22.9	0	9.4	42.2	85.3	0	0	0
Ground or patty - 2.4 oz ckd, 4 oz raw (67gm)	156	17.6	0	8.9	42.6	67.3	0	0	0
Roasted, lean - 3 oz bnls* (78gm)	123	19.7	0	4.3	42	104.7	0	0	0
Roasted, lean/fat - 3 oz bnls (85.2gm)	182	22.9	0	9.4	42.2	85.3	0	0	0
Calf, heart, braised - 1 c chpd/diced (145gm)	302	40.3	2.6	13.2	54.9	397.3	-	17	0
Calf, liver, fried - 3 oz (85.2gm)	222	25.1	3.4	11.2	22.7	372.3	-	8346	31.4
Calf, sweetbreads, braised - 3 oz (85.2gm)	143	27.7	0	2.7	31.2	396.1	-	0	0
Calf, tongue, braised - 1 slice (20gm)	32	4.8	.2	1.2	50	19.8	-	0	0

*3 ounces includes fat, which is trimmed and not eaten.

Wild Game

	Calories (kcal)	Protein (gm)	Carbohydrates (gm)	Fat (gm)	Percent Saturated Fat	Cholesterol (mg)	Dietary Fiber (gm)	Vitamin A (RE)	Vitamin C (mg)
Caribou - 3 oz, bnls (85.2gm)	159	26.5	0	5	36	73.1	0	0	0
Goat - 3 oz, bnls (85.2gm)	177	27.7	0	6.6	41.8	143.6	0	0	0
Moose - 3 oz, bnls (85.2gm)	152	25.3	0	4.8	36	70	0	0	0
Rabbit, domestic, breaded, fried - 3 oz, bnls (85.2gm)	199	23.4	4.9	8.8	36.9	81.8	.1	0	0
Rabbit, wild - 3 oz bnls (85.2gm)	182	24.8	0	8.5	38.5	89.6	0	0	0
Squirrel - 3 oz, bnls (85.2gm)	182	24.8	0	8.5	38.5	89.6	0	0	0
Venison, cured - 3 oz, bnls (85.2gm)	151	24.8	0	5	36.1	68.6	0	0	0
Venison, stewed - 3 oz, bnls (85.2gm)	153	25.2	0	5	36.2	69.8	0	0	0

Thiamin (mg)	Riboflavin (mg)	Niacin (mg)	Vitamin B_6 (mg)	Vitamin B_{12} (mcg)	Folacin (mcg)	Sodium (mg)	Calcium (mg)	Iron (mg)	Potassium (mg)	Zinc (mg)	Magnesium (mg)
.2	2.3	11.2	-	-	-	38.3	7.2	8.1	148.9	-	-
.1	.2	5	.1	1.8	18.6	252.8	10.6	1.5	257.4	3.8	20
.1	.2	3.6	.1	1.8	13.8	186.8	8.5	1.1	188	4.1	16.7
.1	.2	4	.1	2.3	15.2	241.4	9.7	1.4	205.3	4.9	20.9
.1	.3	8.4	.2	1.4	13.5	275.9	32.5	1.1	240	3.7	23.4
.1	.3	5.5	.2	1.3	12.2	301.2	12.7	1	299.6	3.4	22
.1	.3	10.4	.3	1.5	13.2	247	8.2	.8	340.4	2.9	26.1
.1	.2	4.6	.3	1.3	11	252.6	10.6	.7	256.5	2.5	22.6
0	.2	3.6	.1	.8	8	198	8.3	.7	197	2.2	14.5
.1	.2	6.3	.2	1.5	10.9	264	16.7	.8	241.2	3.6	19.2
.1	.2	4.6	.3	1.3	11	252.6	10.6	.7	256.5	2.5	22.6
.4	2.1	11.7	-	-	-	163.9	5.8	6.4	362.5	-	-
.2	3.5	14	-	-	251	100.3	11.1	12.1	385.1	7	8
.1	.1	2.5	-	-	-	98.6	8.5	1.4	368.1	-	-
0	.1	.7	-	-	-	12.2	1.4	.4	32.8	-	-
.1	.5	4.4	.2	4.8	4.1	355.7	12	5.3	222	4	19.8
.1	.3	8.4	.2	1.4	13.5	275.9	32.5	1.1	240	3.7	23.4
.1	.5	4.2	.2	4.6	3.9	340.4	11.5	5.1	212.5	3.9	18.9
.1	.1	9	.3	5.4	6.4	277.1	25.7	1.4	293.9	1.7	21.7
0	.1	9.5	.3	6	3.4	231.1	19	1.2	311	1.8	20.9
0	.1	9.5	.3	6	3.4	231.1	19	1.2	311	1.8	20.9
.1	.5	5.6	.2	5.2	5.6	1141.8	17.5	5	302.1	3.8	26.3
.1	.5	4.2	.2	4.5	3.9	338.3	11.4	5	211.1	3.8	18.8

	Calories (kcal)	Protein (gm)	Carbohydrates (gm)	Fat (gm)	Percent Saturated Fat	Cholesterol (mg)	Dietary Fiber (gm)	Vitamin A (RE)	Vitamin C (mg)
Venison steaks - 3 oz, bnls (85.2gm)	153	25.2	0	5	36.2	69.8	0	0	0
Wild pig - 3 oz, bnls (85.2gm)	197	22.8	0	11	34.4	78.6	0	1.7	.3

MILK AND MILK PRODUCTS

	Calories (kcal)	Protein (gm)	Carbohydrates (gm)	Fat (gm)	Percent Saturated Fat	Cholesterol (mg)	Dietary Fiber (gm)	Vitamin A (RE)	Vitamin C (mg)
Cream, hvy whipping - 1 tbsp (15gm)	52	.3	.4	5.6	62.3	20.6	0	63.1	.1
Cream lt whipping - 1 tbsp (15gm)	44	.3	.4	4.6	62.6	16.6	0	44.3	.1
Cream lt, coffee or table - 1 tbsp (15gm)	29	.4	.5	2.9	62.3	9.9	0	27.3	.1
Cream, med, 25% fat - 1 tbsp (15gm)	37	.4	.5	3.8	62.2	13.1	0	34.8	.1
Cream, half and half - 1 tbsp (15gm)	20	.4	.6	1.7	62.3	5.5	0	16.1	.1
Cream, whipped, topping, pressurized - 1 tbsp (3gm)	8	.1	.4	.7	62.2	2.3	0	6.2	0
Sour cream - 1 tbsp (12gm)	26	.4	.5	2.5	62.3	5.3	0	23.4	.1
Sour cream, half and half - 1 tbsp (15gm)	20	.4	.6	1.8	62.2	5.8	0	16.8	.1
Sour cream, imitn - 1 oz (28.4gm)	59	.7	1.9	5.5	91.1	0	0	0	0
Cream, sbst, lq (w/hydr veg oil and soy pro) - ½ fl oz (15gm)	20	.1	1.7	1.5	19.5	0	0	1.4	0
Cream sbst, lq - ½ fl oz (15gm)	20	.1	1.7	1.5	93.4	0	0	1.4	0
Cream sbst, pwd - 1 tsp (2gm)	11	.1	1.1	.7	91.7	0	0	.4	0
Dessert topping, nondairy, pwd - 1 tbsp prep (4gm)	8	.1	.7	.5	86.1	.4	0	2	0
Dessert topping, nondairy, pres - 1 tbsp (4gm)	10	0	.6	.9	84.8	0	0	1.9	0
Dessert topping, nondairy, froz - 1 tbsp (4gm)	13	.1	.9	1	86.1	0	0	3.4	0

Milk

	Calories (kcal)	Protein (gm)	Carbohydrates (gm)	Fat (gm)	Percent Saturated Fat	Cholesterol (mg)	Dietary Fiber (gm)	Vitamin A (RE)	Vitamin C (mg)
Whole (3.7% fat) - 1 c (244gm)	157	8	11.3	8.9	62.3	34.9	0	83	3.6
Whole (3.3% fat) - 1 c (244gm)	150	8	11.4	8.1	62.2	33.2	0	75.6	2.3
Lowfat (2% fat) - 1 c (244gm)	121	8.1	11.7	4.7	62.2	18.3	0	139.1	2.3
Lowfat (2% fat) pro ftfd - 1 c (246gm)	137	9.7	13.5	4.9	62.2	18.9	0	140.2	2.8
Lowfat (1% fat) - 1 c (244gm)	102	8	11.7	2.6	62.3	9.8	0	144	2.4
Skim - 1 c (245gm)	90	8.7	12.3	.6	-	4.9	0	149.4	2.5

Thiamin (mg)	Riboflavin (mg)	Niacin (mg)	Vitamin B$_6$ (mg)	Vitamin B$_{12}$ (mcg)	Folacin (mcg)	Sodium (mg)	Calcium (mg)	Iron (mg)	Potassium (mg)	Zinc (mg)	Magnesium (mg)
.2	.5	5.7	.2	5.3	5.7	370.7	12.6	5	307.1	3.8	24.3
.6	.3	4.3	.4	.7	6.8	254.8	8	1.1	308.4	2.9	19.2

Source: USDA Food Consumption Survey

Thiamin (mg)	Riboflavin (mg)	Niacin (mg)	Vitamin B$_6$ (mg)	Vitamin B$_{12}$ (mcg)	Folacin (mcg)	Sodium (mg)	Calcium (mg)	Iron (mg)	Potassium (mg)	Zinc (mg)	Magnesium (mg)
0	0	0	0	0	.6	5.6	9.7	0	11.3	0	1.1
0	0	0	0	0	.6	5.1	10.4	0	14.5	0	1.1
0	0	0	0	0	.3	5.9	14.4	0	18.3	0	1.3
0	0	0	0	0	.3	5.6	13.5	0	17.2	0	1.3
0	0	0	0	0	.4	6.1	15.7	0	19.4	.1	1.5
0	0	0	0	0	.1	3.9	3	0	4.4	0	.3
0	0	0	0	0	1.3	6.4	14	0	17.3	0	1.3
0	0	0	0	0	1.6	6.1	15.7	0	19.3	.1	1.5
0	0	0	0	0	0	28.9	.7	.1	45.5	.3	1.8
0	0	0	0	0	0	11.9	1.4	0	28.6	0	0
0	0	0	0	0	0	11.9	1.4	0	28.6	0	0
0	0	0	0	0	0	3.6	.4	0	16.2	0	.1
0	0	0	0	0	.1	2.6	3.6	0	6	0	.4
0	0	0	0	0	0	2.5	.2	0	.8	0	0
0	0	0	0	0	0	1	.3	0	.7	0	.1

Thiamin (mg)	Riboflavin (mg)	Niacin (mg)	Vitamin B$_6$ (mg)	Vitamin B$_{12}$ (mcg)	Folacin (mcg)	Sodium (mg)	Calcium (mg)	Iron (mg)	Potassium (mg)	Zinc (mg)	Magnesium (mg)
.1	.4	.2	.1	.9	12.2	119.1	290.4	.1	368.4	.9	32.7
.1	.4	.2	.1	.9	12.2	119.6	291.3	.1	369.7	.9	32.8
.1	.4	.2	.1	.9	12.4	121.8	296.7	.1	376.7	1	33.4
.1	.5	.2	.1	1.1	14.8	144.6	352	.1	447	1.1	39.6
.1	.4	.2	.1	.9	12.4	123.2	300.1	.1	380.9	1	33.7
.1	.4	.2	.1	.9	13.2	129.9	316.3	.1	418.2	1	35.5

	Calories (kcal)	Protein (gm)	Carbohydrates (gm)	Fat (gm)	Percent Saturated Fat	Cholesterol (mg)	Dietary Fiber (gm)	Vitamin A (RE)	Vitamin C (mg)
Condensed, cnd, swtnd - 1 fl oz (38.2gm)	122	3	20.8	3.3	63.1	12.9	0	30.9	1
Evaporated, cnd, skim - 1 fl oz (31.9gm)	25	2.4	3.6	.1	60.9	1.1	0	37.3	.4
Evaporated, cnd, unswtnd - 1 fl oz (31.5gm)	42	2.1	3.2	2.4	-	9.3	0	17	.6
Dry, skim - 1 oz (28.4gm)	100	10.1	14.7	.1	-	.6	0	.6	1.9
Dry, whole - ¼ c (32gm)	159	8.4	12.3	8.5	62.7	31.1	0	89.6	2.8
Dry, skim, inst, w/vit A - 1 c (68gm)	244	23.9	35.5	.5	-	12.4	0	482.8	3.8
Dry, skim, reg - ¼ c (30gm)	109	10.8	15.6	.2	-	5.9	0	2.4	2
Buttermilk - 1 c (245gm)	99	8.1	11.7	2.2	62.2	8.6	0	19.6	2.4
Chocolate - 1 c (250gm)	208	7.9	25.9	8.5	62.1	30.5	0	72.5	2.3
Chocolate, lowfat, (2% fat) - 1 c (250gm)	179	8	26	5	61.9	17	0	142.5	2.3
Chocolate, lowfat, (1% fat) - 1 c (250gm)	158	8.1	26.1	2.5	61.6	7.3	0	147.5	2.3
Eggnog - 1 c (254gm)	342	9.7	34.4	19	59.4	149.1	0	203.2	3.8
Goat - 1 c (244gm)	168	8.7	10.9	10.1	64.4	27.8	0	136.6	3.1
Human - 1 fl oz (30.8gm)	21	.3	2.1	1.3	45.9	4.3	0	19.7	1.5

Ice Cream And Frozen Desserts

	Calories (kcal)	Protein (gm)	Carbohydrates (gm)	Fat (gm)	Percent Saturated Fat	Cholesterol (mg)	Dietary Fiber (gm)	Vitamin A (RE)	Vitamin C (mg)
Ice cream (and froz cstd), (approx 10% fat) - 1 c (133gm)	269	4.8	31.7	14.3	62.2	59.5	0	133	.7
Ice cream (and froz cstd), (approx 16% fat) - 1 c (148gm)	349	4.1	32	23.7	62.2	87.6	0	219	.6
Ice cream, French, vanilla, soft serve - 1 c (173gm)	377	7	38.3	22.5	60	153.3	0	198.9	.9
Ice milk, vanilla - 1 c (131gm)	184	5.2	29	5.6	62.2	18.2	0	52.4	.8
Ice milk, vanilla, soft serve - 1 c (175gm)	223	8	38.4	4.6	62.3	13.3	0	43.8	1.2
Sherbet, orange - 1 c (193gm)	270	2.2	58.7	3.8	62.3	14.1	0	38.6	3.9
Milk shake, choc - 10.6 oz (301gm)	356	9.1	63.4	8.1	62.2	31.5	0	63	0
Milk shake, vanilla - 11 oz (312.4gm)	350	12.1	55.6	9.5	62.2	36.9	0	87.6	0

Yogurt

	Calories (kcal)	Protein (gm)	Carbohydrates (gm)	Fat (gm)	Percent Saturated Fat	Cholesterol (mg)	Dietary Fiber (gm)	Vitamin A (RE)	Vitamin C (mg)
Plain, whole milk - 4 oz (113.6gm)	70	3.9	5.3	3.7	64.5	14.4	0	34	.6
Plain, skim milk - 4 oz (113.6gm)	63	6.5	8.7	.2	-	2	0	2.3	1
Plain, lowfat - 4 oz (113.6gm)	72	6	8	1.8	64.5	6.9	0	18.1	.9
Coffee and vanilla, lowfat - 4 oz (113.6gm)	97	5.6	15.6	1.4	64.5	5.6	0	14.7	.9

Thiamin (mg)	Riboflavin (mg)	Niacin (mg)	Vitamin B$_6$ (mg)	Vitamin B$_{12}$ (mcg)	Folacin (mcg)	Sodium (mg)	Calcium (mg)	Iron (mg)	Potassium (mg)	Zinc (mg)	Magnesium (mg)
0	.2	.1	0	.2	4.3	48.5	108.3	.1	141.9	.4	9.8
0	.1	.1	0	.1	2.7	36.7	92.4	.1	105.7	.3	8.6
0	.1	.1	0	.1	2.5	33.3	82.2	.1	95.5	.2	7.6
0	.5	.2	.1	1.1	14	646.4	79.4	.1	192.8	1.1	17
.1	.4	.2	.1	1	11.8	118.8	292	.1	425.6	1.1	27
.3	1.2	.6	.2	2.7	33.9	373.1	836.9	.2	1159.7	3	79.6
.1	.5	.3	.1	1.2	15	160.6	377.1	.1	538.2	1.2	33
.1	.4	.1	.1	.5	12.3	257	285.2	.1	370.7	1	26.8
.1	.4	.3	.1	.8	11.8	149	280.2	.6	417.2	1	32.6
.1	.4	.3	.1	.8	12	150.5	284	.6	422	1	33
.1	.4	.3	.1	.9	12	151.7	286.7	.6	425.5	1	33.3
.1	.5	.3	.1	1.1	2.3	138.2	330.2	.5	419.6	1.2	47
.1	.3	.7	.1	.2	1.5	121.5	325.7	.1	498.7	.7	34.1
0	0	.1	0	0	1.6	5.2	9.9	0	15.8	.1	1
.1	.3	.1	.1	.6	2.8	116.1	175.7	.1	256.6	1.4	18.5
0	.3	.1	.1	.5	2.4	108.2	151.1	.1	220.7	1.2	15.9
.1	.4	.2	.1	1	9.2	153.5	235.8	.4	338	2	24.7
.1	.3	.1	.1	.9	3	104.5	176.1	.2	264.6	.6	18.6
.1	.5	.2	.1	1.4	4.7	162.9	274.4	.3	412.3	.9	28.9
0	.1	.1	0	.2	13.9	88.4	103.4	.3	198.4	1.3	15.1
.1	.7	.4	.1	.9	14.7	333	396	.9	672	1.4	48
.1	.6	.5	.1	1.6	20.7	298.6	457.3	.3	571.9	1.2	36.8
0	.2	.1	0	.4	8.4	52.6	136.9	.1	175.3	.7	13.1
.1	.3	.1	.1	.7	13.8	86.8	225.8	.1	289.1	1.1	21.7
.1	.2	.1	.1	.6	12.7	79.6	207.1	.1	265.1	1	19.8
0	.2	.1	.1	.6	11.9	74.6	194.3	.1	248.7	.9	18.6

	Calories (kcal)	Protein (gm)	Carbohydrates (gm)	Fat (gm)	Percent Saturated Fat	Cholesterol (mg)	Dietary Fiber (gm)	Vitamin A (RE)	Vitamin C (mg)
Fruit, lowfat - 4 oz (113.6gm)	115	5	21.6	1.2	64.5	4.8	-	12.5	.7

MISCELLANEOUS (CONDIMENTS, SNACK FOODS, YEAST)

Condiments

Mustard, yellow - 3 tsp (15gm)	11	.7	1	.7	4.5	0	.4	0	0
Olives, green, stuffed - 10 (40gm)	41	.5	.8	4.4	14.1	0	1.6	23.2	5.3
Olives, green - 5 (23gm)	27	.3	.3	2.9	14.1	0	1	6.9	0
Olives, ripe - 5 (23gm)	30	.3	.6	3.2	14.2	0	1	1.4	0
Pickles - ¼ c (39gm)	4	.3	.9	.1	25	0	.6	3.9	2.3
Pickles, dill - 1 lg, appx 4-in lng (135 gm)	14	.7	2.7	.3	0	0	-	-	9.4
Tsukemono, Japanese pickles - ¼ c (34gm)	7	.5	1.5	.1	22.5	0	.9	3.2	.1
Pickles, dill mixed - ¼ c (39gm)	57	.2	14	.2	23.4	0	.8	4.1	2.5
Pickles, mustard - 1/16 c (15gm)	17	.2	4	.1	7.8	0	.2	1.3	.9

Snacks

Corn chips - 10 (18gm)	97	1.2	10.4	5.8	16.6	0	.9	6.8	.4
Corn puffs and twists - 10 (15gm)	85	1.1	7.8	5.5	23.9	0	.6	3.4	0
Corn nuts - 10 (18gm)	80	1.2	13.5	2.5	9.4	0	.7	0	1.1
Soy nuts unsltd - ⅓ c (28gm)	127	10.4	8.6	6.7	13.2	0	1	5.6	.6
Tortilla chips - 10 (18gm)	91	1.3	11.2	4.7	14.9	0	.9	7.7	.4
Popcorn, unpopped - 1 c (205gm)	742	24.4	147.8	9.6	10	0	-	0	0
Popcorn, plain - 1 c popped (8gm)	31	1	6.1	.4	12	0	.6	.9	0
Popcorn, w/butter - 1 c popped (14gm)	64	1.4	8.3	3.1	55.2	6.9	1.1	24.9	0
Popcorn, w/cheese - 1 c popped (26gm)	138	2.7	13.1	8.4	14.9	0	2.1	31.7	1.8
Popcorn, caramel coated - 1 c (35gm)	134	2.1	29.9	1.2	11.4	0	2.1	2.8	0
Popcorn, caramel w/nuts - 1 c (35gm)	137	2.5	28.7	2	12.5	0	2.2	2.7	0
Pretzels, hard - 1 c (45gm)	175	4.4	34.2	2	19.6	0	.9	0	0
Pretzels, soft - 1 (55gm)	190	4.5	38.4	1.7	38.7	1.6	.9	0	0
Pretzels, choc-ctd - 1 (11gm)	47	1	7.8	1.4	48.9	.7	.2	.3	0

Thiamin (mg)	Riboflavin (mg)	Niacin (mg)	Vitamin B$_6$ (mg)	Vitamin B$_{12}$ (mcg)	Folacin (mcg)	Sodium (mg)	Calcium (mg)	Iron (mg)	Potassium (mg)	Zinc (mg)	Magnesium (mg)
0	.2	.1	0	.5	10.5	66.2	172.3	.1	220.6	.8	16.5

Source: USDA Revised *Handbook 8*

Thiamin (mg)	Riboflavin (mg)	Niacin (mg)	Vitamin B$_6$ (mg)	Vitamin B$_{12}$ (mcg)	Folacin (mcg)	Sodium (mg)	Calcium (mg)	Iron (mg)	Potassium (mg)	Zinc (mg)	Magnesium (mg)
0	0	0	0	0	1.2	187.8	12.6	.3	19.5	.2	5.7
0	0	0	0	0	1.6	827	21.4	.6	31.5	.1	7.8
0	0	0	0	0	.7	552	14	.4	12.6	0	5.1
0	0	0	0	0	.5	187	19.3	.4	7.8	0	5.1
0	0	0	0	0	.8	556.9	10.1	.3	78	0	3.1
0	0	0	-	-	-	1826.6	22.9	4.3	270	-	-
0	0	.1	0	0	8.7	181.2	12.9	.1	201.6	.1	3.4
0	0	0	0	0	2.5	292.6	8.2	.4	82.2	.1	1.6
0	0	0	0	0	.7	79	3.4	.2	30	0	3.1

Thiamin (mg)	Riboflavin (mg)	Niacin (mg)	Vitamin B$_6$ (mg)	Vitamin B$_{12}$ (mcg)	Folacin (mcg)	Sodium (mg)	Calcium (mg)	Iron (mg)	Potassium (mg)	Zinc (mg)	Magnesium (mg)
0	0	.3	0	0	1.3	148	22.3	.3	33.3	.2	12.6
0	0	.1	0	0	.9	134.5	9.3	.1	12	0	4.6
0	0	.3	0	0	4.1	121.9	1.8	.4	40.7	.1	18.9
0	0	.5	.1	0	63.3	1.1	38.6	1.2	411.6	1	48.4
0	0	.2	0	0	1.3	109.1	27.7	.3	33.8	.2	14.6
.8	.2	4.3	-	-	-	6.1	20.5	5.1	582.2	-	-
0	0	.2	0	0	1.4	.2	.9	.2	20.5	.3	12.9
.1	0	.2	0	0	2.1	271.6	1.1	.3	35.8	.4	17.6
0	.1	.2	0	0	3.9	169.3	25.7	.6	41.6	.1	19.8
.1	0	.4	0	0	4.9	.3	1.7	.5	89.6	1.1	42.3
.1	0	.6	.1	0	6.5	.6	3.2	.5	97.4	1.1	43.5
.2	.1	2.2	0	0	5.8	756	9.9	2	58.5	.4	10.3
.2	.2	2.3	0	0	7.7	772.2	12.6	2.2	48.4	.5	11.5
0	0	.4	0	0	1.2	135.6	7.7	.4	21.8	.1	3.7

Yeast

	Calories (kcal)	Protein (gm)	Carbohydrates (gm)	Fat (gm)	Percent Saturated Fat	Cholesterol (mg)	Dietary Fiber (gm)	Vitamin A (RE)	Vitamin C (mg)
Yeast, bakers, dry - ¼ oz (7.1gm)	20	2.6	2.7	.1	0	0	-	0	0
Yeast, brewers - 1 tbsp (8gm)	23	3.1	3.1	.1	0	0	-	0	0

MIXED DISHES

	Calories (kcal)	Protein (gm)	Carbohydrates (gm)	Fat (gm)	Percent Saturated Fat	Cholesterol (mg)	Dietary Fiber (gm)	Vitamin A (RE)	Vitamin C (mg)
Beef Bourguignonne - ¾ c (183gm)	194	16	5.4	8	33.8	41.2	.9	38.6	4.1
Beef chow mein or chop suey, w/ndls - 1 c (220gm)	407	25.1	30.8	20.9	23.2	48.4	2.8	131.1	26.7
Beef chow mein or chop suey, wo/ndls - ¾ c (165gm)	204	17.9	8.7	10.9	25.7	38.8	1.6	115.3	23.5
Beef curry - ¾ c (177gm)	345	20.3	9.5	25.7	25	51.2	2.6	345.4	18.5
Beef goulash - ¾ c (187gm)	198	24.2	5.1	8.5	32.1	58.5	.8	42.7	7.3
Beef goulash w/ndls - 1 c (249gm)	330	28.8	21.9	13.6	27.8	82.5	1.3	47.6	7.8
Beef goulash w/potatoes - 1 c (242gm)	291	26.3	18.7	12.1	28.2	59.5	2.7	43.4	17.3
Beef, sloppy joe - ¾ c (188gm)	292	16.1	16.9	18.1	45.3	63.5	4.2	80.4	12.9
Beef stew - 1 c (252gm)	249	22.8	22.2	7.3	41.1	56.7	2.3	20.8	15.8
Beef stroganoff - ¾ c (192gm)	308	19.2	11.4	20.6	40.9	61.4	.8	75.7	1.6
Beef stroganoff w/ndls - 1 c (256gm)	342	19.9	19.9	20.2	40.3	70.6	1.2	73.1	2.3
Beef Wellington - 4 oz (113.6gm)	325	27	11.6	18.2	32.2	92.3	.5	23.3	.7
Bouillabaisse - 1 c (227gm)	228	32.4	4.6	8.4	23.7	105.8	.7	109.9	9.3
Burrito w/chick and bns - 1 (106gm)	236	15.1	27.1	8.1	21.7	29.2	2.7	5.6	0
Burrito w/chick, bns, and chs - 1 (134gm)	350	22.5	27.3	17.4	44	59.9	2.7	90.4	0
Burrito w/beans - 1 (72gm)	149	5.2	22.4	5	17	0	2.8	0	0
Burrito w/bns and chs - 1 (99gm)	286	12.4	27.4	15	46.7	29.4	2.7	85.3	0
Burrito w/beef and bns - 1 (110gm)	291	16.8	26.9	13.5	32.1	43	2.7	.4	0
Burrito w/beef, bns, and chs - 1 (132gm)	388	23.4	24.6	22.3	45.3	72.3	2.6	84.9	0
Cabbage leaves sfd w/beef and rice - 1 roll (106gm)	125	8.6	9.1	6.1	40.1	49.2	2.4	44.6	18.3
Calzone w/meat and chs - ½ (7.5 oz) (213gm)	736	32.1	65	37.9	34.6	105.7	2.5	266.1	0
Chalupas w/chick and chs - 1 (150gm)	311	19.5	20.9	17.1	42.3	51.3	3.6	124.4	6.7

Thiamin (mg)	Riboflavin (mg)	Niacin (mg)	Vitamin B$_6$ (mg)	Vitamin B$_{12}$ (mcg)	Folacin (mcg)	Sodium (mg)	Calcium (mg)	Iron (mg)	Potassium (mg)	Zinc (mg)	Magnesium (mg)
.2	.4	2.6	-	-	-	3.6	3.1	1.1	139.9	-	-
1.2	.3	3	-	-	-	9.7	16.8	1.4	151.5	-	-

Source: USDA Food Consumption Survey and "nonupdated" database

Thiamin (mg)	Riboflavin (mg)	Niacin (mg)	Vitamin B$_6$ (mg)	Vitamin B$_{12}$ (mcg)	Folacin (mcg)	Sodium (mg)	Calcium (mg)	Iron (mg)	Potassium (mg)	Zinc (mg)	Magnesium (mg)
.1	.1	3.3	.2	1.8	14.5	255.8	31.9	2.1	378.2	3.3	29
.2	.2	4.9	.2	1.6	32.2	1027	47	4.2	474.3	4.3	62.9
.1	.2	3.9	.2	1.4	26.1	586.8	31.3	2.6	394	3.5	33.5
.1	.2	5.1	.3	2.2	14.7	999.1	41.3	3.1	701	4.3	45.1
.1	.2	5.4	.2	2.8	14.9	442.5	26.5	2.8	492.2	5.1	34
.2	.3	6.7	.3	3	20.2	475.7	35.5	4.1	557.3	5.8	45.3
.2	.3	6.6	.4	2.8	22.2	454.3	31.9	3.4	830.5	5.5	47.8
.1	.2	5.2	.3	1.9	33.7	1094.5	34.5	2.5	624.7	3.3	39.8
.2	.2	6	.4	2.4	20.2	528.4	26.3	2.7	758	4.7	49.4
.1	.3	4.4	.1	2.2	14.1	927.1	75.1	2.6	398.7	3.9	31
.2	.4	5.2	.1	2.1	17.9	796.3	75	3.1	446	3.9	34
.1	.3	5.9	.2	2.7	23.3	213.7	14.2	3.8	315.4	5.2	29.2
.3	.2	6.5	.4	12.3	27.4	576.2	76.4	3.4	622.4	2.3	64.1
.2	.2	3.6	.1	.1	61.9	158.5	40.1	1.8	224.6	1.4	37.9
.2	.3	3.7	.2	.3	66.4	331.9	241.4	2	254.2	2.3	45.8
.2	.1	1	.1	0	48.8	195.8	34.7	1	156.5	.5	32.9
.2	.2	1.5	.1	.2	64.6	307.5	237.3	1.6	188.6	1.6	38.2
.2	.2	3.9	.2	1.1	62.9	170	38.2	2.4	304.5	3.2	40.3
.2	.3	3.8	.2	1.3	65.7	324.3	236.4	2.5	327	4	46.2
.1	.1	2	.1	.6	26.4	299.1	27.7	1.3	300.3	1.8	20
.6	.8	6.8	.3	.9	127.7	872.8	388.1	5.1	335.7	4	48.4
.2	.2	2.4	.2	.3	61.2	338.1	263.7	1.8	343.5	2	58.2

	Calories (kcal)	Protein (gm)	Carbohydrates (gm)	Fat (gm)	Percent Saturated Fat	Cholesterol (mg)	Dietary Fiber (gm)	Vitamin A (RE)	Vitamin C (mg)
Chicken a la king - ¾ c (181gm)	348	17.8	12.5	25.2	36.3	158.8	1.2	898.6	13.5
Chicken a la king - ¾ c (181gm)	343	18	11.1	25.2	36.2	158.8	.8	297.5	12.9
Chicken cacciatore - ¾ c (183gm)	345	31.4	9.4	19.3	25	95.4	1.5	100.9	18.6
Chicken Creole wo/rice - ¾ c (185gm)	137	19.9	7	3.2	20.4	46.5	2.5	78.1	29.2
Chicken chow mein or chop suey, w/ndls - 1 c (220gm)	286	20.6	22.3	13	20.8	46.4	2	11.8	8
Chicken chow mein or chop suey, wo/ndls - ¾ c (165gm)	145	15.1	7.7	6.2	21.9	36.7	1.2	10.3	7.5
Chicken, Cordon Bleu - 8 oz (227.2gm)	437	39.6	3.3	27	54.6	155.1	.7	218.3	4.9
Chicken or turkey, crmd - ¾ c (181gm)	305	22.8	10.6	18.7	30	71.2	.2	182.9	.9
Chicken w/dumplings - 1 c (244gm)	373	26.9	19.5	20	28.6	94.2	.5	48.8	1.9
Chicken fricassee - ¾ c (183gm)	239	21.1	6.3	13.6	28.9	62.3	.2	10	0
Chicken or turkey hash - 1 c (190gm)	239	19	15.3	11.2	22.1	45.2	2.3	5.6	10.5
Chicken or turkey w/ndls - 1 c (224gm)	300	19.3	23	13.8	28.3	74.6	.7	30.2	.3
Chicken or turkey salad - ¾ c (137gm)	314	22.2	1.9	24	17.7	79.8	.6	36	2.1
Chicken w/sweet and sour sauce - ¾ c (189gm)	172	11.8	21.6	4.6	18	33.4	1.1	47.6	20.3
Chicken teriyaki - ¾ c (183gm)	257	39.3	9	5.1	25.6	114.9	.3	54.5	6.1
Chicken or turkey tetrazini - 1 c (246gm)	351	18.1	24.3	19.6	35.2	49.8	1	116.2	5.4
Chili w/beans - 1 c (254gm)	311	23.3	25.3	13.8	37.5	63.8	6	145	18.2
Chili wo/beans - 1 c (254gm)	331	25.9	17.9	18.2	38.1	86.3	4.5	196.3	24.7
Chow mein or chop suey, meat, wo/ndls - ¾ c (165gm)	216	18.1	8.7	12.3	25.9	46.4	1.6	115.2	23.6
Chimichanga w/beef and chs - 4 oz (113.6gm)	282	16.6	20.3	15.6	48.3	54.4	1.4	67.2	5.4
Chimichanga w/chicken and sour crm - 4 oz (113.6gm)	214	10.2	20	11.1	48.6	34.7	1.1	93.1	4
Codfish ball - 1 (120gm)	227	14.2	15.2	12.4	26.4	75.7	1.4	43.2	4
Crab cake - 1 (120gm)	203	23.2	2	10.8	20	198.9	.1	116.4	.5
Crab, deviled - ¾ c (131gm)	252	15.1	18.5	13	20.7	138.6	1.8	183.4	7.6
Crab imperial - ¾ c (194gm)	281	26.4	7.1	15.8	24	275.8	.3	191.9	11.2
Crab salad - ¾ c (156gm)	205	17.8	9.2	10.7	14.9	107.3	.5	35.5	3.8
Creamed dried beef - ¾ c (186gm)	275	15.1	13	18	34.3	40.2	.2	199.4	1.3

Thiamin (mg)	Riboflavin (mg)	Niacin (mg)	Vitamin B_6 (mg)	Vitamin B_{12} (mcg)	Folacin (mcg)	Sodium (mg)	Calcium (mg)	Iron (mg)	Potassium (mg)	Zinc (mg)	Magnesium (mg)
.1	.3	4.9	.3	.6	17.8	603.3	115.7	1.5	330	1.5	27.5
.1	.3	5.2	.3	.6	17.4	691.2	110.8	1.5	306	1.6	28
.1	.2	10.4	.5	.3	12.4	443.6	44.7	2.2	513.6	2.3	42.8
.1	.1	9.4	.4	.2	12.3	511.6	38.2	1.5	534.1	.9	40.9
.1	.2	6.4	.3	.2	26	1220.3	40.6	2.3	367.6	1.7	45.9
.1	.2	5.1	.3	.2	33.6	725.6	28.1	1.4	314.8	1.2	27.5
.2	.2	14.6	.7	.7	14.9	570.5	173.6	1.7	439.6	2.3	47.1
.1	.3	6.2	.3	.5	9.4	468.3	147.6	1.2	333	1.8	33.2
.2	.3	9.4	.3	.3	9	1006.1	114.7	2.2	299.4	1.9	36.7
.1	.2	5.9	.2	.2	6.9	517.7	16	1.3	217.8	1.5	17.2
.1	.1	4.3	.5	.2	14	627.6	40.3	1.3	614.2	2.1	37.7
.1	.2	4.5	.1	.1	7.5	1063.3	26.5	2.1	158.9	1.5	26.6
0	.1	5	.4	.2	9.6	218.8	27.6	1.2	247.8	1.7	21
.1	.1	4.4	.3	.1	8.2	1037.5	25	1.3	302.4	.9	31.8
.1	.3	12.4	.7	.4	12.9	2669.5	39.2	2.9	519.7	2.7	55.1
.2	.2	4.6	.2	.3	12.5	813.2	145.4	1.9	224.2	1.9	26.7
.1	.3	4.8	.3	1.2	57.7	975.5	58.5	3.9	740.7	4.3	59.4
.1	.3	6	.3	1.7	22.3	1318	51.7	3.6	765.6	5.3	51.6
.2	.2	3.9	.2	1	25.4	592.8	30.2	2.3	405.8	3.2	31.5
.2	.3	3.2	.1	1	33.5	296.7	181.4	1.6	230.8	2.9	28.8
.2	.2	2.7	.1	.2	26.2	158.7	64.4	.9	177.6	.9	23.3
.1	.1	2.8	.3	.5	10.3	269.2	40.2	1.2	449.2	.6	31.5
.1	.1	2.2	.4	10.7	18.9	831.3	66.8	1.3	164.9	5.5	44.3
.2	.2	2.8	.2	6.5	41.6	779.9	69.1	1.7	261.2	3.1	36.1
.3	.3	3.6	.4	12.7	31.2	704.6	115.5	1.9	339.3	5.9	53.2
.2	.1	2.9	.3	10.1	16.2	689.8	57.7	1	261.4	4.4	38.5
.1	.4	1.5	.2	1.5	11.9	1324.8	201.4	1.3	306.9	2.4	31.9

	Calories (kcal)	Protein (gm)	Carbohydrates (gm)	Fat (gm)	Percent Saturated Fat	Cholesterol (mg)	Dietary Fiber (gm)	Vitamin A (RE)	Vitamin C (mg)
Egg roll w/meat - 1 (64gm)	118	5	9.3	6.7	23.9	46.3	.6	12	2.1
Egg roll w/shrimp - 1 (64gm)	106	3.7	10	5.6	21.2	47.2	.7	13.4	2.2
Egg roll w/veg, no meat - 1 (64gm)	102	2.7	9.9	5.9	21.5	38.7	.7	12.2	3.3
Enchilada w/beef, bns, and chs - 1 (129gm)	234	11.8	24.8	10.4	37.6	28	3.5	237.9	14.3
Enchilada w/chick and bns - 1 (113gm)	167	9	22.9	5	16.9	14.5	3.4	179.8	12.4
Enchilada w/chicken, bns, and chs - 1 (126gm)	214	10.5	24.7	8.8	35.5	22.6	3.4	239.2	14.3
Enchilada w/bns - 1 (118gm)	164	6	27.9	3.9	13.6	0	4.6	177.3	12.4
Enchilada w/bns and chs - 1 (131gm)	230	9.2	27.6	10.1	41.3	17.7	4	262.2	14.8
Enchilada w/beef and bns - 1 (116gm)	192	10.5	22.9	7	26.5	21.4	3.4	176.6	12.4
Flounder, filet, stfd w/crab - 7.4 oz (210.gm)	311	38.2	13.7	10.3	22.1	174.1	.5	132.4	2.5
Gnocchi (cheese) - 1 c (70gm)	125	6.3	6	8.4	37.5	59.4	.1	101.2	0
Grape leaves stfd w/rice - 2 oz (56.8gm)	101	1.1	7.6	7.6	13.5	0	.9	133	8.5
Ham salad - ¾ c (137gm)	298	20.4	1.9	23	18.4	57.5	.6	24.1	2.1
Hash, corned beef - 1 c (190gm)	344	16.7	20.3	21.5	48	62.7	.9	0	0
Hash, roast beef - 1 c (190gm)	382	19.4	20.4	24.6	36.1	58	2.1	10.3	7.4
Kidney bean salad - ½ c (116gm)	175	6	23.5	6.9	22.6	9.1	4.3	5.7	1.9
Knish, cheese - 1 (60gm)	209	6.4	18.6	11.9	23.9	71	.5	155.8	0
Knish, meat - 1 (50gm)	186	4	17	11.3	20.9	69.1	.6	148.8	.6
Knish, potato - 1 (61gm)	204	4.5	20	11.7	21.6	69.2	.9	146.7	1.6
Lamb stew - 1 c (252gm)	283	19.6	26.8	11.1	44.3	53.4	5.1	266.6	8
Liver, chick, chpd, w/eggs and onion - ¾ c (156gm)	225	19.2	4.3	14.1	30.7	543.8	.8	3200.9	16.2
Lasagna - approx 2½" × 4" (206gm)	325	19.2	34.3	12.3	52.7	48.4	2.2	132.5	13.1
Lasagna, w/whl-wht ndls - approx 2½ " × 4" (206gm)	325	19.2	34.3	12.3	52.7	48.4	2.2	132.5	13.1
Lasagna, meatless - approx 2½ " × 4" (227gm)	317	16.3	42	9.5	59.3	32.1	2.7	162.4	16.1
Lasagna, meatless, whl-wht ndls - approx 2½ " × 4" (227gm)	317	16.3	42	9.5	59.3	32.1	2.7	162.4	16.1
Lo mein w/meat - 1 c (200gm)	285	15.7	26.6	12.9	22.2	61.1	1.5	22.3	9.1
Lo mein w/veg - 1 c (200gm)	124	6	23.2	1.3	21.6	22	3.1	149.8	12.9
Lobster newburg - ¾ c (183gm)	455	20.7	7.8	38	58.3	312.5	.1	374.5	.6

Thiamin (mg)	Riboflavin (mg)	Niacin (mg)	Vitamin B$_6$ (mg)	Vitamin B$_{12}$ (mcg)	Folacin (mcg)	Sodium (mg)	Calcium (mg)	Iron (mg)	Potassium (mg)	Zinc (mg)	Magnesium (mg)
.1	.1	1.3	.1	.2	8.4	305.8	12.9	.8	126.8	.5	9.9
.1	.1	.8	.1	.1	9.1	325.5	18.2	.9	103.3	.2	10.7
.1	.1	.8	.1	.1	11.9	307.5	13.1	.8	106.4	.3	9.6
.1	.1	2.3	.3	.5	38.5	189.6	175.3	1.8	424.4	2.3	48.2
.1	.1	2.1	.2	0	41	106.8	88	1.5	365.7	1.1	42.9
.1	.1	2	.3	.1	37.8	185.7	175.5	1.5	389.9	1.4	46.8
.1	.1	1.2	.2	0	68.6	95.1	94.2	1.8	412.6	1.1	50.3
.1	.1	1.3	.3	.1	50.6	217.2	223.4	1.7	414.6	1.5	51.4
.1	.1	2.5	.3	.5	41.7	110.8	86.7	1.9	407.5	2.2	44.4
.2	.2	4.6	.4	6	36.7	814.4	86.9	2.6	704.8	2.9	74.1
0	.1	.3	0	.2	8	186.2	136.9	.6	50.6	.6	8.5
0	0	.3	.1	0	6.9	103.9	29.3	1.2	103.2	.2	9.8
.6	.2	4.1	.5	.6	8	1218.1	22	1	356	2.1	21.8
0	.2	4	.2	1.2	15.2	1026	24.7	3.8	380	4.3	28.5
.1	.2	4.3	.4	1.5	16.3	640	24.4	2.3	522	4.5	36
.1	.1	.5	.1	0	98.3	306.3	35.4	1.9	314.9	.9	37
.1	.2	1.1	0	.2	10.7	295.1	26.3	1.3	59.7	.4	8.1
.1	.1	1	0	.2	10.2	222	17.2	1.2	57	.3	7.6
.1	.1	1.3	.1	.2	10.1	239.6	16.9	1.3	106.4	.4	10.6
.2	.3	5.1	.3	1.5	31.3	740.2	34.3	2.2	574.8	3.6	45.8
0	1.2	3	.5	12.7	515.2	1544.8	43.2	6.2	216.8	3.2	26.7
.2	.3	3.1	.2	.6	15.9	625.9	220.8	2.8	433.3	2.7	38.8
.2	.3	3.1	.2	.6	16.5	625.9	221.1	2.7	434.2	2.8	40.5
.2	.3	2.3	.2	.2	17.9	743.7	268.7	2.8	440.1	1.8	41.1
.2	.3	2.3	.2	.2	18.6	743.9	268.9	2.7	441.2	1.8	43.3
.4	.3	3.4	.3	.3	38.8	275.2	25.6	2.2	262.8	1.8	34.6
.2	.2	2.5	.2	0	40.6	623.5	48	2.2	414.9	.9	30.7
.2	.3	1.5	.2	.8	28.7	863.1	187.3	1.4	308.3	2.5	30.9

	Calories (kcal)	Protein (gm)	Carbohydrates (gm)	Fat (gm)	Percent Saturated Fat	Cholesterol (mg)	Dietary Fiber (gm)	Vitamin A (RE)	Vitamin C (mg)
Lobster salad - ¾ c (137gm)	102	7.1	7	5.4	18.7	94.4	1.3	120.2	14.4
Macaroni and cheese - ¾ c (182gm)	384	14.9	35.6	20.1	46.9	40.9	1	206.6	.4
Macaroni salad, wo/egg - ¾ c (133gm)	180	3.2	27.5	6.5	14.5	4.6	1.3	18.8	2.4
Macaroni salad w/egg - ¾ c (133gm)	197	5.6	22.8	9.4	19.1	142	1	57.6	1.9
Macaroni salad w/crab meat - ¾ c (133gm)	181	7.8	18.7	8.4	14.8	38.2	.9	25.4	2.2
Macaroni salad w/shrimp - ¾ c (133gm)	192	7.7	20.7	8.8	14.7	39.2	1	28.4	1.7
Macaroni salad w/tuna - ¾ c (133gm)	291	9.9	14.6	21.4	16.7	31.2	.9	29.8	1.6
Manicotti, chs fill, meat sauce - 1 piece (143gm)	235	14	19.2	11.3	53.3	101.7	1.7	128.2	4.8
Manicotti, chs filled, tom sauce - 1 piece (143gm)	223	12.3	20.5	10.2	55.3	98.3	1.8	136.6	5.1
Matzo ball - 1 (35gm)	50	1.8	6.3	1.8	27.2	46.7	.1	13.3	0
Nachos w/chs and bns - 4 (75gm)	198	8.6	14.4	12	39.9	19.7	2.7	60	.2
Nachos w/bns - 4 (56gm)	122	3.9	14.1	5.8	14.4	0	2.7	3	.2
Paella - 1 c (240gm)	350	20.3	40	11.2	20.7	49.6	1.2	132.7	42
Pasta salad - ¾ c (170gm)	253	3.7	26.3	15.2	14.5	0	1.9	400.4	10.9
Pasta w/carbonara sauce - 1 c (201gm)	372	14.3	49.7	11.2	36.3	115.4	2	34.7	3.6
Pasta w/meat sauce - 1 c (255gm)	307	23	33.2	9.5	39.7	58.6	6.8	157.5	29.8
Pasta, chs, beef, tom sauce - 1 c (242gm)	371	20.2	30.4	18.6	42.7	191.2	2.8	192.8	7.5
Pizza w/meat and veg, thk cst - 1 piece (87gm)	234	9	27.2	9.8	36.3	13.4	1.5	44	12.2
Pizza w/meat and veg, thn cst - 1 piece (79gm)	193	8.7	18.1	9.6	38.9	15.9	1.3	52.3	14.5
Pizza, chs, w/veg, thn cst - 1 piece (⅛ of 12″ dia) (70gm)	148	6.7	17.4	5.8	40.2	8	1.3	51.1	14.2
Pizza w/meat, thk cst - 1 piece (79gm)	244	9.5	28.4	10.1	37.3	14.5	1.3	44.1	5.4
Pizza w/meat, thn cst - 1 piece (71gm)	209	9.6	19.2	10.3	40.3	18.1	1	55.2	6.8
Pizza, chs, thk cst - 1 piece (71gm)	203	7.7	27.6	6.7	37.6	7.3	1.2	43.3	5.3
Pizza, chs, thn cst - 1 piece (63gm)	163	7.5	19	6.2	42.7	9.4	1	55.5	6.8
Pizza, chs, w/veg, thk cst - 1 piece (78gm)	192	7.2	26.1	6.5	36.1	6.6	1.5	42.4	11.8
Pierogies - 1 (57gm)	105	3.8	16.6	2.6	40.1	41.3	.7	22.6	1.2
Pork chow mein or chop suey w/ndls - 1 c (220gm)	432	22.7	30.8	24.7	24	56.2	2.8	130.6	27

Thiamin (mg)	Riboflavin (mg)	Niacin (mg)	Vitamin B_6 (mg)	Vitamin B_{12} (mcg)	Folacin (mcg)	Sodium (mg)	Calcium (mg)	Iron (mg)	Potassium (mg)	Zinc (mg)	Magnesium (mg)
.1	.1	.9	.1	.3	19.6	350.4	34.9	.9	250.9	.9	17
.2	.3	1.6	.1	.3	11.7	791.3	309.6	1.9	241.2	1.7	31.3
.1	.1	1	.1	0	9.7	695.9	26	1.3	141.3	.4	15.6
.1	.1	.8	.1	.4	20.1	608	34.9	1.5	142.8	.7	15.3
.1	.1	1.6	.1	3.3	10.7	250.8	30.2	1.1	162.8	1.7	20.3
.1	.1	1.1	.1	.1	10.8	232.5	43.1	1.3	142.2	.4	21.2
.1	.1	3.8	.3	.6	11.5	369.2	20.4	1.4	195.8	.4	18.8
.1	.3	1.9	.1	.6	16.9	599.1	208.1	1.8	260.9	1.7	24.4
.1	.2	1.5	.1	.4	17.2	629.7	221	1.7	244.1	1.2	23.7
0	0	.3	0	.1	4.7	12.1	6.3	.4	19.8	.2	2.6
.1	.1	.4	.1	.2	44.2	288.7	165.9	.9	165.6	1	35.1
.1	0	.3	.1	0	40.7	171.4	30.3	.8	146.6	.4	29.8
.3	.2	6	.3	17.2	22.6	1210.4	54.3	4.9	343.7	2.4	55.6
.2	.1	1.2	.1	0	13.1	882.4	27.7	1.4	177.4	.5	18.4
.4	.3	2.9	.2	.5	26	355.4	78.4	3.2	229.6	1.4	30.1
.3	.3	6.8	.4	1.1	22.3	1769.3	46	4	924.6	4.6	60.3
.2	.4	4.1	.2	1.2	26.4	1277	142.8	3.3	430.7	3.1	36.5
.2	.2	2.4	.1	.2	27	498.6	117.6	2	177.1	.9	20
.2	.2	1.9	.1	.2	19.2	487.8	135.8	1.5	186.2	1	18.7
.1	.2	1.4	.1	.1	18.4	361.1	131.6	1.3	155.5	.7	16.8
.2	.2	2.5	.1	.2	26.5	515.4	122.5	1.9	154.6	1	19
.2	.2	2	.1	.3	18.5	525.2	148.7	1.4	165.8	1	18
.2	.2	2.1	.1	.1	25.7	400.3	119.3	1.8	127.6	.7	17.3
.1	.2	1.5	.1	.1	18.1	392.7	148.3	1.3	135.7	.7	16.4
.2	.2	2	.1	.1	25.8	385.3	112.7	1.8	148.9	.7	18.1
.1	.1	1	.1	.1	7.5	133.3	34.5	1	86.6	.4	8.9
.5	.3	4.4	.4	.5	31.9	1023.1	44.3	3.2	482.2	2.7	57.9

	Calories (kcal)	Protein (gm)	Carbohydrates (gm)	Fat (gm)	Percent Saturated Fat	Cholesterol (mg)	Dietary Fiber (gm)	Vitamin A (RE)	Vitamin C (mg)
Pork chow mein or chop suey, wo/ndls - ¾ c (165gm)	223	15.7	8.6	14.2	26.3	45.2	1.6	113.7	23.5
Pork w/sweet and sour sauce - ¾ c (170gm)	187	11	19	7.7	27.3	32.1	1	37.2	17.2
Ravioli, chs, no sauce - 1 c (240gm)	433	20.3	48.3	16.8	51.4	302.5	1.4	191.2	.1
Ravioli, chs, w/meat sauce - 1 c (250gm)	358	17.1	34.8	16.6	43	196.4	3.2	221.2	8.6
Ravioli, chs, tom sauce - 1 c (250gm)	338	14.2	37.6	14.6	43.3	195.8	3.4	238.4	9.5
Ravioli, meat, no sauce - 1 c (240gm)	545	33.7	47.8	22.8	38.8	344.4	1.5	79.7	.3
Ravioli, meat, tom sauce - 1 c (250gm)	386	21.4	36.3	17	35	205.6	2.1	178.4	22.6
Rice and beans - ¾ c (179gm)	201	8.3	40.6	.6	14.6	0	4.5	0	0
Rice, fried - ¾ c (123gm)	179	3.5	22	8.5	14.6	40.6	.7	45.1	4.6
Rice, fried w/shrimp - ¾ c (149gm)	216	8.1	25.9	8.7	16.6	104.5	.7	31.9	2.6
Rice pilaf - ¾ c (155gm)	199	3.1	34.6	5.1	19.8	0	.5	65	.6
Salmon loaf - 3.7 oz (105.08gm)	223	17	9.1	12.8	22.7	134.5	.3	130.9	1.9
Salmon salad - ¾ c (156gm)	321	20.6	4.9	24	17	183.3	.9	98.6	3.1
Shepherd's pie - 1 c (243gm)	305	18.4	30.3	12.5	29.3	38.6	3.2	127.7	19.5
Shishkabob - 7 oz (198.8gm)	157	20.2	9.1	4.4	39.3	46.4	2.3	90	33.2
Shrimp chow mein w/ndls - 1 c (220gm)	265	23.4	21.4	9.7	17.4	108.7	2	16.1	6.7
Shrimp chow mein wo/ndls - ¾ c (184gm)	141	19.1	7.4	3.9	14.6	99.2	1.2	14.9	6.3
Shrimp creole w/rice - 1 c (243gm)	301	28.9	25.2	8.7	19	160.9	1.5	162.5	17.8
Shrimp, curried - ¾ c (177gm)	232	21.3	10.1	11.5	32	120.8	.2	141	1.3
Shrimp w/lobster sauce - ¾ c (139gm)	216	26.9	4.9	8.8	20.6	186.3	.4	29.6	.6
Shrimp salad - ¾ c (137gm)	210	20.9	4.1	11.9	15	135.2	.7	31.1	2.5
Shrimp w/sweet and sour sauce - ¾ c (132gm)	358	14.1	30.8	21.1	14.4	78.5	.5	37.6	5.9
Shrimp teriyaki - ¾ c (151gm)	174	27.1	10.2	1.1	-	192.8	.3	45.8	2.8
Spaghetti w/mtbls, meat and tom sauce - 1 c (248gm)	402	25	41	15.3	34	108.1	2.6	126.7	18.8
Spaghetti w/red clam sauce - 1 c (248gm)	226	7.2	33.8	7	14	8.1	2.4	62.3	13.7
Spaghetti w/white clam sauce - 1 c (248gm)	346	10.5	33.9	18.6	14	23.4	1.2	24.4	.5
Spanish rice - ¾ c (182gm)	156	3.3	30.5	2.5	15.5	0	2.4	77.5	29.8
Spinach quiche, wo/meat - 1 piece (143gm)	337	10.9	16.2	25.7	47.5	184	1.5	394.4	4.5

Thiamin (mg)	Riboflavin (mg)	Niacin (mg)	Vitamin B$_6$ (mg)	Vitamin B$_{12}$ (mcg)	Folacin (mcg)	Sodium (mg)	Calcium (mg)	Iron (mg)	Potassium (mg)	Zinc (mg)	Magnesium (mg)
.4	.2	3.5	.3	.4	25.4	1261.5	33	1.7	397.3	2	30.9
.3	.2	2.7	.3	.3	7.3	904.8	20.1	1.2	300.7	1.3	25.3
.4	.5	3	.1	.9	37.6	1426.5	239.3	3.9	182.3	2	30.9
.3	.4	3.4	.2	.8	28.3	1445.8	162.1	3.3	417.7	2.2	36.5
.3	.3	2.7	.2	.5	29.6	1543.9	173.5	3.2	396.4	1.5	35.6
.4	.6	7.4	.3	2.6	38.1	1688.7	88.8	5.6	390.6	5.6	43.5
.3	.4	5.5	.3	1.5	29.2	1239.6	71.4	4	525.6	3.5	43.9
.2	.1	1.5	.2	0	114.4	430.1	53.4	3.6	368.4	1.3	67.7
.1	.1	1.3	.1	.1	12.7	209.5	20.7	1.7	93.6	.6	16.8
.1	.1	1.8	.1	.2	19.4	715.1	37.3	2.4	134.5	.8	26.8
.2	0	1.6	.1	0	5.8	567.9	21.2	1.9	70.6	.7	19.5
.1	.2	4.8	.2	4.3	27.9	731.6	204.7	1.5	303.2	1	29.2
.1	.2	6.4	.4	6	41	532.1	205.4	1.7	399.4	1.3	34.4
.2	.2	4.7	.5	1.3	19.5	636.2	45.9	2.2	728.2	4.1	47.3
.1	.2	4.2	.3	2.4	21.3	452.2	36.7	2.6	548.9	4.2	36.2
.1	.2	3.3	.1	.3	39.8	1047.7	109.5	2.9	351.9	.8	68
.1	.1	2.9	.1	.2	34.5	584.3	94.8	2	315.6	.5	48.2
.2	.1	3.6	.2	.3	24.4	623.9	162.4	4.4	359.1	.7	72.7
.1	.2	1.7	.1	.4	17.4	453.4	211	1.5	263.6	.6	52.2
.1	.1	2.9	.2	.5	29.2	723.8	110.8	2	243.5	.9	53.3
0	0	1.6	.1	.3	17.5	258.4	112.2	1.7	208.6	.3	46.7
0	.1	1.7	.1	.2	10.8	599.2	72.5	1.8	248.2	.4	39.9
.1	.1	5.3	.2	1	16.1	2532.1	99.7	3.5	483.2	2.1	76.2
.3	.4	5.6	.3	1.4	32.4	1538.3	140.5	4.6	660.6	4	59.3
.2	.2	2.3	.2	20.3	16.9	421.9	51.4	3.2	324.7	1.2	39.9
.2	.2	2.2	.1	58.6	20.4	771	59.4	4.9	196	2	55.3
.2	.1	1.9	.2	0	11.8	527.3	50.6	2.2	367.5	.6	30
.2	.3	1	.1	.5	53.4	328.5	245.9	2.3	279	1.4	41.7

	Calories (kcal)	Protein (gm)	Carbohydrates (gm)	Fat (gm)	Percent Saturated Fat	Cholesterol (mg)	Dietary Fiber (gm)	Vitamin A (RE)	Vitamin C (mg)
Stuffed pepper w/rice - ½ (149gm)	198	5	18.3	11.9	33.3	11.8	1.5	179	90.9
Stuffed pepper w/rice and meat - ½ (149gm)	219	11.7	13.4	13.1	45.5	75.9	1.5	48.4	58.4
Stuffed shells, chs-fld, meat sauce - 1 shell (3 oz) (85.2gm)	139	8	12.7	6.2	51.8	61.3	.7	81	7.9
Stuffed shells, chs-fld, tom sauce - 1 shell (3 oz) (85.2gm)	128	6.8	12.9	5.5	53.8	59.1	1.2	77.8	3.3
Steak tartare - ¾ c (168gm)	370	30	.6	26.7	43.5	197.3	.1	32.6	.7
Steak teriyaki - ¾ c (183gm)	317	34.9	8.6	14	34.9	95.8	.1	7.9	11.8
Sukiyaki - ¾ c (122gm)	131	15	4.5	5.8	40.2	134.4	1.3	190.2	3.2
Swedish meatballs w/sauce - ¾ c (186gm)	315	22.8	12.9	18.8	47.2	138	.4	65.4	2.4
Swiss steak - ¾ c (187gm)	192	21.4	7.2	8.3	29	50.4	1.4	228.6	10
Sushi (rice w/vinegar sauce) - ¾ c (109gm)	199	3.4	44.7	.2	-	0	.3	0	0
Sushi w/veg - ¾ c (125gm)	189	3.9	42.1	.3	-	0	1.4	147.6	3.1
Sushi w/veg rolled in seaweed - 4.4 oz roll (124.96gm)	130	2.2	29.6	.1	-	0	.5	50.5	1.9
Sushi w/veg and fish - ¾ c (125gm)	181	6.4	37.1	.4	-	8.9	1.2	133.5	2.8
Taco or tostado w/chick - 1 (72gm)	120	8.8	12.4	4.2	20.8	21.7	1.8	34.6	4.8
Taco or tostado w/chick and chs - 1 (79gm)	148	10.5	12.5	6.5	36.2	29.2	1.8	56.1	4.7
Taco salad - 1 c (122gm)	202	11.5	10.9	12.6	36.1	38	1.8	192	10.4
Taco or tostado w/bns - 1 (80gm)	114	4.3	19.7	2.6	15.8	0	3.6	30.8	4.7
Taco or tostado w/bns and chs - 1 (88gm)	144	6.1	20	5	38.5	7.5	3.7	52.8	4.8
Taco or tostado w/beef - 1 (76gm)	153	10.6	12.4	7	32.7	30.4	1.8	30.8	4.8
Taco or tostado w/beef and chs - 1 (83gm)	182	12.3	12.5	9.4	40.5	37.8	1.8	52.3	4.8
Tamale w/meat - 1 (70gm)	183	7.5	16.2	9.5	38	25.3	1.1	25.2	3.5
Taquito - 1 (72gm)	185	10.5	15.7	9.1	27.3	28.8	1.2	27.1	.7
Tortellini w/tom sauce, meat fld - 1 c (200gm)	262	13	29.8	10	31.5	93	2.2	110.6	5.8
Tuna salad - ¾ c (156gm)	290	24.7	14.6	14.4	23.5	60.3	.8	42.4	3.4
Veal goulash w/carrots - ¾ c (189gm)	211	23.3	5.3	10.3	33.5	80.4	1	415	7.3
Veal goulash wo/carrots - ¾ c (189gm)	205	22.6	5.2	10	33.5	77.8	.8	40.5	7.3
Veal parmigiana w/sauce and chs - approx 6½ oz (182gm)	351	26.9	15.1	20.1	38.6	154.5	2.1	130.3	6.9

Thiamin (mg)	Riboflavin (mg)	Niacin (mg)	Vitamin B$_6$ (mg)	Vitamin B$_{12}$ (mcg)	Folacin (mcg)	Sodium (mg)	Calcium (mg)	Iron (mg)	Potassium (mg)	Zinc (mg)	Magnesium (mg)
.1	.1	1.1	.2	.1	17.6	360.2	103.1	1.9	213.8	.7	22.5
.1	.2	3	.2	1	16.9	905.5	37.2	2.3	301.4	2.4	25.5
.1	.1	1.3	.1	.4	10.4	224.6	109	1.2	171.1	1	15.6
.1	.1	.9	.1	.2	10.3	379.1	116	1.1	149.4	.7	14
.1	.4	8	.1	3.6	19.9	126.4	22.8	3.2	468	6.6	30.7
.1	.3	5.8	.2	2.9	19.7	1117	25.2	4.2	417.5	7.6	38.8
.1	.3	3	.2	1.5	47.2	574.7	52	2.6	359.1	3	37
.2	.4	5.1	.2	1.9	16.7	878.7	90.1	2.3	434	4.1	34.8
.1	.2	5.1	.2	2.4	10.4	473	37	2.7	512.8	4.5	34.2
.2	0	1.8	.1	0	3.5	91.6	14.4	2.2	50	.7	19.1
.2	0	1.8	.1	0	12.2	283.1	18.3	2.1	116.8	.7	22
.1	0	1.1	.1	0	6.9	114.2	16.8	1.5	70.1	.5	15.6
.2	0	1.9	.1	.2	13.7	218.9	18.7	2	150.4	.7	23.6
.1	.1	2.1	.1	.1	17.2	249.8	38.9	.8	168.3	.7	21.7
.1	.1	2.1	.1	.1	18.4	293.5	90	.9	175.1	1	23.7
.1	.2	2.3	.2	.9	22.5	375.1	81.9	1.4	324.1	2.2	26.9
.1	.1	.8	.1	0	60.3	231.1	48.1	1.3	237.7	.6	32.7
.1	.1	.8	.1	.1	62.3	277.9	100.1	1.4	247.3	.8	35
.1	.1	2.6	.2	.7	18.3	255.6	37.4	1.4	227.1	2.2	23.8
.1	.1	2.6	.2	.8	19.6	299.3	88.6	1.4	233.7	2.5	25.7
.1	.1	2	.1	.2	5.7	229.8	7.6	1.3	123.7	1.2	14.8
0	.1	2.5	.2	.7	8.1	214.2	75.6	1.3	168.9	2.4	30.3
.3	.2	2.8	.2	.3	15.5	1229.2	106.9	2.5	282.4	1.5	33.1
.1	.1	10	.4	1.9	19.5	1001.1	22.4	2	356.9	.5	33.7
.1	.3	7.7	.4	1	17.8	460.1	25.4	1.4	497	2.6	35.6
.1	.3	7.4	.4	1	18.9	440.7	25.7	1.3	467.7	2.5	34.4
.2	.4	6.8	.4	1.1	22.7	757	189.3	2.1	540.6	3.1	42.2

	Calories (kcal)	Protein (gm)	Carbohydrates (gm)	Fat (gm)	Percent Saturated Fat	Cholesterol (mg)	Dietary Fiber (gm)	Vitamin A (RE)	Vitamin C (mg)
Veal scallopini w/sauce - approx 3½ oz (96gm)	255	17.6	.8	19.4	29	62.2	.1	165.1	.4
Wontons, fried, meat fld - 4 (76gm)	250	9.7	16.4	16	19.5	62.6	.7	80.1	2

NUTS AND SEEDS

Nuts

	Calories (kcal)	Protein (gm)	Carbohydrates (gm)	Fat (gm)	Percent Saturated Fat	Cholesterol (mg)	Dietary Fiber (gm)	Vitamin A (RE)	Vitamin C (mg)
Almonds, blchd - 1 oz (28.4gm)	166	5.8	5.3	14.9	9.5	-	-	0	.2
Almonds, unblchd - 1 oz (28.4gm)	167	5.7	5.8	14.8	9.5	-	1.3	0	.2
Almonds, dry rstd, sltd - 1 oz (28.4gm)	167	4.6	6.9	14.6	9.5	-	-	0	.2
Almonds, dry rstd, unsltd - 1 oz (28.4gm)	167	4.6	6.9	14.6	9.5	-	-	0	.2
Almonds, oil rstd, sltd - 1 oz (28.4gm)	174	5.4	5.1	16.1	9.5	-	-	0	.3
Almonds, oil rstd, unsltd - 1 oz (28.4gm)	174	5.4	5.1	16.1	9.5	-	-	0	.3
Beechnuts 1 oz (28.4gm)	164	1.8	9.5	14.2	11.4	-	-	0	4.4
Brazilnuts - 1 oz (28.4gm)	186	4.1	3.6	18.8	24.4	-	-	0	.2
Butternuts - 1 oz (28.4gm)	174	7.1	3.4	16.2	2.3	-	-	4	.9
Cashews, dry rstd, sltd - 1 oz (28.4gm)	163	4.4	9.3	13.2	19.8	-	-	0	0
Cashews, dry rstd, unsltd - 1 oz (28.4gm)	163	4.4	9.3	13.2	19.8	-	-	0	0
Cashews, oil rstd, sltd - 1 oz (28.4gm)	163	4.6	8.1	13.7	19.8	-	-	0	0
Cashews, oil rstd, unsltd - 1 oz (28.4gm)	163	4.6	8.1	13.7	19.8	-	-	0	0
Chestnuts, Chinese, stmd - 1 oz (28.4gm)	44	.8	9.6	.2	14.5	-	-	4	7
Chestnuts, Chinese, dried - 1 oz (28.4gm)	103	1.9	22.6	.5	14.9	-	-	9	16.6
Chestnuts, European, rstd - 1 oz (28.4gm)	70	.9	15	.6	19	-	3.3	1	7.4
Coconut meat, raw - 1 piece (2″ × 2″ × ½″) (45gm)	159	1.5	6.9	15.1	88.7	-	-	0	1.5
Coconut, dried - 1 oz (28.4gm)	187	1.9	6.9	18.3	88.7	-	-	0	.4
Coconut, dried, swtnd, flkd, cnd - 4 oz (113.6gm)	505	3.8	46.6	36.1	88.7	0	-	0	0
Coconut, dried, swtnd, shrd - 7 oz (198.8gm)	997	5.7	94.9	70.6	88.7	0	-	0	1.3
Filberts, dried - 1 oz (28.4gm)	179	3.7	4.4	17.8	7.4	-	-	2	.3
Filberts, dry rstd, sltd - 1 oz (28.4gm)	188	2.8	5.1	18.8	7.3	-	-	0	.3

Thiamin (mg)	Riboflavin (mg)	Niacin (mg)	Vitamin B$_6$ (mg)	Vitamin B$_{12}$ (mcg)	Folacin (mcg)	Sodium (mg)	Calcium (mg)	Iron (mg)	Potassium (mg)	Zinc (mg)	Magnesium (mg)
.1	.2	3.6	.2	1	9.8	381	45.2	.7	227.4	1.9	19.3
.3	.2	2.2	.1	.3	15.8	336.7	21.5	1.6	146.9	1.1	17

Source: USDA Food Consumption Survey

Thiamin (mg)	Riboflavin (mg)	Niacin (mg)	Vitamin B$_6$ (mg)	Vitamin B$_{12}$ (mcg)	Folacin (mcg)	Sodium (mg)	Calcium (mg)	Iron (mg)	Potassium (mg)	Zinc (mg)	Magnesium (mg)
0	.2	.9	0	-	10.9	3	70	1	213	.9	81
.1	.2	1	0	-	16.7	3	75	1	208	.8	84
0	.2	.8	0	-	18.1	222	80	1.1	219	1.4	86
0	.2	.8	0	-	18.1	3	80	1.1	219	1.4	86
0	.1	1.1	0	-	18	220	55	1.5	197	.4	82
0	.1	1.1	0	-	18	3	55	1.5	197	.4	82
.1	.1	.2	.2	-	32	11	0	.7	289	.1	0
.3	0	.5	.1	-	1.1	0	50	1	170	1.3	64
.1	0	.3	.2	-	18.8	0	15	1.1	119	.9	67
.1	.1	.4	.1	-	19.7	182	13	1.7	160	1.6	74
.1	.1	.4	.1	-	19.7	4	13	1.7	160	1.6	74
.1	.1	.5	.1	-	19.2	178	12	1.2	151	1.4	72
.1	.1	.5	.1	-	19.2	5	12	1.2	151	1.4	72
0	0	.2	.1	-	13.2	1	3	.3	87	.2	16
.1	.1	.4	.2	-	31.2	2	8	.6	206	.4	39
.1	.1	.4	.1	-	19.9	1	8	.3	168	.2	9
0	0	.2	0	-	11.9	9	6	1.1	160	.5	14
0	0	.2	.1	-	2.6	10	7	.9	154	.6	26
0	0	.3	.3	0	8.1	23	16	2.1	369	1.8	56
.1	0	.9	.5	0	16.2	522	30	3.8	670	3.6	100
.1	0	.3	.2	-	20.4	1	53	.9	126	.7	81
.1	.1	.8	.2	-	21.2	222	55	1	131	.7	84

	Calories (kcal)	Protein (gm)	Carbohydrates (gm)	Fat (gm)	Percent Saturated Fat	Cholesterol (mg)	Dietary Fiber (gm)	Vitamin A (RE)	Vitamin C (mg)
Filberts, dry rstd, unsltd - 1 oz (28.4gm)	188	2.8	5.1	18.8	7.3	-	-	2	.3
Filberts, oil rstd, sltd - 1 oz (28.4gm)	187	4.1	5.4	18.1	7.4	-	-	2	.3
Filberts, oil rstd, unsltd - 1 oz (28.4gm)	187	4.1	5.4	18.1	7.4	-	-	2	.3
Formulated nuts (wht-based), sltd - 1 oz (28.4gm)	177	3.9	6.7	16.4	15.1	-		0	0
Formulated nuts (wht-based), unsltd - 1 oz (28.4gm)	184	3.7	5.9	17.7	15	-	-	0	0
Hickorynuts - 1 oz (28.4gm)	187	3.6	5.2	18.3	10.9	-	-	4	.6
Macadamias - 1 oz (28.4gm)	199	2.4	3.9	20.9	15	-	-	0	0
Macadamias, oil rstd, sltd - 1 oz (10-12 kernels) (28.4gm)	204	2.1	3.7	21.7	15	-	-	0	0
Macadamias, oil rstd, unsltd - 1 oz (10-12 kernels) (28.4gm)	204	2.1	3.7	21.7	15	-	-	0	0
Mixed w/peanuts, dry rstd, sltd - 1 oz (28.4gm)	169	4.9	7.2	14.6	13.4	-	-	0	.1
Mixed w/peanuts, dry rstd, unsltd - 1 oz (28.4gm)	169	4.9	7.2	14.6	13.4	-	-	0	.1
Mixed w/peanuts, oil rstd, sltd - 1 oz (28.4gm)	175	4.8	6.1	16	15.5	-	-	1	.1
Mixed w/peanuts, oil rstd, unsltd - 1 oz (28.4gm)	175	4.8	6.1	16	15.5	-	-	1	.1
Mixed wo/peanuts, oil rstd, sltd - 1 oz (28.4gm)	175	4.4	6.3	15.9	16.2	-	-	1	.2
Mixed wo/peanuts, oil rstd, unsltd - 1 oz (28.4gm)	175	4.4	6.3	15.9	16.2	-	-	1	.2
Peanuts - 1 oz (28.4gm)	161	7.3	4.6	14	13.9	-	-	0	0
Peanuts, oil rstd, sltd - 1 oz (28.4gm)	165	7.6	5.3	14	13.9	-		0	0
Peanuts, oil rstd, unsltd - 1 oz (28.4gm)	165	7.6	5.3	14	13.9	-	-	0	0
Pecans - 1 oz (28.4gm)	190	2.2	5.2	19.2	8	-	-	4	.6
Pecans, dry rstd, sltd - 1 oz (28.4gm)	187	2.3	6.3	18.4	8	-	-	4	.6
Pecans, dry rstd, unsltd - 1 oz (28.4gm)	187	2.3	6.3	18.4	8	-	-	4	.6
Pecans, oil rstd, sltd - 1 oz (28.4gm)	195	2	4.6	20.2	8	-	-	4	.6
Pecans, oil rstd, unsltd - 1 oz (28.4gm)	195	2	4.6	20.2	8	-	-	4	.6
Pine nuts, pignolia - 1 oz (28.4gm)	146	6.8	4	14.4	15.4	-	-	1	.5
Pistachios - 1 oz (28.4gm)	164	5.8	7.1	13.7	12.7	-	-	7	2
Pistachios, dry rstd, sltd - 1 oz (28.4gm)	172	4.2	7.8	15	12.7	-	-	7	2.1

Thiamin (mg)	Riboflavin (mg)	Niacin (mg)	Vitamin B$_6$ (mg)	Vitamin B$_{12}$ (mcg)	Folacin (mcg)	Sodium (mg)	Calcium (mg)	Iron (mg)	Potassium (mg)	Zinc (mg)	Magnesium (mg)
.1	.1	.8	.2	-	21.2	1	55	1	131	.7	84
.1	.1	.8	.2	-	21.3	223	56	1	132	.7	85
.1	.1	.8	.2	-	21.3	1	56	1	132	.7	85
.1	.1	.4	.1	-	40.4	143	7	.7	90	.8	17
.1	.1	.4	.1	-	35.4	26	6	.7	91	.8	17
.2	0	.3	.1	-	11.4	0	17	.6	124	1.2	49
.1	0	.6	.1	-	4.5	1	20	.7	104	.5	33
.1	0	.6	.1	-	4.5	74	13	.5	94	.3	33
.1	0	.6	.1	-	4.5	2	13	.5	94	.3	33
.1	.1	1.3	.1	-	14.3	190	20	1.1	169	1.1	64
.1	.1	1.3	.1	-	14.3	3	20	1.1	169	1.1	64
.1	.1	1.4	.1	-	23.6	185	31	.9	165	1.4	67
.1	.1	1.4	.1	-	23.6	3	31	.9	165	1.4	67
.1	.1	.6	.1	-	16	199	30	.7	154	1.3	71
.1	.1	.6	.1	-	16	3	30	.7	154	1.3	71
.2	0	4	.1	-	28.6	5	17	.9	204	.9	51
.1	0	4.2	.1	-	30	123	24	.5	200	1.9	53
.1	0	4.2	.1	-	30	4	24	.5	200	1.9	53
.2	0	.3	.1	-	11.1	0	10	.6	111	1.6	36
.1	0	.3	.1	-	11.6	222	10	.6	105	1.6	38
.1	0	.3	.1	-	11.6	0	10	.6	105	1.6	38
.1	0	.3	.1	-	11.2	215	10	.6	102	1.6	37
.1	0	.3	.1	-	11.2	0	10	.6	102	1.6	37
.2	.1	1	0	-	16.3	1	7	2.6	170	1.2	66
.2	0	.3	.1	-	16.5	2	38	1.9	310	.4	45
.1	.1	.4	.1	-	16.8	222	20	.9	275	.4	37

	Calories (kcal)	Protein (gm)	Carbohydrates (gm)	Fat (gm)	Percent Saturated Fat	Cholesterol (mg)	Dietary Fiber (gm)	Vitamin A (RE)	Vitamin C (mg)
Pistachio, dry rstd, unsltd - 1 oz (28.4gm)	172	4.2	7.8	15	12.7	-	-	7	2.1
Soybeans, rstd, sltd - 1 oz (28.4gm)	129	10.5	8.7	6.8	13.2	-	-	6	.6
Soybeans, rstd, unsltd - 1 oz (28.4gm)	129	10.5	8.7	6.8	13.2	-	-	6	.6
Walnuts, black - 1 oz (28.4gm)	172	6.9	3.4	16.1	6.4	-	-	8	.9
Walnuts, English or Persian - 1 oz (28.4gm)	182	4.1	5.2	17.6	9	-	-	4	.9

Seeds

Pumpkin and squash kernels, rstd, std - 1 oz (28.4gm)	148	9.4	3.8	12	18.9	-	-	11	.5
Pumpkin and squash kernels, rstd, unstd - 1 oz (28.4gm)	148	9.4	3.8	12	18.9	-	-	11	.5
Sunflower kernels, dried - 1 oz (28.4gm)	162	6.5	5.3	14.1	10.5	-	-	1	.4
Watermelon kernels, dried - 1 oz (28.4gm)	158	8.1	4.4	13.4	20.6	-	-	0	0

Nut and Seed Products

Almond butter, std - 1 tbsp (16gm)	101	2.4	3.4	9.5	9.5	-	-	0	.1
Almond butter, unstd - 1 tbsp (16gm)	101	2.4	3.4	9.5	9.5	-	-	0	.1
Almond butter, honey and cinn, std - 1 tbsp (16gm)	96	2.5	4.3	8.4	9.5	-	-	0	.1
Almond meal, partly defatted, - 1 oz (28.4gm)	116	11.2	8.2	5.2	9.5	-	-	0	.2
Almond paste - 1 oz (28.4gm)	127	3.4	12.4	7.7	9.5	-	-	0	.2
Cashew butter, std - 1 oz (28.4gm)	167	5	7.8	14	19.8	-	-	0	0
Cashew butter, unstd - 1 oz (28.4gm)	167	5	7.8	14	19.8	-	-	0	0
Coconut cream, cnd - 1 tbsp (19gm)	36	.5	1.6	3.4	88.6	-	-	0	.3
Coconut cream, raw (lq expressed from grated meat) - 1 tbsp (15gm)	49	.5	1	5.2	88.7	-	-	0	.4
Peanut butter, std - 1 tbsp (16gm)	95	4.6	2.5	8.2	16.7	-	-	0	0
Peanut butter, unstd - 1 tbsp (16gm)	95	4.6	2.5	8.2	16.7	-	-	0	0
Sesame butter (tahini) - 1 oz (28.4gm)	169	4.8	6	15.3	14	-	-	2	0

Thiamin (mg)	Riboflavin (mg)	Niacin (mg)	Vitamin B$_6$ (mg)	Vitamin B$_{12}$ (mcg)	Folacin (mcg)	Sodium (mg)	Calcium (mg)	Iron (mg)	Potassium (mg)	Zinc (mg)	Magnesium (mg)
.1	.1	.4	.1	-	16.8	2	20	.9	275	.4	37
0	0	.5	.1	-	64	46	39	1.3	417	1	49
0	0	.5	.1	-	64	1	39	1.3	417	1	49
.1	0	.2	.2	-	18.6	0	16	.9	149	1	57
.1	0	.3	.2	-	18.7	3	27	.7	142	.8	48
.1	.1	.5	0	-	16.3	163	12	4.2	229	2.1	152
.1	.1	.5	0	-	16.3	5	12	4.2	229	2.1	152
.6	.1	1.3	.2	-	64.6	1	33	1.9	196	1.4	100
.1	0	1	0	-	16.4	28	15	2.1	184	2.9	146
0	.1	.5	0	-	10.4	72	43	.6	121	.5	48
0	.1	.5	0	-	10.4	2	43	.6	121	.5	48
0	.1	.5	0	-	10.3	27	43	.6	120	.5	48
.1	.5	1.8	0	-	16.2	212	120	2.4	398	.8	82
.1	.2	.8	0	-	15.8	3	65	.9	184	.7	73
.1	.1	.5	.1	-	19.4	174	12	1.4	155	1.5	73
.1	.1	.5	.1	-	19.4	4	12	1.4	155	1.5	73
0	0	0	0	-	2.7	10	0	.1	19	.1	3
0	0	.1	0	-	3.4	1	2	.3	49	.1	4
0	0	2.2	.1	-	13.1	75	5	.3	110	.5	28
0	0	2.2	.1	-	13.1	3	5	.3	110	.5	28
.3	.1	1.5	0	-	27.8	33	121	2.5	118	1.3	27

Source: USDA Revised *Handbook 8*

PORK

Pork, Fresh

Note: 3 oz = a piece about 2½ × 2½" × ¾". Chops = about 3 per lb w/bone, raw, or 5.3 oz each before cooking. Lean means the lean portions after all separable fat has been trimmed. Lean/fat means both lean and fat as trimmed at time of purchase.

	Calories (kcal)	Protein (gm)	Carbohydrates (gm)	Fat (gm)	Percent Saturated Fat	Cholesterol (mg)	Dietary Fiber (gm)	Vitamin A (RE)	Vitamin C (mg)
Leg, lean/fat, rstd - 3 oz (85.2gm)	250	21.3	.1	17.6	-	79	0	2	.3
Leg, lean, rstd - 3 oz (85.2gm)	187	24.1	.1	9.4	-	80	0	2	.3
Loin, lean/fat, rstd - 3 oz (85.2gm)	271	20	.1	20.7	-	77	0	2	.2
Loin, lean, rstd - 3 oz (85.2gm)	204	22.9	.1	11.9	-	77	0	2	.3
Shoulder, lean/fat, rstd - 3oz (85.2gm)	277	18.8	.1	21.9	-	81	0	2	.2
Shoulder, lean, rstd - 3 oz (85.2gm)	207	21.6	.1	12.8	-	82	0	2	.3
Spareribs, lean/fat, brsd - 3 oz (yield from abt 5 oz raw) (85.2gm)	338	24.7	.1	25.8	-	103	0	3	-
Steak, shoulder, lean/fat, brld - 1 (abt 5" × 5" × 1½") (185gm)	647	40.5	0	52.6	35.9	190	0	5	.5
Steak, shoulder, lean/fat, brsd - 1 (abt 5" × 5" × 1½") (160gm)	594	42.2	0	45.9	36	178	0	5	.5
Chop, loin, lean/fat, brsd - 1 (75gm)	266	22.1	0	19	36.2	81	0	2	.2
Chop, loin lean/fat, brld - 1 (87gm)	275	23.9	0	19.2	36.3	84	0	2	.3
Chop, loin lean/fat, pan-frd - 1 (89gm)	333	20.7	0	27.2	36	92	0	2	.3
Chop, loin, lean, brsd - 1 (61gm)	166	21.2	0	8.4	34.4	68	0	2	.2
Chop, loin, lean, brld - 1 (72gm)	166	23	0	7.5	34.5	71	0	2	.3
Pork fat, ckd - 1 oz (28.4gm)	200	1.9	.1	21.3	-	26	0	1	.1
Brains, brsd - 3 oz (85.2gm)	117	10.4	.1	8.1	-	2169	0	.1	11.9
Feet, smrd - 2.5 oz (71gm)	138	13.7	.1	8.8	-	71	0	.1	.1
Kidneys, brsd - 3 oz (85.2gm)	128	21.6	.1	4	-	408	0	66	9
Liver, brsd - 3 oz (85.2gm)	141	22.2	3.2	3.8	-	302	0	4589	20
Tongue, brsd - 3 oz (85.2gm)	230	20.5	.1	15.9	-	124	0	.1	1.4
Chitterlings, smrd - 3 oz (85.2gm)	258	8.8	.1	24.5	-	122	0	.1	.1

Thiamin (mg)	Riboflavin (mg)	Niacin (mg)	Vitamin B₆ (mg)	Vitamin B₁₂ (mcg)	Folacin (mcg)	Sodium (mg)	Calcium (mg)	Iron (mg)	Potassium (mg)	Zinc (mg)	Magnesium (mg)
.6	.3	3.9	.4	.6	9	51	5	.9	280	2.5	18
.6	.3	4.2	.4	.7	10	55	6	1	317	2.8	21
.7	.3	4.6	.4	.8	4	53	7	.9	271	2.3	16
.7	.4	5.1	.4	.8	5	59	7	1	312	2.6	19
.5	.3	3.4	.3	.8	4	58	6	1.2	258	3.1	15
.5	.4	3.7	.4	.8	4	65	6	1.3	299	3.6	17
.4	.4	4.7	.3	1	4	79	40	1.6	272	4	21
1.2	.7	7.4	.5	1.9	8	138	10	2.2	649	6.7	44
.8	.5	6.4	.4	1.3	2	107	11	2.8	557	7.4	30
.6	.2	4.5	.3	.5	3	38	4	.6	238	1.9	14
.9	.2	4.3	.3	.6	4	61	4	.7	312	1.7	22
.9	.2	4.6	.4	.7	4	64	4	.7	323	1.7	23
.5	.2	4.1	.3	.4	3	33	4	.6	227	1.8	14
.8	.2	4	.3	.5	4	56	3	.7	302	1.6	21
.1	.1	.8	.1	.2	.1	9	1	.1	23	.2	2
.1	.2	2.9	.2	1.3	4	77	8	1.6	166	1.3	10
.1	.1	.4	.1	.2	1	21	32	.4	104	.8	4
.4	1.4	5	.4	6.7	35	68	11	4.5	121	3.6	15
.3	1.9	7.2	.5	15.9	139	42	9	15.3	128	5.8	12
.3	.5	4.6	.2	2.1	3	93	16	4.3	201	3.9	17
.1	.1	.1	.1	.9	3	33	23	3.2	7	4.3	9

Pork, Cured

	Calories (kcal)	Protein (gm)	Carbohydrates (gm)	Fat (gm)	Percent Saturated Fat	Cholesterol (mg)	Dietary Fiber (gm)	Vitamin A (RE)	Vitamin C (mg)
Bacon, ckd - 3 slices (19gm)	109	5.8	.2	9.4	-	16	0	.1	6.4
Bacon, raw - 3 slices (68gm)	378	5.9	.1	39.2	-	46	0	.1	14.8
Breakfast strips, ckd - 3 slices (34gm)	156	9.9	.4	12.5	-	36	0	.1	14.8
Canadian-style bacon, grld - 2 slices (46.5gm)	86	11.3	.7	4	-	27	0	.1	10
Feet, pickled - 1 oz (28.4gm)	58	3.9	.1	4.6	-	26	0	.1	-
Ham, bnls, rstd - 3 oz (85.2gm)	140	18.7	.5	6.6	34	48	0	.1	18.7
Ham, bnls, cold - 1 slice (28.4gm)	46	5.2	.7	2.4	34	15	0	.1	7.7
Ham, bnls, rstd - 1 c (140gm)	231	30.8	.7	10.7	34	80	0	0	30.8
Ham, cnd, reg (approx 13% fat), rstd - 3 oz (85.2gm)	192	17.5	.4	13	34	52	0	.1	11.9
Ham, cnd (approx 13% fat) cold - 1 oz (28.4gm)	54	4.9	.1	3.7	34	11	0	.1	6.2
Ham, cnd, ex lean (approx 4% fat), rstd - 3 oz (85.2gm)	116	18	.5	4.2	34	25	0	.1	23.4
Ham, cnd, ex lean (approx 4% fat, cold) - 1 oz (28.4gm)	34	5.3	.1	1.3	34	11	0	.1	7.6
Ham, canned, rstd - 1 c (140gm)	234	29.3	.7	11.8	33.4	57	0	0	32
Ham, cntr slice, lean/fat, cold - 1 oz (28.4gm)	57	5.7	0	3.7	35.5	15	0	0	-
Ham, cntr slice, lean, raw - 1 oz (28.4gm)	55	7.9	.1	2.4	33.5	20	0	0	-
Ham, cntr slice, lean/fat, cold - 4 oz (113.6gm)	229	22.8	.1	14.6	34	61	0	.1	-
Ham patty, grld - 1 (59.5gm)	203	8	1.1	18.4	34	43	0	.1	.1
Ham steak, bnls, ex lean - 1 oz (28.4gm)	35	5.6	0	1.2	34	13	0	0	9.2
Ham, whole, lean/fat, rstd - 3 oz (85.2gm)	207	18.4	.1	14.3	34	52	0	.1	-
Ham, whole, lean, rstd - 3 oz (85.2gm)	133	21.3	.1	4.7	34	47	0	.1	-
Salt pork, raw - 1 oz (28.4gm)	212	1.5	.1	22.9	34	25	0	.1	.1

Thiamin (mg)	Riboflavin (mg)	Niacin (mg)	Vitamin B$_6$ (mg)	Vitamin B$_{12}$ (mcg)	Folacin (mcg)	Sodium (mg)	Calcium (mg)	Iron (mg)	Potassium (mg)	Zinc (mg)	Magnesium (mg)
.2	.1	1.4	.1	.4	1	303	2	.4	92	.7	5
.3	.1	1.9	.1	.7	1	497	5	.5	104	.8	6
.3	.2	2.6	.2	.6	1	714	5	.7	158	1.3	9
.4	.1	3.3	.3	.4	2	719	5	.4	181	.8	10
.1	.1	.2	.2	.2	1	262	9	.2	67	.4	1
.7	.3	4.6	.3	.6	3	1177	7	1.2	308	2.3	16
.3	.1	1.5	.2	.3	1	362	2	.3	84	.6	5
1	.4	7.5	.5	.9	5	1938	11	1.9	507	3.7	26
.7	.3	4.6	.3	.9	4	800	7	1.2	304	2.2	14
.3	.1	1	.2	.3	2	352	2	.3	90	.5	4
.9	.3	4.2	.4	.6	5	965	5	.8	296	1.9	18
.3	.1	1.6	.2	.3	2	356	2	.3	103	.6	5
1.3	.4	7	.6	1.2	7	1495	10	1.5	491	3.3	27
.2	.1	1.4	.1	.2	1	393	2	.2	95	.5	5
.2	.1	1.1	.1	.3	2	764	3	.3	145	.8	7
1	.3	5.5	.6	.9	4	1566	8	.9	380	2.2	18
.3	.2	2	.1	.5	2	632	5	1	145	1.2	6
.2	.1	1.4	.1	.2	1	360	1	.3	92	.6	5
.6	.2	3.8	.4	.6	3	1009	6	.8	243	2	16
.6	.3	4.3	.4	.6	3	1128	6	.8	269	2.2	19
.1	.1	.5	.1	.1	.1	404	2	.2	19	.3	2

Source: USDA Revised *Handbook 8*

POULTRY

Chicken, Broilers or Fryers (average 3.3 lb chicken)

	Calories (kcal)	Protein (gm)	Carbohydrates (gm)	Fat (gm)	Percent Saturated Fat	Cholesterol (mg)	Dietary Fiber (gm)	Vitamin A (RE)	Vitamin C (mg)
Fried, batter - ½ chicken (466gm)	1347	105	43.9	80.8	26.6	404	-	130	0
Fried, flour - ½ chicken (314gm)	844	89.7	9.9	46.8	27.2	283	-	84	0
Roasted, meat and skin, - ½ chicken (299gm)	715	81.6	0	40.7	27.8	263	0	140	0
Stewed, meat and skin, - ½ chicken (334gm)	730	82.4	0	42	27.8	262	0	141	0
Back, meat and skin, frd, batter - ½ (120gm)	397	26.4	12.3	26.3	26.6	105	-	43	0
Back, meat and skin, rstd - ½ (53gm)	159	13.8	0	11.1	27.8	46	0	53	0
Back, meat and skin, stewed - ½ (61gm)	158	13.5	0	11.1	27.6	48	0	54	0
Back, meat only, rstd - ½ (40gm)	96	11.3	0	5.3	27.4	36	0	11	0
Breast, meat and skin, raw -½ (145gm)	250	30.2	0	13.4	28.8	92	0	35	1.5
Breast, meat and skin, frd, batter - ½ (140gm)	364	34.8	12.6	18.5	26.7	119	-	28	0
Breast, meat and skin, frd, flour - ½ (98gm)	218	31.2	1.6	8.7	27.6	88	-	15	0
Breast, meat and skin, rstd - ½ (98gm)	193	29.2	0	7.6	28.2	83	0	26	0
Breast, meat and skin, stwd - ½ (110gm)	202	30.1	0	8.2	28.1	83	0	26	0
Breast, meat only, rstd - ½ (86gm)	142	26.7	0	3.1	28.3	73	0	5	0
Drumstick, meat and skin, raw - 1 (73gm)	117	14.1	0	6.3	27.6	59	0	21	2
Drumstick, meat and skin, frd, batter - 1 (72gm)	193	15.8	6	11.3	26.3	62	-	18	0
Drumstick, meat and skin, frd, flour - 1 (49gm)	120	13.2	.8	6.7	26.6	44	-	12	0
Drumstick, meat and skin, rstd - 1 (52gm)	112	14.1	0	5.8	27.2	48	0	15	0
Drumstick, meat and skin, stwd - 1 (57gm)	116	14.4	0	6.1	27.4	48	0	15	0
Drumstick, meat only, rstd - 1 (44gm)	76	12.4	0	2.5	26.1	41	0	8	0
Neck, meat and skin, frd, flour - 1 (36gm)	119	8.6	1.5	8.5	26.8	34	-	21	0
Neck, meat and skin, smrd - 1 (38gm)	94	7.4	0	6.9	27.6	27	0	18	0
Neck, meat only, smrd - 1 (18gm)	32	4.4	0	1.5	25.9	14	0	7	0

Thiamin (mg)	Riboflavin (mg)	Niacin (mg)	Vitamin B_6 (mg)	Vitamin B_{12} (mcg)	Folacin (mcg)	Sodium (mg)	Calcium (mg)	Iron (mg)	Potassium (mg)	Zinc (mg)	Magnesium (mg)
.5	.9	32.8	1.4	1.3	35	1360	97	6.4	863	7.8	96
.3	.6	28.2	1.3	1	20	264	52	4.3	735	6.4	79
.2	.5	25.4	1.2	.9	16	244	45	3.8	667	5.8	70
.2	.5	18.7	.7	.7	16	224	44	3.9	556	5.9	64
.1	.3	7	.3	.3	10	380	31	1.8	216	2.4	23
0	.1	3.6	.1	.1	3	46	11	.8	111	1.2	11
0	.1	2.6	.1	.1	3	39	11	.7	89	1.2	10
0	.1	2.8	.1	.1	3	38	10	.6	95	1.1	9
.1	.1	14.4	.8	.5	6	91	16	1.1	319	1.2	36
.2	.2	14.7	.6	.4	8	385	28	1.8	282	1.3	34
.1	.1	13.5	.6	.3	4	75	16	1.2	253	1.1	29
.1	.1	12.5	.5	.3	3	69	14	1	240	1	27
0	.1	8.6	.3	.2	3	68	14	1	195	1.1	24
.1	.1	11.8	.5	.3	3	63	13	.9	220	.9	25
.1	.1	4	.2	.3	6	61	8	.8	151	1.5	16
.1	.2	3.7	.2	.2	6	194	12	1	134	1.7	14
0	.1	3	.2	.2	4	44	6	.7	112	1.4	11
0	.1	3.1	.2	.2	4	47	6	.7	119	1.5	12
0	.1	2.4	.1	.1	4	43	7	.8	105	1.5	11
0	.1	2.7	.2	.1	4	42	5	.6	108	1.4	11
0	.1	1.9	.1	.1	2	29	11	.9	65	1.1	7
0	.1	1.3	0	.1	1	20	10	.9	41	1	5
0	.1	.7	0	0	1	12	8	.5	25	.7	3

	Calories (kcal)	Protein (gm)	Carbohydrates (gm)	Fat (gm)	Percent Saturated Fat	Cholesterol (mg)	Dietary Fiber (gm)	Vitamin A (RE)	Vitamin C (mg)
Thigh, meat and skin, raw - 1 (94gm)	199	16.2	0	14.3	28.5	79	0	40	2.1
Thigh, meat and skin, frd, batter - 1 (86gm)	238	18.6	7.8	14.2	26.7	80	-	25	0
Thigh, meat and skin, frd, flour - 1 (62gm)	162	16.6	2	9.3	27.3	60	-	18	0
Thigh, meat and skin, rstd - 1 (62gm)	153	15.5	0	9.6	27.9	58	0	30	0
Thigh, meat and skin, stwd - 1 (68gm)	158	15.8	0	10	27.8	57	0	30	0
Thigh, meat only, rstd - 1 (52gm)	109	13.5	0	5.7	27.7	49	0	10	0
Wing, meat and skin, raw - 1 (49gm)	109	9	0	7.8	28	38	0	21	.3
Wing, meat and skin, frd, batter - 1 (49gm)	159	9.7	5.4	10.7	26.7	39	-	17	0
Wing, meat and skin, frd, flour - 1 (32gm)	103	8.4	.8	7.1	27.4	26	-	12	0
Wing, meat and skin, rstd - 1 (34gm)	99	9.1	0	6.6	27.9	29	0	16	0
Wing, meat and skin, stwd - 1 (40gm)	100	9.1	0	6.7	27.9	28	0	16	0
Wing, meat only, rstd - 1 (21gm)	43	6.4	0	1.7	27.5	18	0	4	0

Roasters

Dark meat, meat only, rstd - 3 oz (85.2gm)	150	19	0	7.3	27.8	63	0	14	0
Light meat, meat only, rstd - 3 oz (85.2gm)	128	23	0	3.4	26.5	63	0	5	0

Stewing Chicken

Dark meat, meat only, stwd - 1 c (140 gm)	361	39.4	0	21.4	26.6	132	0	61	0
Light meat, meat only, stwd - 1 c (140 gm)	298	46.3	0	11.2	24.8	98	0	31	0
Canned, meat only, boned, w/broth - 5 oz (142gm)	234	30.9	0	11.3	27.6	88	0	48	2.8

Organs

Giblets smrd - 1 c (145gm)	228	37.5	1.4	6.9	31.2	570	-	3232	11.6
Giblets (roaster) smrd - 1 c (145gm)	239	38.8	1.2	7.6	31.4	517	-	3539	9.5
Gizzard, smrd - 1 c (145gm)	222	39.4	1.6	5.3	28.4	281	0	82	2.4
Heart, smrd - 1 c (145gm)	268	38.3	.1	11.5	28.5	350	0	12	2.6
Liver, smrd - 1 c (140gm)	219	34.1	1.2	7.6	33.8	883	0	6878	22.2

Thiamin (mg)	Riboflavin (mg)	Niacin (mg)	Vitamin B$_6$ (mg)	Vitamin B$_{12}$ (mcg)	Folacin (mcg)	Sodium (mg)	Calcium (mg)	Iron (mg)	Potassium (mg)	Zinc (mg)	Magnesium (mg)
.1	.1	5.1	.2	.3	7	71	9	.9	181	1.5	19
.1	.2	4.9	.2	.2	8	248	16	1.2	165	1.8	18
.1	.2	4.3	.2	.2	5	55	8	.9	147	1.6	15
0	.1	3.9	.2	.2	4	52	8	.8	137	1.5	14
0	.1	3.3	.1	.1	4	49	8	.9	115	1.5	13
0	.1	3.4	.2	.2	4	46	6	.7	124	1.3	12
0	0	2.9	.2	.1	2	36	6	.5	76	.6	9
.1	.1	2.6	.1	.1	3	157	10	.6	68	.7	8
0	0	2.1	.1	.1	1	25	5	.4	57	.6	6
0	0	2.3	.1	.1	1	28	5	.4	62	.6	7
0	0	1.8	.1	.1	1	27	5	.4	56	.6	6
0	0	1.5	.1	.1	1	19	3	.2	44	.4	4
.1	.2	5	.3	.3	5.4	80	9	.9	187	2	16
.1	.1	11.8	.5	.3	3	64	13	.9	720	.7	21
.2	.5	6.4	.3	.4	12	133	17	2.3	285	4.4	30
.1	.3	12	.5	.4	5	81	19	1.7	279	1.2	32
0	.2	9	.5	.4	6	714	20	2.3	196	2	17
.1	1.4	5.9	.5	14.7	545	85	18	9.3	229	6.6	30
.1	1.2	5.8	.4	12.3	439	86	18	8.8	232	6.7	29
0	.4	5.8	.2	2.8	77	97	14	6	259	6.4	29
.1	1.1	4.1	.5	10.6	116	69	27	13.1	192	10.6	29
.2	2.4	6.2	.8	27.1	1077	71	20	11.9	196	6.1	29

	Calories (kcal)	Protein (gm)	Carbohydrates (gm)	Fat (gm)	Percent Saturated Fat	Cholesterol (mg)	Dietary Fiber (gm)	Vitamin A (RE)	Vitamin C (mg)
Pâté de Foie Gras, cnd (Goose Liver) - 1 oz (28gm)	131	3.2	1.3	12.4	33	43	-	284	.6
Pâté, Chicken Liver, cnd - 1 oz (28gm)	57	3.8	1.9	3.7	30.5	111	-	62	2.8

Turkey

Light meat and skin, rstd - 3½ oz (100gm)	197	28.6	0	8.3	28.1	76	0	0	0
Light meat, meat only, rstd - 3½ oz (100gm)	157	29.9	0	3.2	32	69	0	0	0
Light meat, roasted - 1 c (140gm)	219	41.9	0	4.5	32	97	0	0	0
Canned, meat only, w/broth - 5 oz (142gm)	231	33.6	0	9.7	29.2	94	0	0	2.8
Dark meat, and skin, rstd - 3½ oz (100gm)	221	27.5	0	11.5	30.2	89	0	0	0
Dark meat, meat only, rstd - 3½ oz (100gm)	187	28.6	0	7.2	33.5	85	0	0	0
Dark meat, rstd - 1 c (140gm)	262	40	0	10.1	33.6	119	0	0	0
Roll, light meat - 1 oz (28.4gm)	42	5.3	.2	2.1	-	12	0	.1	.1
Roll, light and dark meat - 1 oz (28.4gm)	42	5.2	.6	2	-	16	0	.1	.1
Gizzard, ckd, - 1 c (145gm)	236	42.7	.9	5.6	28.6	336	0	80	2.3
Heart, ckd - 1 c (145gm)	257	38.8	3	8.8	28.7	327	0	12	2.5
Liver, ckd - 1 c (140gm)	237	33.6	4.8	8.3	31.6	876	0	5238	2.6

Game

Duck, meat and skin, rstd - ½ (382gm)	1287	72.6	0	108.3	34.1	320	0	241	0
Duck, meat only, rstd - ½ (221gm)	445	51.9	0	24.8	37.3	198	0	51	0
Goose, meat and skin, rstd - ½ (774gm)	2362	194.7	0	169.7	31.4	708	0	162	0
Goose, meat only, rstd - ½ (591gm)	1406	171.2	0	74.9	36	569	0	71	0
Goose, liver, raw - 1 (94gm)	125	15.4	5.9	4	37	484	0	8728	4.2
Quail, meat and skin, raw - 1 (109gm)	210	21.4	0	13.1	28.1	83	0	80	6.6
Pheasant, raw, meat and skin - ½ (400gm)	723	90.8	0	37.2	29	284	0	212	21.1
Squab (pigeon), meat and skin, raw - 1 (199gm)	584	36.8	0	47.4	35.4	189	0	145	10.3

Thiamin (mg)	Riboflavin (mg)	Niacin (mg)	Vitamin B$_6$ (mg)	Vitamin B$_{12}$ (mcg)	Folacin (mcg)	Sodium (mg)	Calcium (mg)	Iron (mg)	Potassium (mg)	Zinc (mg)	Magnesium (mg)
0	.1	.7	0	2.7	17	198	20	1.6	39	.3	4
0	.4	2.1	.1	2.3	91	109	3	2.6	27	.6	4
.1	.1	6.3	.5	.4	6	63	21	1.4	285	2	26
.1	.1	6.8	.5	.4	6	64	19	1.4	305	2	28
.1	.2	9.6	.8	.5	8	89	27	1.9	426	2.9	39
0	.2	9.4	.5	.4	9	663	17	2.6	318	3.4	28
.1	.2	3.5	.3	.4	9	76	33	2.3	274	4.2	23
.1	.2	3.6	.4	.4	9	79	32	2.3	290	4.5	24
.1	.3	5.1	.5	.5	13	110	45	3.3	406	6.3	34
.1	.1	2	.1	.1	1	139	11	.4	71	.5	5
.1	.1	1.4	.1	.1	1	166	9	.4	77	.6	5
0	.5	4.5	.2	2.8	75	79	22	7.9	306	6	27
.1	1.3	4.7	.5	10.4	114	79	19	10	265	7.6	32
.1	2	8.3	.7	66.5	932	89	15	10.9	272	4.3	21
.7	1	18.4	.7	1.1	25	227	43	10.3	780	7.1	62
.6	1	11.3	.6	.9	22	143	26	6	557	5.8	44
.6	2.5	32.3	2.9	3.1	17	543	104	21.9	2546	20.3	169
.5	2.3	24.1	2.8	2.9	71	447	84	17	2291	18.7	148
.5	.8	6.1	.7	50.8	694	132	40	28.7	216	2.9	23
.3	.3	8.2	.6	.5	8	58	14	4.3	235	2.6	25
.3	.6	25.7	2.6	3.1	24	161	50	4.6	971	3.9	78
.4	.4	12	.8	.8	12	107	24	7	396	4.4	44

Source: USDA Revised *Handbook 8*

SAUCES

Note: All sauce mixes are prepared with water unless noted, and according to package directions.

	Calories (kcal)	Protein (gm)	Carbohydrates (gm)	Fat (gm)	Percent Saturated Fat	Cholesterol (mg)	Dietary Fiber (gm)	Vitamin A (RE)	Vitamin C (mg)
Barbecue - 1 c (250gm)	188	4.5	32	4.5	14.9	0	-	218	17.5
Bearnaise, mix, dry - 1 c (16.5gm)	60	2.3	9.9	1.5	14.8	0	-	0	.3
Bearnaise, mix, prep w/milk and btr - 1 c (254.8gm)	701	8.3	17.5	68.2	61.2	189	-	757	1.8
Cheese, mix, dry - 1 pkt (35gm)	158	8	11.9	8.9	47.4	18	-	25	.4
Cheese, mix, prep w/milk - 1 c (279gm)	307	16	23.2	17.1	54.5	53	-	117	2.2
Curry, mix, dry - 1 c (28gm)	121	2.6	14.3	6.5	14.8	0	-	3	.6
Curry, mix prep w/milk - 1 c (272gm)	270	10.7	25.7	14.7	41.2	35	-	41	2.7
Hollandaise, w/butter, mix, dry - 1 c (44.9gm)	249	4.9	14.4	20.7	58.7	53	-	229	.4
Hollandaise, w/butter, mix, prep - 1 c (259.2gm)	237	4.7	13.8	19.7	58.8	51	-	220	.3
Hollandaise, w/veg oil, mix, dry - 1 c (16.5gm)	62	2.3	10.3	1.5	20.9	0	-	0	.2
Hollandaise, w/veg oil, mix, prep w/milk and btr - 1 c (254.8gm)	703	8.3	17.9	68.3	61.3	189	-	696	1.5
Mushroom, mix, dry - 1 c (22.7gm)	97	4	15.2	2.6	14.8	0	-	0	0
Mushroom, mix, prep w/milk - 1 c (266.7gm)	228	11.3	23.8	10.3	52.4	35	-	93	1.9
Sour cream, mix, dry - 1 c (70.4gm)	360	11.1	34	22.1	49.8	56	-	68	.3
Sour cream, mix, prep w/milk - 1 c (314.4gm)	509	19.1	45.4	30.3	53.2	91	-	145	2.5
Soy sauce - 1 tbsp (18gm)	11	1.6	1.5	0	-	0	-	0	0
Stroganoff, mix, dry - 1 c (55.6gm)	195	6.7	32.1	5.3	64.9	14	-	81	.4
Stroganoff, mix, prep w/milk and water - 1 c (296gm)	271	11.7	33.9	10.7	63.3	38	-	127	1.5
Sweet and sour, mix, dry - 1 c (75.6gm)	294	.8	72.7	.1	12.5	-	-	0	0
Sweet and sour, mix, prep - 1 c (313.3gm)	294	.8	72.7	.1	12.5	0	-	0	0
Teriyaki, mix, dry - 1 pkt (46gm)	130	4.1	27.6	.9	14.1	0	-	0	0
Teriyaki, mix, prep - 1 c (283gm)	131	4.1	27.6	.9	14.1	0	-	0	0
Teriyaki, btld - 1 tbsp (18gm)	15	1.1	2.9	0	-	0	-	0	0

Thiamin (mg)	Riboflavin (mg)	Niacin (mg)	Vitamin B$_6$ (mg)	Vitamin B$_{12}$ (mcg)	Folacin (mcg)	Sodium (mg)	Calcium (mg)	Iron (mg)	Potassium (mg)	Zinc (mg)	Magnesium (mg)
.1	.1	2.3	.2	0	10	2038	48	2.3	435	.5	45
0	0	.1	0	.1	2.1	559	27	.1	48	.1	5
.1	.3	.3	.1	.5	10.2	1265	229	.3	298	.8	25
.1	.2	.1	0	.3	4.6	1447	280	.1	183	.9	16
.1	.6	.3	.1	1.1	12.6	1566	570	.3	554	1	47
0	.1	.2	0	.1	2.5	1155	50	.9	100	.3	12
.1	.5	.5	.1	1.1	16.3	1276	485	1.1	496	1.1	46
0	.2	.1	.5	.8	22	1639	130	.9	131	.7	8
.1	.2	.1	.5	.8	20.7	1565	124	.9	124	.8	8
0	.1	.1	0	.1	2.3	429	42	.1	62	.1	4
.1	.3	.2	.1	.5	10.2	1134	240	.2	308	.8	25
0	.1	1.3	0	0	7.5	1726	2	.3	120	.2	5
.2	.8	4.8	.2	.8	40	1533	293	.5	493	1.3	37
0	.3	.4	0	.2	2.8	887	256	.5	363	1.3	15
.1	.7	.6	.1	.9	15.7	1007	546	.6	733	1.4	44
0	0	.6	0	0	1.9	1029	3	.5	64	0	8
1	.6	.8	.1	.3	4.4	2252	371	1.6	481	1.3	23
.9	.8	.8	.1	.6	8.9	1829	521	1.3	672	1.1	38
0	.1	.8	.4	0	2.3	779	41	1.6	66	.1	9
0	.1	.9	.3	0	1.9	779	41	1.6	66	.1	9
0	.1	1.3	.1	0	27.6	4784	112	2.8	215	.1	83
0	.1	1.3	.1	0	28.3	4791	112	2.8	215	.1	85
0	0	.2	0	0	3.6	690	4	.3	41	0	11

	Calories (kcal)	Protein (gm)	Carbohydrates (gm)	Fat (gm)	Percent Saturated Fat	Cholesterol (mg)	Dietary Fiber (gm)	Vitamin A (RE)	Vitamin C (mg)
White, mix, dry - 1 c (19.8gm)	92	2.2	10	5.3	25	0	-	0	.6
White, mix, prep w/milk - 1 c (273.8gm)	241	10.2	21.4	13.4	47.6	34	-	92	2.6

SEA FOOD

Note: Weight given is for seafood *cooked* and boneless or without shell unless otherwise noted. It is assumed that salt and, in some cases, fat have been added during cooking, accounting for a higher sodium and fat content. If you cook without salt, assume that raw fresh fish contains from 10 to 20 mg of sodium per ounce, and raw shellfish, from 35 to 80 mg of sodium per ounce. For the fat content of raw seafood, see page 52.

	Calories (kcal)	Protein (gm)	Carbohydrates (gm)	Fat (gm)	Percent Saturated Fat	Cholesterol (mg)	Dietary Fiber (gm)	Vitamin A (RE)	Vitamin C (mg)
Abalone - 3 oz (85.2gm)	120	18.6	3.7	3	21	54.6	0	47.8	1.5
Abalone, floured, frd - 3 oz (85.2gm)	155	18.2	6.9	5.5	25.2	52	.1	13.5	0
Anchovy, cnd - 1 oz (28.4gm)	49	5.4	.1	2.9	28.2	15.4	0	10.9	0
Barracuda, bkd/brld - 3 oz (85.2gm)	135	20.9	.3	5.1	25.3	54.6	0	47.1	1.5
Barracuda, breaded/floured, frd - 3 oz (85.2gm)	169	20.4	3.7	7.5	26.8	52	.1	12.1	0
Carp, bkd/brld - 3 oz (85.2gm)	161	19.4	.5	8.5	20.6	59.2	0	103.1	3.3
Carp, floured/breaded, frd - 3 oz (85.2gm)	226	17.7	10.2	12.3	24.4	83.8	.2	47.6	.7
Carp, smoked - 1 oz (28.4gm)	50	7.9	0	1.8	-	24.2	0	20.2	.4
Catfish, bkd/brld - 3 oz (85.2gm)	149	19.1	.5	7.4	22.4	59.5	0	84	2.5
Catfish, floured/breaded, frd - 3 oz (85.2gm)	218	17.4	10.3	11.5	25.6	84.3	.2	32.8	0
Clams, raw - 3 oz (85.2gm)	65	10.7	1.7	1.4	25	42.5	0	25.5	8.5
Clams, stmd/bld - 3 oz (85.2gm)	93	10.1	1.6	4.8	21.1	40	0	69.4	6.4
Clams, breaded, frd - 3 oz (85.2gm)	158	12.4	9.6	7.4	25.5	70.4	.1	32.2	6.6
Clams, cnd - ½ c (80gm)	76	12.6	2	1.6	-	50	0	27	8
Clams, smoked, cnd in oil - 3 oz (85.2gm)	151	11.9	1.9	10.4	25	47.3	0	28.4	9
Cod, bkd/brld - 3 oz (85.2gm)	100	17.5	.3	3.2	19.2	49.6	0	47.1	3.1
Cod, dried, sltd - 1 oz (28.4gm)	36	8.1	0	.2	-	23	0	11.2	0
Cod, floured/breaded, frd - 3 oz (85.2gm)	175	16	6.7	9.3	24.9	65.5	.1	17.8	1.3
Cod, sltd - 2.5 oz, dried, soaked in water (85gm)	91	19.8	0	.7	-	56.2	0	13.6	0
Cod, smoked - 3 oz (85.2gm)	87	19.7	0	.3	-	64.6	0	12.7	0

Thiamin (mg)	Riboflavin (mg)	Niacin (mg)	Vitamin B$_6$ (mg)	Vitamin B$_{12}$ (mcg)	Folacin (mcg)	Sodium (mg)	Calcium (mg)	Iron (mg)	Potassium (mg)	Zinc (mg)	Magnesium (mg)
0	.1	.1	0	.2	2.8	675	133	.1	73	.2	8
.1	.4	.5	.1	1.1	15.8	796	425	.3	443	.5	264

Source: USDA Revised *Handbook 8*

Thiamin (mg)	Riboflavin (mg)	Niacin (mg)	Vitamin B$_6$ (mg)	Vitamin B$_{12}$ (mcg)	Folacin (mcg)	Sodium (mg)	Calcium (mg)	Iron (mg)	Potassium (mg)	Zinc (mg)	Magnesium (mg)
.2	.1	1.2	.1	82.7	4.7	515.5	39.4	2.4	398.4	1.4	45.6
.2	.1	1.4	.1	78.8	4.6	459.4	37.2	2.5	379.1	1.4	44.2
0	.1	1.5	0	2	4.5	230.4	47	.8	165.2	.5	2.8
0	.1	4.9	.4	.1	11.2	302.2	18.6	1.6	296.2	.2	32.7
.1	.1	5.1	.4	.1	10.7	256.1	17.3	1.7	281.7	.2	32
0	0	1.5	.2	.2	15.3	472.6	58.1	1	316.6	5.4	23.1
0	.1	1.9	.2	.2	19.1	442.1	66.7	1.5	272.5	4.4	23.9
0	0	.7	.1	.1	6.3	107.1	22.5	.4	125.7	2.2	9.1
0	0	1.8	.2	2.1	15.4	491.8	29.2	.4	365.7	.9	39.5
.1	.1	2	.2	1.8	19.2	456.2	44.4	1	309.6	.9	36.6
.1	.2	1.1	.1	51	13.6	102	58.6	5.2	153.8	1.7	55.2
.1	.1	.9	.1	43.3	9.7	326	57.8	4.4	132.4	1.6	52.8
.1	.2	1.5	.1	41.9	16.6	353.8	75.6	5.6	173.9	1.8	58.7
.1	.2	1.2	.1	54	12	120	69	5.5	162.9	2	65
.1	.2	1.2	.1	56.7	15.1	333.2	66.6	5.8	171.1	1.9	62.1
.1	.1	2.1	.2	.7	2.3	331.9	12.6	.4	384.5	.5	28.8
0	.1	3.1	.2	.6	1.4	1960	63	1	44.8	.3	19.6
.1	.1	2.2	.2	.6	6.6	320.7	24.4	.8	332.1	.5	27.5
0	.1	2.2	.1	.2	1.7	437.8	23.9	.9	33	.5	22.4
.1	0	3.6	.2	.9	8.5	680	19.5	.6	340	.8	21.2

	Calories (kcal)	Protein (gm)	Carbohydrates (gm)	Fat (gm)	Percent Saturated Fat	Cholesterol (mg)	Dietary Fiber (gm)	Vitamin A (RE)	Vitamin C (mg)
Crab, hard shell, stmd - 2 med blue (96.6gm)	89	16.5	.5	1.8	-	95.4	0	9.5	1.9
Crab, soft shell, frd - 1 crab (65.3gm)	213	11.7	11.6	13.1	24.8	87.4	.3	15.9	.9
Crab, cnd - 3 oz (85.2gm)	86	14.8	.9	2.1	16	85.8	0	8.5	0
Crayfish, bld/stmd - 3 oz (85.2gm)	88	17.1	.6	1.4	-	95.2	0	11.3	0
Croaker, bkd/brld - 3 oz (85.2gm)	154	20.2	.6	7.4	20.7	62.1	0	84.3	3
Croaker, floured/breaded, frd - 3 oz (85.2gm)	233	17.9	11.9	12.2	25.1	89.9	.2	25.9	0
Eel - 3 oz (85.2gm)	286	15.5	5.3	22	23.8	51	.2	358.4	0
Eel, smoked - 3oz (85.2gm)	280	15.8	0	23.6	23.4	54.4	0	410.5	0
Fish sticks - 2 oz (56.8gm)	109	8.7	6	5.5	25.1	42.6	.1	11.8	.7
Flounder, fillet, brld/bkd - 3 oz (85.2gm)	101	16.6	.3	3.3	20.9	49.6	0	47.1	1.5
Flounder, fillet, breaded, frd - 3 oz (85.2gm)	176	15.3	6.7	9.3	25.4	65.5	.1	17.8	0
Frog legs, frd - 2 legs (48.3gm)	121	8.3	8.6	5.7	25.9	78.2	.2	22.1	1.6
Gefilte fish - 1 c (227gm)	267	38.6	2	10.5	20.1	170.3	.1	158.7	.7
Haddock, fillet, brld/bkd - 3 oz (85.2gm)	102	18.2	.4	3.2	19.3	59.5	0	53.6	1.6
Haddock, floured/breaded, frd - 3 oz (85.2gm)	194	16	10.6	9.7	25.2	82.8	.2	21	0
Haddock, smoked - 3 oz (85.2gm)	87	19.7	0	.3	17.5	64.6	0	12.7	0
Halibut, fillet, batter-frd - 3 oz (85.2gm)	153	17.4	6	6.1	19.7	54.4	.2	142.5	0
Halibut, smoked - 3 oz (85.2gm)	190	17.7	0	12.7	17.3	42.5	0	112.2	0
Herring, bkd/brld - 3 oz (85.2gm)	222	19.4	.4	15.4	29.6	94.9	0	69	4.4
Herring, plain - 3 oz (85.2gm)	189	17.3	0	12.8	32.5	85	0	7.6	0
Herring, pickled - 1 oz (28.4gm)	62	5.7	0	4.2	32.5	28	0	2.5	0
Herring, pickled, w/crm sauce - 1 oz (28.4gm)	62	4.7	.2	4.6	40.2	24.9	0	13.1	0
Herring, smoked, kippered - 3 oz (85.2gm)	179	18.9	0	11	32.2	92.6	0	7.6	0
Herring, dried, sltd - 1 oz (28.4gm)	72	6.3	0	5	32.2	30.6	0	2.5	0
Herring, floured/breaded, frd - 3 oz (85.2gm)	279	17.1	10.3	18.3	28.8	109.4	.2	34.9	2
Lobster, bkd/brld w/fat - 3 oz (85.2gm)	111	14.9	.2	5.2	51.1	78.5	0	47.1	0
Lobster, floured/breaded, frd - 3 oz (85.2gm)	185	15.5	7.1	10.2	23.1	87.4	.1	16.7	0

Thiamin (mg)	Riboflavin (mg)	Niacin (mg)	Vitamin B$_6$ (mg)	Vitamin B$_{12}$ (mcg)	Folacin (mcg)	Sodium (mg)	Calcium (mg)	Iron (mg)	Potassium (mg)	Zinc (mg)	Magnesium (mg)
.2	.1	2.7	.3	9.5	11.5	422.3	42.5	.8	171.8	4.1	33.1
.1	.1	2.1	.2	4.6	11.6	300.1	40.5	1.2	126.3	2.5	23.8
.1	.1	1.6	.3	8.5	10.2	510	38.2	.7	93.5	3.7	28.9
.1	.1	1.5	.2	3	12.5	269.2	63.7	.9	116.7	1.9	29.5
.1	.1	5.9	.3	2	16.2	613.1	16.6	.5	274.9	.8	35.8
.1	.1	5.3	.2	1.6	20.3	540.3	37.3	1.2	233.7	.8	33.4
.2	.4	1.6	.2	5.3	13.2	179.7	18.5	1	396.2	2.8	18.5
.2	.3	1.2	.3	6.8	7.6	88.4	15.3	.6	358.7	3.4	21.2
0	.1	1.3	.1	.4	5.3	223.3	18.4	.6	175.8	.3	15.6
0	0	1.6	.2	1.1	10.3	339.9	14.6	.8	344.8	.5	30.8
.1	.1	1.8	.1	.9	13.2	327.2	26.1	1.1	299.6	.5	29.1
.1	.1	.9	.1	.3	14	238.9	27	1.2	131.5	.6	12.9
.3	.3	4.3	.4	2.3	31.4	605.4	63.2	1.3	548.9	3.9	38.9
0	.1	2.8	.2	1.2	9.5	322.7	25.7	.7	309.3	.8	25
.1	.1	2.8	.1	1	14.6	388.9	42	1.2	254.7	.8	24.7
.1	0	3.6	.2	.9	8.5	680	19.5	.6	340	.8	21.2
.1	.1	6.7	.3	.8	10.9	139.6	32.2	.9	366.8	.4	24.3
.1	.1	7.1	.3	.6	13.6	4250	11	.6	850	.8	25.5
0	.2	4	.4	.6	15.6	376.6	53.3	1.2	475.2	1	34.6
0	.2	2.8	.1	5.9	8.5	1190	56.1	1.2	119	.8	8.5
0	.1	.9	0	2	2.8	392	18.5	.4	39.2	.3	2.8
0	.1	.7	0	1.6	2.8	315.7	21.3	.3	39.4	.2	2.9
0	.2	2.8	.2	1.3	8.5	765	56.1	1.2	399.5	.8	34
0	.1	1.1	.1	2	3	1465.9	21.7	.5	59.3	.3	9.9
.1	.2	3.6	.3	.7	19.2	467.9	62.8	1.6	385	1	32.4
.1	.1	1.2	.1	.3	13.7	398.4	54.1	.6	144.5	1.8	16.6
.3	.1	1.6	.2	.4	18.4	434.6	39.9	1	167.9	1.6	22.6

	Calories (kcal)	Protein (gm)	Carbohydrates (gm)	Fat (gm)	Percent Saturated Fat	Cholesterol (mg)	Dietary Fiber (gm)	Vitamin A (RE)	Vitamin C (mg)
Lobster, stmd/bld/cnd - 3 oz (85.2gm)	81	15.9	.3	1.3	13.3	72.2	0	10.2	0
Mackerel, dried - 1 oz (28.4gm)	85	5.2	0	7	25.9	26.6	0	13.2	0
Mackerel, fillet, brld - 3 oz (85.2gm)	213	18.9	.3	14.6	25.1	94.3	0	147.5	3.9
Mackerel, smoked - 3 oz (85.2gm)	186	20.2	0	11	26.2	80.7	0	39.9	0
Mackerel, cnd - 3 oz (85.2gm)	182	21.4	0	10.1	26	95.1	0	127.5	0
Mullet, bkd/brld - 3 oz (85.2gm)	195	21.3	.5	11.5	27.6	59.5	0	101.6	2.5
Mullet, breaded, frd - 3 oz (85.2gm)	254	19.1	10.3	14.7	28.1	84.3	.2	47.7	0
Mussels - 3 oz, ckd (85.2gm)	138	14.2	3.3	7.1	20.6	49.2	0	93.2	0
Mussels, tom sauce - ¾ c (180gm)	218	27	17.1	4.1	24	90	2.7	79.2	7.2
Ocean perch, bkd/brld - 3 oz (85.2gm)	110	17.9	.3	3.7	18.9	54.6	0	47.1	1.5
Ocean perch, batter-frd - 3 oz (85.2gm)	172	14.4	5.7	9.9	23.8	55.4	.2	14	0
Ocean perch, floured/ breaded, frd - 3 oz (85.2gm)	183	16.4	6.7	9.7	24.6	69.5	.1	17.8	0
Octopus, frd - 3 oz (85.2gm)	150	14.7	6.9	6.7	25.8	109.8	.1	19	0
Octopus, smoked - 3 oz (85.2gm)	106	22.2	0	1.2	27.5	144.8	0	19.5	0
Oysters, raw - 3 oz (85.2gm)	56	7.1	2.9	1.5	33.3	42.5	0	79	4.2
Oysters, brld/bkd - 3 oz (85.2gm)	133	8.9	9.8	6.2	23.5	45.9	.1	136.7	3.7
Oysters, batter-frd - 3 oz (85.2gm)	181	8.8	12.1	10.5	26.5	94.9	.2	80.9	2.9
Oysters, breaded, frd - 3 oz (85.2gm)	165	8.5	9.5	10.1	26.5	65.5	.1	79.2	3.3
Oysters, cnd - 3 oz (85.2gm)	81	9	5.2	2.3	31.8	47.8	0	98.8	5.3
Oysters, smoked - 3 oz (85.2gm)	91	11.6	4.7	2.5	33.3	69	0	128.3	6.9
Perch, fillet, brld/bkd - 3 oz (85.2gm)	113	19.4	.3	3.4	23.2	54.6	0	60.5	3.9
Perch fillet, batter-frd - 3 oz (85.2gm)	154	16	5.9	7	25.1	57.3	.2	24.1	1.8
Perch, breaded, frd - 3 oz (85.2gm)	221	19.2	11.3	10.6	26.1	87.8	.2	33.8	2
Pike, bkd/brld - 3 oz (85.2gm)	110	18.2	.3	3.6	19.2	54.6	0	151.5	1.5
Pike, fillet, breaded, frd - 3 oz (85.2gm)	183	16.6	6.7	9.6	24.7	69.5	.1	98.6	0
Pompano, bkd/brld - 3 oz (85.2gm)	218	20.5	.5	14.4	33.5	59.8	0	85.6	4.6
Pompano, floured/breaded, frd - 3 oz (85.2gm)	271	18.4	10.3	16.8	31.9	84.3	.2	34.9	2

Thiamin (mg)	Riboflavin (mg)	Niacin (mg)	Vitamin B₆ (mg)	Vitamin B₁₂ (mcg)	Folacin (mcg)	Sodium (mg)	Calcium (mg)	Iron (mg)	Potassium (mg)	Zinc (mg)	Magnesium (mg)
.1	.1	1.3	.2	.3	14.4	178.5	55.2	.7	153	1.9	17
0	.1	.9	.1	3.4	4.2	1246	18.5	.4	145.6	.3	16.8
.1	.3	8.1	.6	6.7	13.9	335.9	7.6	1	422.2	.6	28.8
0	.2	2.8	.4	5.9	8.5	238	56.1	1.2	255	.6	25.5
0	.3	8.9	.3	7.6	7.1	607.1	263.1	2.2	425	.5	30.4
.1	.1	5.6	.4	.1	15.4	514.5	32.5	2	324.6	.7	36.2
.1	.1	5	.3	.2	19.2	473.8	46.9	2.2	277.8	.7	34.1
.2	.2	1.2	0	17.7	11.9	569.1	89.8	3	281.4	3.9	23.5
.3	.4	2.8	.2	32.4	42.3	1122.3	167.4	5.9	676.8	7.3	46.8
.1	.1	1.8	.2	.9	8.5	340.9	22.5	1	272.4	.5	30.8
.1	.1	1.7	.2	.8	8.4	107.9	34.3	1.1	216.6	.5	24.5
.1	.1	1.9	.2	.8	11.7	328.1	32.6	1.3	240.2	.5	29.1
0	.1	1.9	.3	15.2	17.4	335.4	41.3	1.1	327.8	1.6	25.9
0	.1	2.6	.5	27.5	22	107.2	42	1	525.6	2.5	36.2
.1	.2	2.1	0	15.3	8.5	62	79.9	4.7	102.8	63.5	27.2
.1	.2	2.6	0	14	10.7	372.3	99.9	5.4	126.8	68.4	33.5
.1	.2	2.3	0	11.3	13.5	335.1	83.5	4.8	116.9	54.5	28.8
.1	.2	2.3	0	12.5	11.6	323.2	92.7	4.9	119.9	60.9	30.7
0	.2	.8	0	15.9	8.5	403.7	29.7	5.9	74.4	74.4	31.9
.2	.2	3.4	.1	24.8	13.8	100.7	129.7	7.6	167	103.1	44.2
.1	.2	1.6	.1	1.8	13.9	329.9	14.6	.6	233.7	1.2	18.9
.1	.2	1.6	.1	1.5	12.7	103.4	29.5	.8	194.9	1	16.3
.1	.2	2.1	.1	1.6	19.9	501.7	37.5	1.3	228.6	1.2	23
.2	.2	2.2	.1	1.8	13.9	313.1	15.6	.4	322	1.1	18.9
.2	.2	2.3	.1	1.5	16.1	305.3	26.9	.8	280.9	1	19.4
.4	.2	3.9	.2	1.1	15.2	480.4	53.3	1.2	215.9	.5	34.2
.3	.3	3.6	.2	.9	19.2	445.3	62.8	1.6	193.2	.6	32.4

	Calories (kcal)	Protein (gm)	Carbohydrates (gm)	Fat (gm)	Percent Saturated Fat	Cholesterol (mg)	Dietary Fiber (gm)	Vitamin A (RE)	Vitamin C (mg)
Porgy, bkd/brld - 3 oz (85.2gm)	172	21.5	.6	8.7	21.3	62.1	0	96.5	3
Porgy, breaded, frd - 3 oz (85.2gm)	246	18.9	11.9	13.2	25.1	89.9	.2	34.4	0
Roe, cod, shad - ½ oz (14.2gm)	22	3.4	.3	.8	18.7	49.3	0	9.9	1.8
Roe, herring - 1 tbsp (14gm)	18	3.4	.2	.3	17.4	50.4	0	3.8	1.7
Roe, sturgeon (caviar) - 1 tbsp (16gm)	46	4.9	.7	2.5	30	54.7	0	96	0
Salmon, bkd/brld - 3 oz (85.2gm)	149	20.5	.4	6.8	19.2	35.7	0	100.2	1.8
Salmon, stmd/pchd - 3 oz (85.2gm)	126	21.2	0	3.9	18.9	37.2	0	62.3	0
Salmon, cnd - 3 oz (85.2gm)	130	17.4	0	6.1	16	29.9	0	33.5	0
Salmon, dried - 1 oz (28.4gm)	42	7	0	1.3	18.9	12.2	0	20.5	0
Salmon, smoked - 3 oz (85.2gm)	150	18.4	0	7.9	24.7	32.3	0	7.6	0
Sardines, cnd, mustard sauce - 2 sardines (22.7gm)	47	4.5	.4	2.9	32.5	26.4	0	2.2	0
Sardines, cnd in oil - 3 oz (85.2gm)	172	20.4	0	9.4	18.9	102	0	56.1	0
Sardines, cnd, tom sauce - 2 sardines (22.7gm)	47	4.5	.4	2.9	29.5	26.4	0	13.4	0
Scallops, stmd/bld - 3 oz (85.2gm)	85	12.6	2.7	2.7	18.4	28.7	0	49.9	0
Scallops, brld/bkd - 3 oz (85.2gm)	106	15.7	3.4	3.4	18.4	35.8	0	63.9	0
Scallops, breaded, frd - 3 oz (85.2gm)	177	14.2	9.4	9.4	24.6	53.3	.1	30.6	0
Sea bass, bkd/brld - 3 oz (85.2gm)	117	19.8	.4	3.5	19.7	56.2	0	65.1	1.8
Sea bass, floured/breaded, frd - 3 oz (85.2gm)	176	18.3	8	7.4	25.3	76	.2	28.2	0
Shrimp, stmd/bld - 3 oz (85.2gm)	102	20.2	1.7	.9	-	167.8	0	12.1	0
Shrimp, brld - 3 oz (85.2gm)	116	18.6	1.6	3.4	18.8	153.6	0	46.4	0
Shrimp, floured/breaded, frd - 3 oz (85.2gm)	199	15.9	10.7	9.8	25	167.6	.2	25	0
Shrimp, cnd - 3 oz (85.2gm)	99	20.6	.6	.9	-	127.5	0	15.3	0
Shrimp, dried - 1 oz (28.4gm)	82	17.2	.5	.8	-	106.3	0	12.8	0
Smelts, brld/bkd - 3 oz (85.2gm)	144	20.3	.5	6.4	20.3	59.8	0	69.8	2.5
Smelts, breaded, frd - 3 oz (85.2gm)	214	18.2	10.3	10.6	24.9	84.3	.2	22.1	0
Snails (escargots) - 1 oz (28.4gm)	37	5.5	.7	1.2	-	19	0	16.6	0
Squid, raw - 3 oz (85.2gm)	67	13.5	.6	.7	-	119	0	12.7	0
Squid, bld - 3 oz (85.2gm)	82	16	1.5	.9	-	175.8	0	12.5	0

Thiamin (mg)	Riboflavin (mg)	Niacin (mg)	Vitamin B$_6$ (mg)	Vitamin B$_{12}$ (mcg)	Folacin (mcg)	Sodium (mg)	Calcium (mg)	Iron (mg)	Potassium (mg)	Zinc (mg)	Magnesium (mg)
.1	.1	2	.3	2	16.2	586	66.2	.7	334.7	.8	58.4
.1	.1	2.3	.2	1.6	20.3	520.2	74	1.3	278	.8	50.2
0	.1	.2	0	1.3	9.4	58.3	4.6	.1	19.1	.1	2.9
0	.1	.2	0	1.1	10.6	10.2	4.2	.1	18.5	.1	2.8
0	.2	.4	.1	3.2	8	352	44.2	1.9	28.8	.2	6.4
.1	.1	7.4	.2	2.3	24.5	379.5	132.9	.8	319	.5	31.8
.1	.1	7.6	.2	2.4	24.9	68	134.9	.8	325.1	.5	31.9
0	.1	6.5	.3	5.9	17	376.2	190.7	.8	299.7	.8	25.5
0	0	2.5	.1	.8	8.2	22.4	44.4	.3	107.1	.2	10.5
0	.2	2.8	.6	5.9	17	2677.5	11.9	1.2	357	.3	11.9
0	0	1.3	0	1.7	3.8	182.4	72.7	1.2	62.4	.1	2.4
0	.3	6.3	.1	6.8	6.8	699.5	371.4	2.5	501.5	2.5	25.5
0	.1	1.3	.1	1.4	5.8	96	107.8	1	76.8	.6	14.6
.1	0	1	.1	.9	9.9	425.7	23.3	1.3	293.1	1.6	33.4
.1	.1	1.3	.1	1	14	530.8	29.2	1.8	407	2	41.8
.1	.1	1.4	.1	.9	15.5	471.2	37.5	1.9	343.4	1.8	37.2
.2	.1	2.9	.3	1.8	14.3	376.4	26.7	.7	317	.3	42
.2	.1	3	.2	1.6	17.5	368.3	38.9	1.1	281.3	.4	39.3
0	0	2.7	.1	.6	9.2	133.1	70.5	1.6	172.2	1.7	39.9
0	0	3.1	.1	.8	9.6	414.3	67.1	1.6	226.7	1.5	43.8
.1	.1	2.8	.1	.7	14.1	383.8	61	1.9	188.9	1.3	36.1
0	0	1.5	0	.3	12.7	119	97.7	1.4	103.7	.2	42.5
0	0	1.3	0	.2	10.6	99.2	81.5	1.2	86.5	.1	35.4
0	.1	1.5	.1	2.9	4.7	505.4	15.3	.4	424.3	1.1	34.2
0	.2	1.8	.1	2.4	10.9	464.6	33.5	1	353.2	1	32.4
0	0	.5	0	.1	1.8	31.4	3.6	1.2	130.4	.3	85.2
0	.1	2	.3	17	11.9	62.9	17.4	.5	308.5	2.4	21.2
0	.1	2.3	.3	14.7	8.8	292.2	13.2	.5	283.7	3.9	22.7

	Calories (kcal)	Protein (gm)	Carbohydrates (gm)	Fat (gm)	Percent Saturated Fat	Cholesterol (mg)	Dietary Fiber (gm)	Vitamin A (RE)	Vitamin C (mg)
Squid, frd - 3 oz (85.2gm)	159	15.6	8.2	6.7	25.2	177.2	.1	19	0
Squid, dried - 1.5 oz (42.6gm)	130	25.3	2.3	1.4	-	278.1	0	20.9	0
Squid, pickled - 1 oz (28.4gm)	23	4.4	.8	.2	-	48.5	0	3.6	0
Sturgeon, stmd - 3 oz (85.2gm)	99	19.1	0	2	23.7	58.1	0	125.5	0
Sturgeon, smoked - 3 oz (85.2gm)	135	26.1	0	2.7	23.7	79.2	0	171	0
Swordfish, steak, brld - 3 oz (85.2gm)	148	19.7	.4	7.1	22.7	56.2	0	475.9	1.8
Swordfish, fillet, breaded, frd - 3 oz (85.2gm)	207	17.3	6.7	11.9	25.3	69.5	.1	334.9	0
Terrapin (turtle), baked - ½ c (80gm)	107	19.1	0	2.9	20.7	48.2	0	58.7	0
Trout, brld - 3 oz (85.2gm)	217	21.4	.3	13.8	22.2	54.6	0	84.3	1.5
Trout, breaded, bkd - 3 oz (85.2gm)	138	19.1	7.4	2.9	24.2	71.1	.1	31	2.2
Trout, smoked - 3 oz (85.2gm)	153	29.1	0	3.2	21.9	74.3	0	40.9	3.9
Tuna, raw - 3 oz (85.2gm)	113	21	0	2.5	26.7	47.6	0	22.9	0
Tuna, fresh, brld - 3 oz (85.2gm)	155	24.5	.3	5.5	23.5	55.6	0	57.8	1.5
Tuna, cnd in oil, drnd - 3 oz (85.2gm)	167	24.5	0	7	32.9	55.2	0	20.4	0
Tuna, cnd in water, drnd - 3 oz (85.2gm)	135	29.7	0	.8	-	66.9	0	28.7	0
Whiting, brld/bkd - 3 oz (85.2gm)	97	16.4	.3	3.8	20.8	54.6	0	47.1	1.5
Whiting, floured/breaded, frd - 3 oz (85.2gm)	171	15.1	6.7	9.7	25.1	69.5	.1	17.8	0
Yellowtail, raw - 3.5 oz (99.4gm)	138	21	0	5.4	37	55	-	33	0

SOUPS

Note: All soups are prepared with water unless noted, and according to package directions.

	Calories (kcal)	Protein (gm)	Carbohydrates (gm)	Fat (gm)	Percent Saturated Fat	Cholesterol (mg)	Dietary Fiber (gm)	Vitamin A (RE)	Vitamin C (mg)
Bean w/bacon, cnd, prep - 1 c (253gm)	173	7.9	22.8	5.9	25.8	3	-	89	1.6
Bean w/frnkfrtr, cnd, prep - 1 c (250gm)	187	10	22	7	30.4	13	-	88	.9
Bean w/ham, cnd, chky, r-t-s- 1 c (8 fl oz) (243gm)	231	12.6	27.1	8.5	39.1	22	-	396	4.4
Beef broth/bouillon, pwdr - 1 c (3gm)	19	1.3	1.9	.7	-	1	-	1	0
Beef broth/bouillon, pwdr, prep - 1 c (244gm)	19	1.3	1.9	.7	-	1	-	2	0
Beef broth/bouillon, cnd, r-t-s - 1 c (240gm)	16	2.7	.1	.5	-	0	-	0	0

Thiamin (mg)	Riboflavin (mg)	Niacin (mg)	Vitamin B$_6$ (mg)	Vitamin B$_{12}$ (mcg)	Folacin (mcg)	Sodium (mg)	Calcium (mg)	Iron (mg)	Potassium (mg)	Zinc (mg)	Magnesium (mg)
0	.1	2.9	.3	15.2	14.4	335.4	27	.9	327.8	3.5	25.9
0	.2	4.6	.5	29.4	17.6	294	19.7	.8	560.9	6.2	39.2
0	0	.8	.1	5.1	2.7	399.6	5.7	.1	98.8	1.1	9.5
.1	.1	8.3	.2	2.2	14.3	291.2	12.6	.6	379.4	.7	30.3
.1	.1	11.9	.3	3	20.5	412.5	20.9	1	646.3	1.2	51.4
0	.1	7.8	.5	.9	14.3	369.3	22.6	.9	465	.6	31.8
.1	.1	6.9	.4	.8	16.1	307.7	31.8	1.2	386.5	.6	29.1
.1	.1	1	.1	.9	12.3	320.5	116.1	1.4	223	1	20.1
.1	.2	8.3	.2	3	15.3	342.8	28.5	.8	295.2	1.3	20.8
.1	.1	3.4	.2	2.5	17.7	332.3	28.7	1	308.9	.6	23.1
.1	.1	5	.3	4.3	21.6	365	20.1	.8	483.5	.8	31.2
0	.1	11.3	.8	2.5	12.7	31.4	13.6	1.1	237.1	.8	25.5
0	.1	12.5	.8	2.7	13.9	299.2	18.6	1.3	282.3	1	30.8
0	.1	10.1	.4	1.9	12.7	680	6.8	1.6	255.8	.3	29.7
0	.1	14.4	.4	2.3	15.9	929.7	17	1.7	296.4	.4	36.1
.1	.2	2.8	.1	.8	13	335.9	43.4	.7	365.6	.3	30.8
.1	.2	2.8	.1	.7	15.3	324	49.7	1	316.6	.4	29.1
.1	.1	1.9	-	-	-	74	23	.6	420	-	-

Source: USDA Food Consumption Survey

.1	0	.6	0	.1	31.9	952	81	2.1	403	1	44
.1	.1	1.	.1	.1	30	1092	86	2.3	477	1.2	49
.1	.1	1.7	.1	.1	29.2	972	79	3.2	425	1.1	46
0	0	.4	0	.1	2.6	1359	5	.1	36	0	4
0	0	.4	0	0	2.4	1358	5	.1	36	0	4
0	.1	1.9	0	.2	4.8	782	15	.4	130	0	5

	Calories (kcal)	Protein (gm)	Carbohydrates (gm)	Fat (gm)	Percent Saturated Fat	Cholesterol (mg)	Dietary Fiber (gm)	Vitamin A (RE)	Vitamin C (mg)
Beef broth/bouillon/consomme, prep - 1 c (241gm)	29	5.4	1.8	0	-	0	-	0	1
Beef broth, (bouillon cubes) prep - 1 c (241.3gm)	8	.9	.8	.2	-	0	-	0	0
Beef mushroom, cnd, cdsd - 1 c (251gm)	153	11.6	13.1	6	49.8	13	-	0	0
Beef mushroom, cnd, prep - 1 c (244gm)	73	5.8	6.3	3	49.5	7	-	0	4.7
Beef ndl, cnd, prep - 1 c (244gm)	84	4.8	9	3.1	37.3	5	-	63	.3
Beef ndl, mix, prep - 1 c (251gm)	41	2.2	6	.8	-	3	-	0	.5
Beef, cnd, chky, r-t-s - 1 c (240gm)	170	11.7	19.6	5.1	49.4	14	-	262	7
Black bean, cnd, cdsd - 1 c (257gm)	235	12.4	39.6	3.4	25.7	0	-	116	.5
Black bean, cnd, prep - 1 c (247gm)	117	5.6	19.8	1.5	-	0	-	49	.7
Cauliflower, mix, prep - 1 c (256.1gm)	68	2.9	10.7	1.7	-	0	-	1	2.6
Cheese, cnd, cdsd - 1 c (257gm)	311	10.9	21.1	20.9	63.6	59	-	218	0
Cheese, cnd, prep w/milk - 1 c (251gm)	230	9.4	16.2	14.6	62.6	48	-	148	1.2
Cheese, cnd, prep w/water - 1 c (247gm)	155	5.4	10.5	10.5	63.6	30	-	109	0
Chicken broth cubes, prep - 1 c (243gm)	13	.9	1.5	.3	-	1	-	5	0
Chicken broth/bouillon, mix, prep - 1 c (244gm)	21	1.3	1.4	1.1	-	1	-	12	.1
Chicken broth, cnd, cdsd - 1 c (251gm)	78	11.1	1.9	2.6	29.9	3	-	0	0
Chicken broth, cnd, prep - 1 c (244gm)	39	4.9	.9	1.4	-	1	-	0	0
Chicken gumbo, cnd, cdsd - 1 c (251gm)	113	5.3	16.7	2.9	22.7	8	-	28	10
Chicken gumbo, cnd, prep - 1 c (244gm)	56	2.6	8.4	1.4	-	5	-	15	4.9
Chicken mushroom, cnd, cdsd - 1 c (251gm)	274	8.8	19.1	18.3	26.3	20	-	226	0
Chicken mushroom, cnd, prep - 1 c (244gm)	132	4.4	9.3	9.2	26.2	10	-	112	0
Chicken ndl mix - 1 pkt (74.4gm)	257	14.3	36	5.7	22.5	10	-	31	1.5
Chicken ndl, cnd, chky, r-t-s - 1 c (240gm)	175	12.7	17	6	23.2	18	-	122	0
Chicken ndl, cnd, cdsd - 1 c (246gm)	150	7.9	18.7	4.6	26.3	12	-	130	.1
Chicken, ndl, cnd, prep - 1 c (241gm)	75	4.1	9.3	2.5	-	7	-	72	.2

Thiamin (mg)	Riboflavin (mg)	Niacin (mg)	Vitamin B6 (mg)	Vitamin B12 (mcg)	Folacin (mcg)	Sodium (mg)	Calcium (mg)	Iron (mg)	Potassium (mg)	Zinc (mg)	Magnesium (mg)
0	0	.7	0	0	3	637	8	.5	153	.4	0
0	0	.2	0	0	2.4	1158	2	.1	20	0	2
.1	.2	2.3	.1	.4	17.6	1940	10	1.8	316	2.8	18
0	.1	1	0	.2	9.8	942	5	.9	154	1.5	10
.1	.1	1.1	0	.2	4.4	952	15	1.1	99	1.5	6
.1	.1	.7	0	0	1.6	1041	5	.3	81	.1	9
.1	.2	2.7	.1	.6	13.4	866	32	2.3	336	2.6	5
.1	.1	1.1	.2	0	51.4	2493	90	3.9	643	2.8	85
.1	.1	.5	.1	0	24.7	1198	45	2.1	274	1.4	42
.1	.1	.5	0	.2	2.6	843	9	.5	105	.3	3
0	.3	.8	.1	0	7.7	1920	284	1.5	308	1.3	8
.1	.3	.5	.1	.4	10	1020	288	.8	340	.7	20
0	.1	.4	0	0	4.9	959	142	.8	154	.6	4
0	0	.3	0	0	2.4	792	12	.1	24	0	4
0	0	.2	0	0	2.4	1484	15	.1	25	0	4
0	.1	5.6	.1	.5	10	1571	14	1	427	.5	5
0	.1	3.3	0	.3	4.9	776	10	.5	210	.2	3
.5	.8	1.3	.1	.1	12.6	1910	49	1.8	151	.8	8
0	0	.7	.1	0	4.9	955	24	.9	75	.4	4
.1	.2	3.3	.1	.1	5	1940	58	1.8	316	2	18
0	.1	1.6	0	.1	.2	942	29	.9	154	1	10
.3	.3	4.3	.4	0	6.8	6243	154	2.4	153	1	34
.1	.2	4.3	0	.3	4.8	850	24	1.4	108	1	10
.1	.1	3	.1	.3	4.3	1863	27	1.5	111	.6	10
.1	.1	1.4	0	.1	2.2	1106	17	.8	55	.4	5

	Calories (kcal)	Protein (gm)	Carbohydrates (gm)	Fat (gm)	Percent Saturated Fat	Cholesterol (mg)	Dietary Fiber (gm)	Vitamin A (RE)	Vitamin C (mg)
Chicken ndl, mix, prep - 1 c (252.3gm)	53	2.9	7.4	1.2	-	3	-	5	.3
Chicken ndl, w/mtbls, cnd, chky, r-t-s - 1 c (248gm)	99	8.1	8.4	3.6	30	10	-	233	7.8
Chicken rice, cnd, chky, r-t-s - 1 c (240gm)	127	12.3	13	3.2	29.8	12	-	586	3.8
Chicken rice, mix, prep - 1 c (252.8gm)	60	2.4	9.3	1.4	-	3	-	0	0
Chicken veg, cnd, chky, r-t-s - 1 c (240gm)	167	12.3	18.9	4.8	29.8	17	-	600	5.5
Chicken veg, cnd, cdsd - 1 c (246gm)	149	7.2	17.2	5.7	29.8	17	-	534	2.1
Chicken veg, cnd, prep - 1 c (241gm)	74	3.6	8.6	2.8	29.9	10	-	265	1
Chicken veg, mix, prep - 1 c (250.7gm)	49	2.7	7.8	.8	-	3	-	3	1.2
Chicken w/dplgs, cnd, cdsd - 1 c (246gm)	195	11.3	12.1	11.1	23.7	66	-	103	0
Chicken w/dplgs, cnd, prep - 1 c (241gm)	97	5.6	6	5.5	23.7	34	-	53	0
Chicken w/rice, cnd, cdsd - 1 c (246gm)	120	7.1	14.4	3.8	23.7	12	-	133	.3
Chicken w/rice, cnd, prep - 1 c (241gm)	60	3.5	7.1	1.9	-	7	-	65	.1
Chicken, cnd, chky, r-t-s - 1 c (251gm)	178	12.7	17.3	6.6	29.9	30	-	131	1.3
Chili beef, cnd, cdsd - 1 c (263gm)	339	13.4	42.9	13.2	49.8	26	-	302	8.1
Chili beef, cnd, prep - 1 c (250gm)	169	6.7	21.5	6.6	50.5	13	-	150	4.1
Clam chowder, cnd, New Eng, prep w/milk - 1 c (248gm)	163	9.5	16.6	6.6	44.7	22	-	40	3.5
Clam chowder, cnd, New Eng, prep - 1 c (244gm)	95	4.8	12.4	2.9	14.2	5	-	0	2
Clam chowder, Mnhtn, cnd, chky, r-t-s - 1 c (240gm)	133	7.3	18.8	3.4	62.1	14	-	329	12.2
Clam chowder, Mnhtn, cnd, w/tom, prep - 1 c (244gm)	77	4.2	12.2	2.3	-	2	-	93	3.2
Consomme, mix, prep - 1 c (249gm)	17	2.2	2.1	0	-	0	-	2	0
Crab, cnd, r-t-s - 1 c (244gm)	76	5.5	10.3	1.5	25.2	10	-	51	0
Cream of asparagus, cnd, cdsd - 1 c (251gm)	173	4.6	21.4	8.2	-	10	-	90	5.5
Cream of asparagus, cnd, prep w/milk - 1 c (248gm)	161	6.3	16.4	8.2	40.7	22	-	84	3.9
Cream of asparagus, cnd, prep - 1 c (244gm)	87	2.3	10.7	4.1	25.4	5	-	44	2.8
Cream of asparagus, dehy, prep - 1 c (250.8gm)	58	2.2	8.9	1.7	-	0	-	28	.8

Thiamin (mg)	Riboflavin (mg)	Niacin (mg)	Vitamin B_6 (mg)	Vitamin B_{12} (mcg)	Folacin (mcg)	Sodium (mg)	Calcium (mg)	Iron (mg)	Potassium (mg)	Zinc (mg)	Magnesium (mg)
.1	.1	.9	0	0	1.4	1284	32	.5	31	.2	7
.1	.1	2.5	.1	.3	5	1039	30	1.7	154	.5	10
0	.1	4.1	0	.3	3.8	888	35	1.9	108	1	10
0	0	.4	0	.1	.5	980	8	0	10	.1	0
0	.2	3.3	.1	.2	12	1068	25	1.5	367	2.2	10
.1	.1	2.5	.1	.3	9.8	1896	35	1.8	309	.7	12
0	.1	1.2	0	.1	4.8	944	18	.9	154	.4	6
.1	0	.7	.1	.1	2.5	808	15	.6	68	.2	21
0	.1	3.5	.1	.3	4.9	1728	29	1.3	234	.7	7
0	.1	1.8	0	.2	2.4	861	15	.6	116	.4	4
0	0	2.3	0	.3	2.1	1635	34	1.5	202	.5	0
0	0	1.1	0	.1	1.1	814	17	.8	100	.3	1
.1	.2	4.4	.1	.3	4.6	887	24	1.7	176	1	8
.1	.2	2.1	.3	.6	36.8	2071	87	4.3	1051	2.8	61
.1	.1	1.1	.2	.3	17.5	1035	43	2.1	525	1.4	30
.1	.2	1	.1	10.3	9.7	992	187	1.5	300	.8	23
0	0	1	.1	8	3.6	915	44	1.5	146	.8	8
.1	.1	1.8	.3	7.9	9.3	1000	67	2.6	384	1.7	19
.1	0	1.3	.1	2.2	9.5	1808	34	1.9	261	.9	10
0	0	.6	0	.1	4	3299	7	.1	57	0	7
.2	.1	1.3	.1	.2	14.6	1234	65	1.2	326	1.5	15
.1	.2	1.6	0	.1	47.7	1963	58	1.6	346	1.8	8
.1	.3	.9	.1	.5	29.8	1041	175	.9	359	.9	20
.1	.1	.8	0	.1	22	981	29	.8	173	.9	4
.1	.1	.5	0	0	7.5	800	23	.5	133	.7	3

	Calories (kcal)	Protein (gm)	Carbohydrates (gm)	Fat (gm)	Percent Saturated Fat	Cholesterol (mg)	Dietary Fiber (gm)	Vitamin A (RE)	Vitamin C (mg)
Cream of celery, cnd, cdsd - 1 c (251gm)	180	3.3	17.6	11.2	25.1	28	-	60	.4
Cream of celery, cnd, prep w/milk - 1 c (248gm)	165	5.7	14.5	9.7	40.8	32	-	67	1.4
Cream of celery, cnd, prep - 1 c (244gm)	90	1.7	8.8	5.6	25	15	-	32	.2
Cream of celery, mix, prep - 1 c (254gm)	63	2.6	9.8	1.6	-	1	-	28	.2
Cream of chick, cnd, cdsd - 1 c (251gm)	233	6.9	18.5	14.7	28.2	20	-	113	.3
Cream of chicken, cnd, prep - 1 c (244gm)	116	3.4	9.3	7.4	28.3	10	-	56	.2
Cream of chicken, mix, prep - 1 c (261.1gm)	107	1.8	13.4	5.3	63.6	3	-	123	.5
Cream of mushroom, cnd, cdsd - 1 c (251gm)	257	4	18.6	19	27.1	3	-	0	2.4
Cream of mushroom, cnd, prep w/milk - 1 c (248gm)	203	6.1	15	13.6	37.7	20	-	37	2.3
Cream of mushroom, cnd, prep - 1 c (244gm)	129	2.3	9.3	9	27.2	2	-	0	1
Cream of onion, cnd, cdsd - 1 c (251gm)	221	5.5	26.1	10.5	27.9	30	-	60	2.5
Cream of onion, cnd, prep w/milk - 1 c (248gm)	186	6.8	18.4	9.4	43.1	32	-	67	2.4
Cream of onion, cnd, prep - 1 c (244gm)	107	2.8	12.7	5.3	27.9	15	-	29	1.3
Cream of potato, cnd, cdsd - 1 c (251gm)	147	3.5	22.9	4.7	51.5	13	-	58	0
Cream of potato, cnd, prep w/milk - 1 c (248gm)	148	5.8	17.2	6.4	58.3	22	-	67	1.2
Cream of potato, cnd, prep - 1 c (244gm)	73	1.7	11.5	2.4	51.7	5	-	29	0
Cream of shrimp, cnd, cdsd - 1 c (251gm)	180	5.6	16.4	10.4	62.3	33	-	33	0
Cream of shrimp, cnd, prep w/milk - 1 c (248gm)	165	6.8	13.9	9.3	62.3	35	-	55	1.2
Cream of shrimp, cnd, prep - 1 c (244gm)	90	2.8	8.2	5.2	62.2	17	-	15	0
Cream of veg, mix, prep - 1 c (260.1gm)	105	1.9	12.3	5.7	25.1	0	-	3	3.9
Escarole, cnd, r-t-s - 1 c (248gm)	27	1.5	1.8	1.8	-	2	-	218	4.5
Gazpacho, cnd, r-t-s - 1 c (244gm)	57	8.7	.8	2.2	12.9	0	-	20	3.1
Leek, mix, prep - 1 c (253.9gm)	71	2.1	11.4	2.1	49.5	3	-	0	2.5
Lentil w/ham, cnd, r-t-s - 1 c (248gm)	139	9.3	20.2	2.8	40.3	7	-	35	4.2
Minestrone, cnd, cdsd - 1 c (246gm)	167	8.6	22.6	5	21.6	2	-	470	2.2

Thiamin (mg)	Riboflavin (mg)	Niacin (mg)	Vitamin B_6 (mg)	Vitamin B_{12} (mcg)	Folacin (mcg)	Sodium (mg)	Calcium (mg)	Iron (mg)	Potassium (mg)	Zinc (mg)	Magnesium (mg)
.1	.1	.7	0	.1	4.7	1899	80	1.3	246	.3	13
.1	.2	.4	.1	.5	8.5	1010	186	.7	309	.2	22
0	0	.3	0	.2	2.4	949	40	.6	123	.2	6
0	.1	.3	0	.1	2	839	36	.5	109	.1	5
.1	.1	1.6	0	.2	3.2	1973	68	1.2	174	1.3	5
0	.1	.8	0	.1	1.6	986	34	.6	87	.6	3
.1	.2	2.6	.1	.3	5.2	1184	76	.3	215	1.6	5
.1	.2	1.6	0	.3	7.5	2032	64	1.1	167	1.2	9
.1	.3	.9	.1	.5	9.9	1076	178	.6	270	.6	20
0	.1	.7	0	.1	4.9	1032	46	.5	100	.6	4
.1	.2	1	.1	.1	14.3	1908	68	1.3	246	.3	13
.1	.3	.6	.1	.5	12.4	1004	180	.7	310	.6	22
.1	.1	.5	0	.1	6.8	927	34	.6	120	.1	5
.1	.1	1.1	.1	.1	6.1	2000	40	.9	274	1.3	3
.1	.2	.6	.1	.5	9.2	1060	166	.5	323	.7	17
0	0	.5	0	.1	3	1000	20	.5	137	.6	1
0	.1	.9	.1	1.2	7.5	1953	36	1.1	118	1.5	18
.1	.2	.5	.4	1	9.9	1036	164	.6	248	.8	22
0	0	.4	0	.6	3.7	976	18	.5	59	.8	10
1.2	.1	.5	0	.1	7.8	1171	31	.5	96	.3	10
.1	.1	2.3	.2	.5	34.7	3865	32	.7	265	2.2	5
0	0	.9	.1	0	9.8	1183	24	1	224	.2	7
.1	0	.3	0	0	7.6	965	30	.5	89	.2	10
.2	.1	1.4	.2	.3	49.6	1319	42	2.6	357	.7	22
.1	.1	1.9	.2	0	32.2	1830	69	1.9	627	1.5	15

	Calories (kcal)	Protein (gm)	Carbohydrates (gm)	Fat (gm)	Percent Saturated Fat	Cholesterol (mg)	Dietary Fiber (gm)	Vitamin A (RE)	Vitamin C (mg)
Minestrone, cnd, prep - 1 c (241gm)	83	4.3	11.2	2.5	21.9	2	-	234	1.1
Minestrone, cnd, chky, r-t-s - 1 c (240gm)	127	5.1	20.7	2.8	52.8	5	-	434	4.8
Minestrone, mix, prep - 1 c (253.9gm)	79	4.4	11.9	1.7	47.4	3	-	30	1
Mushroom barley, cnd, cdsd - 1 c (251gm)	153	3.8	24.1	4.5	19.7	0	-	40	0
Mushroom barley, cnd, prep - 1 c (244gm)	73	1.9	11.7	2.3	19.5	0	-	20	0
Mushroom w/beef stock, cnd, cdsd - 1 c (251gm)	171	6.3	18.6	8.1	38.6	15	-	251	2
Mushroom w/beef stock, cnd, prep - 1 c (244gm)	85	3.1	9.3	4	38.5	7	-	124	1
Mushroom, mix, prep - 1 c (253gm)	96	2.2	11.1	4.9	16.7	0	-	0	1
Onion, mix, dry - 1 pkt (39gm)	115	4.5	20.9	2.3	-	2	-	1	.9
Onion, cnd, cdsd - 1 c (246gm)	114	7.5	16.4	3.5	14.9	0	-	0	2.5
Onion, cnd, prep - 1 c (241gm)	57	3.8	8.2	1.7	-	0	-	0	1.2
Onion, mix, prep - 1 c (246gm)	28	1.1	5.1	.6	22.8	0	-	0	.2
Oxtail, mix, prep - 1 c (253.1gm)	71	2.8	9	2.6	49.6	3	-	0	0
Oyster stew, cnd, cdsd - 1 c (246gm)	119	4.2	8.2	7.7	65.3	27	-	15	6.3
Oyster stew, cnd, prep w/milk - 1 c (245gm)	134	6.1	9.8	7.9	63.7	32	-	44	4.4
Oyster stew, cnd, prep - 1 c (241gm)	59	2.1	4.1	3.8	65.3	14	-	7	3.1
Pea, green, cnd, cdsd - 1 c (263gm)	328	17.2	53.1	5.9	48	0	-	39	3.4
Pea, green, cnd, prep w/milk - 1 c (254gm)	239	12.6	32.2	7	56.9	18	-	58	2.9
Pea, green, cnd, prep - 1 c (250gm)	164	8.6	26.5	2.9	48	0	-	20	1.7
Pea, green, mix, dry - 1 pkt (113gm)	402	23.2	68.6	4.8	36.4	1	-	15	1.1
Pea, green, mix, prep - 1 c (271gm)	133	7.7	22.7	1.6	-	3	-	5	0
Pea split, w/ham, cnd, chky, r-t-s - 1 c (240gm)	184	11.1	26.8	4	39.9	7	-	487	7
Pea, split w/ham, cnd, cdsd - 1 c (269gm)	379	20.6	56	8.8	40	16	-	89	2.9
Pea, split w/ham, cnd, prep - 1 c (253gm)	189	10.3	27.9	4.4	40	8	-	46	1.4
Pepperpot, cnd, cdsd - 1 c (246gm)	208	12.8	18.8	9.3	44.5	20	-	175	2.8

Thiamin (mg)	Riboflavin (mg)	Niacin (mg)	Vitamin B6 (mg)	Vitamin B12 (mcg)	Folacin (mcg)	Sodium (mg)	Calcium (mg)	Iron (mg)	Potassium (mg)	Zinc (mg)	Magnesium (mg)
.1	0	.9	.1	0	16.1	911	34	.9	312	.7	7
.1	.1	1.2	.2	0	31.2	864	61	1.8	612	1.4	14
.1	.1	1	.1	0	17.8	1026	38	1	340	.8	8
.1	.2	1.8	.4	0	12.6	1832	25	1	191	1	18
0	.1	.9	.2	0	4.9	891	13	.5	93	.5	10
.1	.2	2.4	.1	0	18.4	1940	21	1.7	316	2.8	18
0	.1	1.2	0	0	9.2	970	10	.8	158	1.4	9
.3	.1	.5	0	.3	5.1	1020	66	.5	200	.1	5
.1	.2	2	0	0	6.3	3493	55	.6	260	.2	25
.1	0	1.2	.1	0	30.6	2116	53	1.4	138	1.2	5
0	0	.6	0	0	15.2	1053	26	.7	69	.6	2
0	.1	.5	0	0	1.5	848	13	.1	63	.1	6
0	0	.8	0	.3	5.1	1210	10	.3	84	0	10
0	.1	.5	0	4.4	4.9	1968	43	2	98	20.7	10
.1	.2	.3	.1	2.6	9.8	1040	167	1	235	10.3	21
0	0	.2	0	2.2	2.4	980	22	1	49	10.3	5
.2	.1	2.5	.1	0	3.6	1977	54	3.9	381	3.4	79
.2	.3	1.3	.1	.4	7.9	1048	173	2	377	1.8	55
.1	.1	1.2	.1	0	1.8	987	27	1.9	190	1.7	39
.7	.5	4.1	.1	1.1	45.4	3687	68	3	718	1.8	140
.2	.2	1.3	0	.3	42	1220	22	1	238	.6	46
.1	.1	2.5	.2	.2	4.7	965	33	2.1	305	3.1	38
.3	.2	3	.1	.5	5.1	2018	43	4.6	800	2.6	96
.1	.1	1.5	.1	.3	2.5	1008	22	2.3	399	1.3	48
.1	.1	2.5	.1	.3	19.7	1948	47	1.8	305	2.5	10

	Calories (kcal)	Protein (gm)	Carbohydrates (gm)	Fat (gm)	Percent Saturated Fat	Cholesterol (mg)	Dietary Fiber (gm)	Vitamin A (RE)	Vitamin C (mg)
Pepperpot, cnd, prep - 1 c (241gm)	103	6.4	9.4	4.6	44.5	10	-	87	1.4
Scotch broth, cnd, cdsd - 1 c (246gm)	161	10	19	5.3	42.6	10	-	438	1.7
Scotch broth, cnd, prep - 1 c (241gm)	80	5	9.5	2.6	42.4	5	-	217	.9
Stockpot, cnd, cdsd - 1 c (257gm)	199	9.7	23	7.8	22.2	8	-	797	4.2
Stockpot, cnd, prep - 1 c (247gm)	100	4.9	11.5	3.9	22.1	5	-	398	2.1
Tomato beef w/ndl, cnd cdsd - 1 c (251gm)	280	8.9	42.3	8.6	37.1	8	-	105	0
Tomato beef w/ndl, cnd, prep - 1 c (244gm)	140	4.4	21.2	4.3	37.1	5	-	54	0
Tomato bisque, cnd, cdsd - 1 c (257gm)	247	4.5	47.5	5	21.5	10	-	144	11.8
Tomato bisque, cnd, prep w/milk - 1 c (251gm)	198	6.3	29.4	6.6	47.6	23	-	110	7
Tomato bisque, cnd, prep - 1 c (247gm)	123	2.3	23.7	2.5	21.5	5	-	72	5.9
Tomato rice, cnd, cdsd - 1 c (257gm)	240	4.2	43.9	5.4	18.9	3	-	152	29.7
Tomato rice, cnd, prep - 1 c (247gm)	120	2.1	21.9	2.7	19.1	2	-	77	14.8
Tomato veg, mix - 1 c (253gm)	55	2	10.2	.9	-	0	-	20	6
Tomato, cnd, cdsd - 1 c (251gm)	171	4.1	33.2	3.8	19	0	-	141	133
Tomato, cnd, prep w/milk - 1 c (248gm)	160	6.1	22.3	6	48.3	17	-	109	67.7
Tomato, cnd, prep - 1 c (244gm)	86	2.1	16.6	1.9	-	0	-	68	66.5
Tomato, mix, prep - 1 c (265gm)	102	2.4	19.4	2.4	45.6	1	-	82	4.6
Turkey ndl, cnd, cdsd - 1 c (251gm)	138	7.8	17.3	4	27.9	10	-	58	.3
Turkey ndl, cnd, prep - 1 c (244gm)	69	3.9	8.6	2	28.1	5	-	29	.2
Turkey, veg, cnd, cdsd - 1 c (246gm)	140	6.2	17.3	6.1	29.6	2	-	492	0
Turkey veg, cnd, prep - 1 c (241gm)	74	3.1	8.6	3	29.8	2	-	243	0
Turkey, chky, r-t-s - 1 c (236gm)	136	10.2	14.1	4.4	27.7	9	-	715	6.4
Vegetable beef, cnd, cdsd - 1 c (251gm)	158	11.2	20.4	3.8	44.9	10	-	379	4.7
Vegetable beef, mix, prep - 1 c (253.1gm)	53	2.9	8	1.1	-	1	-	23	1.3
Vegetable beef, prep - 1 c (244gm)	79	5.6	10.2	1.9	-	5	-	190	2.4

Thiamin (mg)	Riboflavin (mg)	Niacin (mg)	Vitamin B$_6$ (mg)	Vitamin B$_{12}$ (mcg)	Folacin (mcg)	Sodium (mg)	Calcium (mg)	Iron (mg)	Potassium (mg)	Zinc (mg)	Magnesium (mg)
.1	0	1.2	.1	.2	9.6	970	23	.9	152	1.2	5
0	.1	2.3	.1	.5	19.7	2032	30	1.7	320	3.2	7
0	0	1.2	.1	.3	9.6	1012	15	.8	159	1.6	4
.1	.1	2.4	.2	0	20.6	2097	43	1.7	475	2.3	8
0	.1	1.2	.1	0	9.9	1048	22	.9	238	1.2	4
.2	.2	3.7	.2	.4	15.1	1835	35	2.2	442	1.5	15
.1	.1	1.9	.1	.2	7.3	917	18	1.1	221	.8	8
.1	.1	2.3	.2	0	30.8	2097	81	1.6	835	1.2	18
.1	.3	1.3	.1	.4	21.3	1108	186	.9	604	.6	25
.1	.1	1.1	.1	0	14.8	1048	40	.8	417	.6	9
.1	.1	2.1	.2	0	28.3	1632	46	1.6	661	1	10
.1	0	1.1	.1	0	13.6	815	23	.8	330	.5	5
.1	0	.8	.1	0	10.1	1146	8	.6	103	.2	20
.2	.1	2.8	.2	0	29.5	1744	27	3.5	527	.5	15
.1	.2	1.5	.2	.4	20.9	932	159	1.8	450	.3	23
.1	.1	1.4	.1	0	14.7	872	13	1.8	263	.2	8
.1	0	.8	.1	.1	6.7	943	54	.4	295	.2	15
.1	.1	2.8	.1	.3	4.5	1632	23	1.9	151	1.2	10
.1	.1	1.4	0	.1	2.2	815	12	.9	75	.6	5
.1	.1	2	.1	.3	9.8	1818	33	1.5	352	1.2	7
0	0	1	0	.2	4.8	905	17	.8	175	.6	4
0	.1	3.6	.3	2.1	11.1	923	50	1.9	361	2.1	24
.1	.1	2.1	.2	.6	21.2	1914	33	2.2	346	3.1	12
0	0	.5	.1	.3	7.6	1002	13	.9	76	.3	23
0	0	1	.1	.3	10.6	957	17	1.1	173	1.5	6

	Calories (kcal)	Protein (gm)	Carbohydrates (gm)	Fat (gm)	Percent Saturated Fat	Cholesterol (mg)	Dietary Fiber (gm)	Vitamin A (RE)	Vitamin C (mg)
Vegetable w/beef broth, cnd, cdsd - 1 c (246gm)	162	5.9	26.3	3.8	23.2	2	-	421	4.7
Vegetable w/beef broth, cnd, prep - 1 c (241gm)	81	3	13.1	1.9	-	2	-	210	2.4
Vegetable, cnd, chky, r-t-s - 1 c (240gm)	122	3.5	19	3.7	14.9	0	-	588	6
Vegetarian veg, cnd, cdsd - 1 c (246gm)	145	4.2	24.1	3.9	14.9	0	-	603	2.9
Vegetarian veg, cnd, prep - 1 c (241 gm)	72	2.1	12	1.9	-	0	-	301	1.4

SPICES AND HERBS

	Calories (kcal)	Protein (gm)	Carbohydrates (gm)	Fat (gm)	Percent Saturated Fat	Cholesterol (mg)	Dietary Fiber (gm)	Vitamin A (RE)	Vitamin C (mg)
Allspice, ground - 1 tsp (1.9gm)	5	.1	1.4	.2	-	0	-	1	.7
Anise seed - 1 tsp (2.1gm)	7	.4	1.1	.3	-	0	-	-	-
Basil, ground - 1 tsp (1.4gm)	3	.2	.9	.1	-	0	-	13.1	.9
Bay leaf, crumbled - 1 tsp (.6gm)	2	0	.4	.1	-	0	-	3.7	.3
Caraway seed - 1 tsp (2.1gm)	7	.4	1	.3	-	0	-	.8	-
Cardamon, ground - 1 tsp (2gm)	6	.2	1.4	.1	-	0	-	0	-
Celery seed - 1 tsp (2gm)	8	.4	.8	.5	-	0	-	.1	.3
Chervil, dried - 1 tsp (.6gm)	1	.1	.3	0	-	0	-	-	-
Chili powder - 1 tsp (2.6gm)	8	.3	1.4	.4	-	0	-	90.8	1.7
Cinnamon, ground - 1 tsp (2.3gm)	6	.1	1.8	.1	-	0	-	.6	.7
Cloves, ground - 1 tsp (2.1gm)	7	.1	1.3	.4	-	0	-	1.1	1.7
Coriander leaf, dried - 1 tsp (.6gm)	2	.1	.3	0	-	0	-	-	3.4
Coriander seed - 1 tsp (1.8gm)	5	.2	1	.3	5.6	0	-	0	-
Cumin seed - 1 tsp (2.1gm)	8	.4	.9	.5	-	0	-	2.7	.2
Curry powder - 1 tsp (2gm)	6	.3	1.2	.3	-	0	-	2	.2
Dill seed - 1 tsp (2.1gm)	6	.3	1.2	.3	4.9	0	-	.1	-
Dill weed, dried - 1 tsp (1gm)	3	.2	.6	0	-	0	-	-	-
Fennel seed - 1 tsp (2gm)	7	.3	1	.3	3.4	0	-	.3	-
Fenugreek seed - 1 tsp (3.7gm)	12	.9	2.2	.2	-	0	-	-	.1
Garlic powder - 1 tsp (2.8gm)	9	.5	2	0	-	0	-	0	-
Ginger, ground - 1 tsp (1.8gm)	6	.2	1.3	.1	32.7	0	-	.3	-
Mace, ground - 1 tsp (1.7gm)	8	.1	.9	.6	29.5	0	-	1.4	-
Marjoram, dried - 1 tsp (.6gm)	2	.1	.4	0	-	0	6	4.8	.3

Thiamin (mg)	Riboflavin (mg)	Niacin (mg)	Vitamin B$_6$ (mg)	Vitamin B$_{12}$ (mcg)	Folacin (mcg)	Sodium (mg)	Calcium (mg)	Iron (mg)	Potassium (mg)	Zinc (mg)	Magnesium (mg)
.1	.1	1.9	.1	0	20.9	1626	35	1.9	386	1.6	13
.1	0	1	.1	0	9.6	810	18	1	192	.8	7
.1	.1	1.2	.2	0	16.5	1010	56	1.6	396	3.1	7
.1	.1	1.8	.1	0	21.2	1652	43	2.2	421	.9	14
.1	0	.9	.1	0	10.6	823	21	1.1	209	.5	7

Source: USDA Revised *Handbook 8*

Thiamin (mg)	Riboflavin (mg)	Niacin (mg)	Vitamin B$_6$ (mg)	Vitamin B$_{12}$ (mcg)	Folacin (mcg)	Sodium (mg)	Calcium (mg)	Iron (mg)	Potassium (mg)	Zinc (mg)	Magnesium (mg)
0	0	.1	-	0	-	1.5	12.6	.1	19.8	0	2.6
-	-	-	-	0	-	.3	13.6	.8	30.3	.1	3.6
0	0	.1	-	0	-	.5	29.6	.6	48.1	.1	5.9
0	0	0	-	0	-	.1	5	.3	3.2	0	.7
0	0	.1	-	0	-	.4	14.5	.3	28.4	.1	5.4
0	0	0	-	0	-	.4	7.7	.3	22.4	.1	4.6
-	-	-	-	0	-	3.2	35.3	.9	28	.1	8.8
-	-	-	0	0	-	.5	8.1	.2	28.4	.1	.8
0	0	.2	-	0	-	26.3	7.2	.4	49.8	.1	4.4
0	0	0	-	0	-	.6	28.3	.9	11.5	0	1.3
0	0	0	-	0	-	5.1	13.6	.2	23.1	0	5.5
0	0	.1	-	0	-	1.3	7.5	.3	26.9	-	4.2
0	0	0	-	0	0	.6	12.8	.3	22.8	.1	5.9
0	0	.1	-	0	-	3.5	19.5	1.4	37.5	.1	7.7
0	0	.1	-	0	-	1	9.6	.6	30.9	.1	5.1
0	0	.1	-	0	-	.4	31.8	.3	24.9	.1	5.4
0	0	0	0	0	-	2.2	18.6	.5	34.4	0	4.7
0	0	.1	-	0	-	1.8	23.9	.4	33.9	.1	7.7
0	0	.1	-	0	2.1	2.5	6.5	1.2	28.5	.1	7.1
0	0	0	-	0	-	.7	2.2	.1	30.8	.1	1.6
0	0	.1	-	0	-	.6	2.1	.2	24.2	.1	3.3
0	0	0	-	0	-	1.4	4.3	.2	7.9	0	2.8
0	0	0	-	0	-	.5	11.9	.5	9.1	0	2.1

	Calories (kcal)	Protein (gm)	Carbohydrates (gm)	Fat (gm)	Percent Saturated Fat	Cholesterol (mg)	Dietary Fiber (gm)	Vitamin A (RE)	Vitamin C (mg)
Mustard seed, yellow - 1 tsp (3.3gm)	15	.8	1.2	.9	-	0	-	.2	-
Nutmeg, ground - 1 tsp (2.2gm)	11	.1	1.1	.8	-	0	-	.2	-
Onion powder - 1 tsp (2.1gm)	7	.2	1.7	0	-	0	-	0	.3
Oregano, ground - 1 tsp (1.5gm)	5	.2	1	.2	-	0	-	10.4	-
Paprika - 1 tsp (2.1gm)	6	.3	1.2	.3	-	0	-	127.3	1.5
Parsley, dried - 1 tsp (.3gm)	1	.1	.2	0	-	0	-	7	.4
Pepper, black - 1 tsp (2.1gm)	5	.2	1.4	.1	-	0	-	.4	-
Pepper, red or cayenne - 1 tsp (1.8gm)	5	.2	1	.3	-	0	-	74.9	1.4
Pepper, white - 1 tsp (2.4gm)	7	.3	1.6	.1	-	0	-	0	-
Poppy seed - 1 tsp (2.8gm)	15	.5	.7	1.3	-	0	-	0	-
Poultry seasoning - 1 tsp (1.5gm)	5	.1	1	.1	-	0	-	3.9	.2
Pumpkin pie spice - 1 tsp (1.7gm)	6	.1	1.2	.2	-	0	-	.4	.4
Rosemary, dried - 1 tsp (1.2gm)	4	.1	.8	.2	-	0	-	3.8	.7
Saffron - 1 tsp (.7gm)	2	.1	.5	0	-	0	-	-	-
Sage, ground - 1 tsp (.7gm)	2	.1	.4	.1	-	0	-	4.1	.2
Savory, ground - 1 tsp (1.4gm)	4	.1	1	.1	-	0	-	7.2	-
Tarragon, ground - 1 tsp (1.6gm)	5	.4	.8	.1	-	0	-	6.7	-
Thyme, ground - 1 tsp (1.4gm)	4	.1	.9	.1	-	0	-	5.3	-
Tumeric, ground - 1 tsp (2.2gm)	8	.2	1.4	.2	-	0	-	0	.6
Sesame seed - 1 tsp (2.7gm)	16	.8	.3	1.5	-	.1	-	.2	.1

VEGETABLES

Note: Fresh vegetables are without added salt unless noted.

	Calories (kcal)	Protein (gm)	Carbohydrates (gm)	Fat (gm)	Percent Saturated Fat	Cholesterol (mg)	Dietary Fiber (gm)	Vitamin A (RE)	Vitamin C (mg)
Alfalfa sprouts - 1 c (33gm)	10	1.3	1.3	.2	-	0	.7	5	2.7
Amaranth, ckd - ½ c (66gm)	14	1.4	2.7	.1	-	0	-	183	27.1
Artichokes, bld - 1 (120gm)	53	2.8	12.4	.2	-	0	-	17	8.9
Artichokes, froz, ckd - ½ c (80gm)	36	2.5	7.3	.4	-	0	.7	13	4
Asparagus, raw - ½ c (67gm)	15	2.1	2.5	.1	-	0	.7	60	22.1
Asparagus, ckd, - ½ c (90gm)	22	2.3	4	.3	-	0	-	75	24.4
Asparagus, cnd - ½ c spears (121gm)	24	2.6	3	.8	-	0	-	64	22.3
Asparagus, froz, ckd - 4 spears (60gm)	17	1.7	2.3	.2	-	0	-	49	14.7

Thiamin (mg)	Riboflavin (mg)	Niacin (mg)	Vitamin B6 (mg)	Vitamin B12 (mcg)	Folacin (mcg)	Sodium (mg)	Calcium (mg)	Iron (mg)	Potassium (mg)	Zinc (mg)	Magnesium (mg)
0	0	.3	-	0	-	.1	17.2	.3	22.5	.2	9.8
0	0	0	-	0	-	.4	4.1	.1	7.7	0	4
0	0	0	-	0	-	1.1	7.6	.1	19.8	0	2.6
0	-	.1	-	0	-	.2	23.6	.7	25	.1	4.1
0	0	.3	-	0	-	.7	3.7	.5	49.2	.1	3.9
0	0	0	0	0	-	1.4	4.4	.3	11.4	0	.7
0	0	0	-	0	-	.9	9.2	.6	26.4	0	4.1
0	0	.2	-	0	-	.5	2.7	.1	36.3	0	2.7
0	0	0	-	0	-	.1	6.4	.3	1.7	0	2.2
0	0	0	0	0	-	.6	40.6	.3	19.6	.3	9.3
0	0	0	-	0	-	.4	14.9	.5	10.3	0	3.4
0	0	0	-	0	-	.9	11.6	.3	11.3	0	2.3
0	-	0	-	0	-	.6	15.4	.4	11.5	0	2.6
-	-	-	-	0	-	1	.8	.1	12.1	-	-
0	0	0	-	0	-	.1	11.6	.2	7.5	0	3
0	-	.1	-	0	-	.3	29.8	.5	14.7	.1	5.3
0	0	.1	-	0	-	1	18.2	.5	48.3	.1	5.5
0	0	.1	-	0	-	.8	26.5	1.7	11.4	.1	3.1
0	0	.1	-	0	0	.8	4	.9	55.6	.1	4.3
.1	.1	.2	.1	.1	.1	1.1	3.6	.3	11	.3	9.4

Source: USDA Revised *Handbook 8*

Thiamin (mg)	Riboflavin (mg)	Niacin (mg)	Vitamin B6 (mg)	Vitamin B12 (mcg)	Folacin (mcg)	Sodium (mg)	Calcium (mg)	Iron (mg)	Potassium (mg)	Zinc (mg)	Magnesium (mg)
0	0	.2	0	0	11.9	2	10	.3	26	.3	9
0	.1	.4	.1	0	37.5	14	138	1.5	423	.6	36
.1	.1	.7	.1	0	53.4	79	47	1.6	316	.4	47
.1	.1	.7	.1	0	95	42	17	.4	218	.3	25
.1	.1	.8	.1	0	80	1	14	.4	202	.5	12
.1	.1	.9	.1	0	88.2	4	22	.6	279	.4	17
.1	.1	1.2	.1	0	115.7	472	19	2.2	208	.5	12
-	-	.6	.1	0	80.8	2	14	.4	131	.3	8

	Calories (kcal)	Protein (gm)	Carbohydrates (gm)	Fat (gm)	Percent Saturated Fat	Cholesterol (mg)	Dietary Fiber (gm)	Vitamin A (RE)	Vitamin C (mg)
Bamboo shoots, raw - ½ c (½" slices) (76gm)	21	2	3.9	.2	-	0	2	2	3
Bamboo shoots, ckd - 1 c (½" slices) (120gm)	14	1.8	2.3	.3	-	0	-	0	0
Bamboo shoots, cnd - 1 c (⅛" slices) (131gm)	25	2.3	4.2	.5	-	0	-	1	1.4
Beans, lima, green, raw - ½ c (78gm)	88	5.3	15.7	.7	-	0	2.9	24	18.3
Beans, lima, grn, ckd - ½ c (85gm)	104	6	20	.3	-	-	-	315	8.6
Beans, mung, sprouts, raw - ½ c (52gm)	16	1.6	3.1	.1	-	0	.6	1	6.8
Beans, mung, sprouts, ckd - ½ c (62gm)	13	1.3	2.6	.1	-	0	-	1	7
Beans, mung, sprouts, cnd - ½ c (62gm)	8	.9	1.3	0	-	0	-	1	.2
Beans, navy sprouts, raw - ½ c (52gm)	35	3	7	.4	-	0	1.3	0	10
Beans, shellie, cnd - ½ c (122gm)	37	2.1	7.6	.2	-	0	-	28	3.7
Beans, snap, grn, raw - ½ c (55gm)	17	1	3.9	.1	-	0	1.2	37	8.9
Beans, snap, grn, ckd - ½ c (62gm)	22	1.2	4.9	.2	-	0	1.1	41	6
Beans, snap, grn, cnd - ½ c (68gm)	13	.8	3.1	.1	-	0	.9	24	3.2
Beans, snap, grn, froz, ckd - ½ c (68gm)	18	.9	4.2	.1	-	0	1.1	36	5.6
Beans, snap, ylw, raw - ½ c (55gm)	17	1	3.9	.1	-	0	1.2	6	8.9
Beans, snap, ylw, ckd - ½ c (62gm)	22	1.2	4.9	.2	-	0	1.1	5	6
Beans, snap, ylw, cnd - ½ c (68gm)	13	.8	3.1	.1	-	0	.9	7	3.2
Beans, snap, ylw, froz, ckd - ½ c (68gm)	18	.9	4.2	.1	-	0	1.1	8	5.6
Beet grns, ckd - ½ c (1" pieces) (72gm)	20	1.9	3.9	.1	-	0	-	367	17.9
Beets, raw - ½ c slices (68gm)	30	1	6.8	.1	-	0	-	1	7.5
Beets, ckd - ½ c slices (85gm)	26	.9	5.7	0	-	0	-	1	4.7
Beets, cnd - ½ c (123gm)	36	1	8.3	.1	-	0	-	1	4.8
Beets, Harvard, cnd - ½ c slices (123gm)	89	1	22.4	.1	-	0	-	1	2.9
Beets, pickled, cnd - ½ c slices (114gm)	75	.9	18.6	.1	-	0	-	1	2.6
Broadbeans, grn, raw - 1 bean (8gm)	6	.4	.9	.1	-	0	-	3	2.7

Thiamin (mg)	Riboflavin (mg)	Niacin (mg)	Vitamin B6 (mg)	Vitamin B12 (mcg)	Folacin (mcg)	Sodium (mg)	Calcium (mg)	Iron (mg)	Potassium (mg)	Zinc (mg)	Magnesium (mg)
.1	.1	.5	.2	0	5.4	3	10	.4	405	.8	2
0	.1	.4	.1	0	2.8	5	14	.3	640	.6	3
0	0	.2	.2	0	4.2	9	10	.4	104	.9	6
.2	.1	1.1	.2	0	26.5	6	27	2.4	365	.6	45
.1	-	.1	.2	0	-	14	27	2	485	.1	63
0	.1	.4	0	0	31.6	3	7	.5	77	.2	11
0	.1	.5	0	0	18.2	6	7	.4	63	.3	9
0	0	.1	0	0	6	87	9	.3	17	.2	5
.1	-	.6	-	0	-	-	8	1	159	-	53
0	.1	.3	.1	0	22	408	36	1.2	133	.3	18
0	.1	.4	0	0	20.1	3	21	.6	115	.1	14
0	.1	.4	0	0	20.6	2	29	.8	185	.2	16
0	0	.1	0	0	21.6	170	18	.6	74	.2	9
0	.1	.3	0	0	5.6	9	31	.6	76	.4	15
0	.1	.4	0	0	20.1	3	21	.6	115	.1	14
0	.1	.4	0	0	20.6	2	29	.8	185	.2	16
0	0	.1	0	0	21.6	170	18	.6	74	.2	9
0	.1	.3	0	0	5.6	9	31	.6	76	.4	15
.1	.2	.4	.1	0	10.3	173	82	1.4	654	.4	49
0	0	.3	0	0	63	49	11	.6	220	.3	14
0	0	.2	0	0	45.2	42	9	.5	266	.2	31
0	0	.2	.1	0	35.7	324	17	.8	175	.3	20
0	.1	.1	.1	0	35.7	199	13	.4	201	.3	24
0	.1	.3	.1	0	30.2	301	13	.5	169	.3	18
0	0	.1	0	0	7.8	4	2	.1	20	.1	3

	Calories (kcal)	Protein (gm)	Carbohydrates (gm)	Fat (gm)	Percent Saturated Fat	Cholesterol (mg)	Dietary Fiber (gm)	Vitamin A (RE)	Vitamin C (mg)
Broccoli, raw - ½ c chopped (44gm)	12	1.3	2.3	.1	-	0	.6	68	41
Broccoli, ckd - ½ c chopped (78gm)	23	2.3	4.3	.2	-	0	-	110	49
Broccoli, froz, ckd - ½ c (92gm)	25	2.9	4.9	.1	-	0	2	174	36.9
Brussels sprouts, ckd - 1 sprout (21gm)	8	.5	1.8	.1	-	0	.3	15	13
Brussels sprouts, froz, ckd - ½ c (78gm)	33	2.8	6.5	.3	-	0	1.4	46	35.6
Cabbage, Chinese (bok-choi), raw - ½ c shrd (35gm)	5	.5	.8	.1	-	0	-	105	15.8
Cabbage, Chinese (bok-choi), ckd - ½ c shrd (85gm)	10	1.3	1.5	.1	-	0	-	218	22.1
Cabbage, common, raw - ½ c shrd (35gm)	8	.4	1.9	.1	-	0	.4	4	16.5
Cabbage, common, ckd - ½ c shrd (75gm)	16	.7	3.6	.2	-	0	-	6	18.2
Carrots - 1 med (72gm)	31	.7	5.6	.1	-	-	1.2	2025	6.7
Carrots, raw - ½ c shrd (55gm)	24	.6	5.6	.1	-	0	.8	1547	5.1
Carrots, ckd - ½ c slices (78gm)	35	.9	8.2	.1	-	0	1.5	1915	1.8
Carrots, cnd - ½ c slices (73gm)	17	.5	4	.1	-	0	.9	1005	2
Carrots, froz, ckd - ½ c slices (73gm)	26	.9	6	.1	-	0	1.3	1292	2
Carrot juice, cnd - ½ c (123gm)	49	1.2	11.4	.2	-	0	-	3167	10.5
Cauliflower, raw - ½ c (1" pieces) (50gm)	12	1	2.5	.1	-	0	-	1	35.8
Cauliflower, ckd - ½ c (1" pieces) (62gm)	15	1.2	2.9	.1	-	0	1	1	34.3
Celeriac, raw - ½ c (78gm)	31	1.2	7.2	.2	-	0	-	0	6.2
Celery, raw - 1 stalk (1½ oz) (42.6gm)	6	.3	1.4	.1	-	0	.4	5	2.5
Celery, ckd - ½ c dice (75gm)	11	.4	2.6	.1	-	0	-	8	3.5
Chard, swiss, raw - ½ c chpd (18gm)	3	.3	.7	0	-	0	-	59	5.4
Chard, swiss, ckd - ½ c chpd (88gm)	18	1.6	3.6	.1	-	0	-	276	15.8
Chives, raw - 1 tsp chpd (1gm)	-	0	0	0	-	0	-	6	.8
Collards, raw - ½ c chpd (93gm)	18	1.5	3.5	.2	-	0	-	310	21.7
Collards, ckd - ½ c chpd (95gm)	13	1.1	2.5	.1	-	0	-	211	9.3
Collards, froz, ckd - ½ c chpd (85gm)	31	2.5	6.1	.4	-	0	-	508	22.5

Thiamin (mg)	Riboflavin (mg)	Niacin (mg)	Vitamin B$_6$ (mg)	Vitamin B$_{12}$ (mcg)	Folacin (mcg)	Sodium (mg)	Calcium (mg)	Iron (mg)	Potassium (mg)	Zinc (mg)	Magnesium (mg)
0	.1	.3	.1	0	31.2	12	21	.4	143	.2	11
.1	.2	.6	.2	0	53.3	8	89	.9	127	.1	47
.1	.1	.4	.1	0	51.9	22	47	.6	166	.3	19
0	0	.1	0	0	12.6	4	7	.3	67	.1	4
.1	.1	.4	.2	0	79	18	19	.6	254	.3	19
0	0	.2	.1	0	23	23	37	.3	88	.1	7
0	.1	.4	.1	0	34.5	29	79	.9	315	.1	9
0	0	.1	0	0	19.8	6	16	.2	86	.1	5
0	0	.2	0	0	15.2	14	25	.3	154	.1	11
.1	-	.7	.1	0	10	25	19	.4	233	.1	11
.1	0	.5	.1	0	7.7	19	15	.3	178	.1	8
0	0	.4	.2	0	10.8	52	24	.5	177	.2	10
0	0	.4	.1	0	6.7	176	19	.5	131	.2	6
0	0	.3	.1	0	7.9	43	21	.4	115	.2	7
.1	.1	.5	.3	0	4.7	36	29	.6	360	.2	17
0	0	.3	.1	0	33.1	7	14	.3	178	.1	7
0	0	.3	.1	0	31.7	4	17	.3	200	.1	7
0	0	.5	.1	0	5.9	78	34	.6	234	.3	16
0	0	.1	0	0	3.6	35	15	.2	114	.1	5
0	0	.2	0	0	5	48	27	.1	266	.1	9
0	0	.1	0	0	2.5	38	9	.3	68	.1	15
0	.1	.3	.1	0	7.6	157	51	2	483	.3	76
0	0	0	0	0	.1	0	1	0	3	0	1
0	.1	.3	.1	0	10.7	26	109	.6	137	.9	16
0	0	.2	0	0	6.2	18	74	.4	88	.6	10
0	.1	.5	.1	0	64.7	42	179	.9	214	.2	26

	Calories (kcal)	Protein (gm)	Carbohydrates (gm)	Fat (gm)	Percent Saturated Fat	Cholesterol (mg)	Dietary Fiber (gm)	Vitamin A (RE)	Vitamin C (mg)
Coriander, raw - ¼ c (4gm)	1	.1	.1	0	-	0	-	11	.4
Corn, white, ckd - ½ c cut (82gm)	89	2.7	20.6	1.1	-	0	-	0	5.1
Corn, white, cnd, crm style - ½ c (128gm)	93	2.2	23.2	.5	-	0	-	-	-
Corn, white, cnd, vac pk - ½ c (105gm)	83	2.5	20.4	.5	-	0	-	0	8.5
Corn, white, froz, ckd - ½ c (82gm)	67	2.5	16.8	.1	-	0	1.7	0	2.1
Corn, ylw, ckd - ½ c cut (82gm)	89	2.7	20.6	1.1	-	0	-	18	5.1
Corn, ylw, cnd, crm style - ½ c (128gm)	93	2.2	23.2	.5	-	0	-	12	5.9
Corn, ylw, cnd, vac pk - ½ c (105gm)	83	2.5	20.4	.5	-	0	-	25	8.5
Corn, ylw, froz, ckd - ½ c (82gm)	67	2.5	16.8	.1	-	0	1.7	20	2.1
Corn w/red and grn peppers, cnd - ½ c (114gm)	86	2.6	20.7	.6	-	0	-	26	10
Cress, garden, raw - 1 sprig (1gm)	-	0	.1	0	-	0	-	9	.7
Cress, garden, ckd - ½ c (68gm)	16	1.3	2.6	.4	-	0	-	524	15.6
Cucumber, w/skin, raw - ½ c slices (52gm)	7	.3	1.5	.1	-	0	.3	2	2.4
Dandelion grns, raw - ½ c chpd (28gm)	13	.8	2.6	.2	-	0	-	392	9.8
Dandelion grns, ckd - ½ c chpd (52gm)	17	1	3.3	.3	-	0	-	608	9.4
Eggplant, ckd - ½ c (1" cubes) (48gm)	13	.4	3.2	.1	-	0	-	3	.6
Endive, raw - ½ c chpd (25gm)	4	.3	.8	.1	-	0	-	51	1.6
Garlic, raw - 1 clove (3gm)	4	.2	1	0	-	0	-	0	.9
Ginger root, raw - 5 slices (11gm)	8	.2	1.7	.1	-	0	-	0	.6
Gourd (calabash), ckd - ½ c (1" cubes) (73gm)	11	.4	2.7	0	-	0	-	0	6.2
Kale, raw - ½ c chpd (34gm)	17	1.1	3.4	.2	-	0	-	303	40.8
Kale, ckd - ½ c chpd (65gm)	21	1.2	3.7	.3	-	0	-	481	26.7
Kale, froz, ckd - ½ c chpd (65gm)	19	1.9	3.4	.3	-	0	-	413	16.4
Leeks, raw - ¼ c chpd (26gm)	16	.4	3.7	.1	-	0	.3	2	3.1
Leeks, ckd - ¼ c chpd (26gm)	8	.2	2	.1	-	0	-	1	1.1
Lettuce, btrhead (inc Boston and bibb), raw - 2 leaves (15gm)	2	.2	.4	0	-	0	.1	15	1.2
Lettuce, cos/romaine, raw - 1 inner leaf (10gm)	2	.2	.2	0	-	0	-	26	2.4

Thiamin (mg)	Riboflavin (mg)	Niacin (mg)	Vitamin B6 (mg)	Vitamin B12 (mcg)	Folacin (mcg)	Sodium (mg)	Calcium (mg)	Iron (mg)	Potassium (mg)	Zinc (mg)	Magnesium (mg)
0	0	0	0	0	.4	1	4	.1	22	0	1
.2	.1	1.3	0	0	38.1	14	2	.5	204	.4	26
-	-	-	-	-	-	365	4	.5	172	.7	22
0	.1	1.2	.1	0	51.8	286	5	.4	195	.5	24
.1	.1	1.1	.1	0	18.7	4	2	.3	114	.3	15
.2	.1	1.3	0	0	38.1	14	2	.5	204	.4	26
0	.1	1.2	.1	0	57.3	365	4	.5	172	.7	22
0	.1	1.2	.1	0	51.8	286	5	.4	195	.5	24
.1	.1	1.1	.1	0	18.7	4	2	.3	114	.3	15
0	.1	1.1	.1	0	38.6	396	5	.9	174	.4	29
0	0	0	0	0	.8	0	1	0	6	0	0
0	.1	.5	.1	0	25.2	5	41	.5	240	.1	18
0	0	.2	0	0	7.2	1	7	.1	78	.1	6
.1	.1	.2	.1	0	7.6	21	52	.9	111	.1	10
.1	.1	.3	.1	0	6.5	23	73	.9	121	.1	12
0	0	.3	0	0	6.9	2	3	.2	119	.1	6
0	0	.1	0	0	35.5	6	13	.2	79	.2	4
0	0	0	0	0	.1	1	5	.1	12	0	1
0	0	.1	0	0	1.2	1	2	.1	46	0	5
0	0	.3	0	0	3.1	1	18	.2	124	.5	8
0	0	.3	.1	0	10	15	46	.6	152	.1	12
0	0	.3	.1	0	8.6	15	47	.6	148	.1	12
0	.1	.4	.1	0	9.3	10	90	.6	209	.1	12
0	0	.1	.1	0	16.7	5	15	.6	47	0	7
0	0	.1	0	0	6.3	3	8	.3	23	0	4
0	0	0	0	0	11	1	5	0	39	0	2
0	0	.1	0	0	13.6	1	4	.1	29	0	1

	Calories (kcal)	Protein (gm)	Carbohydrates (gm)	Fat (gm)	Percent Saturated Fat	Cholesterol (mg)	Dietary Fiber (gm)	Vitamin A (RE)	Vitamin C (mg)
Lettuce, iceberg, raw - 1 large leaf (¾ oz) (20gm)	3	.2	.4	0	-	0	.2	7	.8
Lettuce, looseleaf, raw - 1 leaf (10gm)	2	.1	.4	0	-	0	-	19	1.8
Mixed, veg, cnd - ½ c (82gm)	38	2.1	7.6	.2	-	0	2	955	4.1
Mixed veg, froz, ckd - ½ c (91gm)	54	2.6	11.9	.1	-	0	2.1	389	2.9
Mushrooms, raw - 1 (18gm)	5	.4	.8	.1	-	0	-	0	.6
Mushrooms, ckd - 1 (12gm)	3	.3	.6	.1	-	0	-	0	.5
Mushrooms, cnd - 1 (12gm)	3	.2	.6	0	-	0	-	0	0
Mushrooms, shiitake, ckd - 4 (72gm)	40	1.1	10.3	.2	-	0	-	0	.2
Mushrooms, shiitake, dried - 1 (3.6gm)	11	.3	2.7	0	-	0	-	0	.1
Mustard grns, raw - ½ c chpd (28gm)	7	.8	1.4	.1	-	0	.2	148	19.6
Mustard grns, ckd - ½ c chpd (70gm)	11	1.6	1.5	.2	-	0	-	212	17.7
Mustard grns, froz, ckd - ½ c chpd (75gm)	14	1.7	2.3	.2	-	0	-	335	10.4
Okra, raw - ½ c slices (50gm)	19	1	3.8	.1	-	0	-	33	10.5
Okra, ckd - ½ c slices (80gm)	25	1.5	5.8	.1	-	0	-	46	13.1
Okra, froz, ckd - ½ c slices (92gm)	34	1.9	7.5	.3	-	0	-	47	11.2
Onions, raw - 1 tbsp chpd (10gm)	3	.1	.7	0	-	0	.1	0	.8
Onions, bld - 1 tbsp chpd (15gm)	4	.1	.9	0	-	0	-	0	.9
Onions, cnd - 1 (63gm)	12	.5	2.5	.1	-	0	.7	0	2.7
Onions, froz, whole - ⅓ of 10-oz pkg (94gm)	33	.8	7.9	.1	-	0	-	2	7.5
Onions, spring, raw - 1 tbsp chpd (6gm)	2	.1	.3	0	-	0	-	30	2.7
Onion rings, breaded, froz - 2 rings (20gm)	81	1.1	7.6	5.3	32.2	0	-	5	.3
Parsley, raw - 10 sprigs (10gm)	3	.2	.7	0	-	0	-	52	9
Parsnips, raw - ½ c slices (67gm)	50	.8	12.1	.2	-	0	-	0	11.4
Parsnips, ckd - ½ c slices (78gm)	63	1	15.2	.2	-	0	2.1	0	10.1
Peas, blackeye, bld - ½ c (82gm)	89	7	15	.7	-	0	-	52	1
Peas, grn, raw - ½ c (78gm)	63	4.2	11.3	.3	-	0	2.7	50	31.2
Peas, grn, ckd - ½ c (80gm)	67	4.3	12.5	.2	-	0	3	48	11.4
Peas, grn, cnd - ½ c (85gm)	59	3.8	10.7	.3	-	0	3.5	65	8.1
Peas, grn, froz, ckd - ½ c (80gm)	63	4.1	11.4	.2	-	0	3	53	7.9

Thiamin (mg)	Riboflavin (mg)	Niacin (mg)	Vitamin B$_6$ (mg)	Vitamin B$_{12}$ (mcg)	Folacin (mcg)	Sodium (mg)	Calcium (mg)	Iron (mg)	Potassium (mg)	Zinc (mg)	Magnesium (mg)
0	0	0	0	0	11.2	2	4	.1	32	0	2
0	0	0	0	0	5	1	7	.1	26	0	1
0	0	.5	.1	0	19.4	122	22	.9	239	.3	13
.1	.1	.8	.1	0	17.3	32	22	.8	154	.4	20
0	.1	.7	0	0	3.8	1	1	.2	67	.1	2
0	0	.5	0	0	2.2	0	1	.2	43	.1	1
0	0	.2	0	0	1.5	51	1	.1	15	.1	2
0	.1	1.1	.1	0	15	3	2	.3	85	1	10
0	0	.5	0	0	5.9	0	0	.1	55	.3	5
0	0	.2	.1	0	52.5	7	29	.4	99	.1	9
0	0	.3	.1	0	51.4	11	52	.5	141	.1	10
0	0	.2	.1	0	52.1	19	75	.8	104	.1	10
.1	0	.5	.1	0	43.9	4	41	.4	151	.3	28
.1	0	.7	.1	0	36.5	4	50	.4	257	.4	46
.1	.1	.7	0	0	134	3	88	.6	215	.6	47
0	0	0	0	0	2	0	2	0	16	0	1
0	0	0	0	0	1.9	1	4	0	23	0	2
0	0	0	.1	0	6.1	234	29	.1	70	.2	3
0	0	.2	.1	0	19.9	9	34	.4	133	.1	10
0	0	0	0	0	.8	0	4	.1	15	0	1
.1	0	.7	0	0	2.6	75	6	.3	26	.1	4
0	0	.1	0	0	18.3	4	13	.6	54	.1	4
.1	0	.5	.1	0	44.8	7	24	.4	251	.4	19
.1	0	.6	.1	0	45.4	8	29	.4	287	.2	23
.1	.1	.9	-	0	86	4	23	1	344	.6	41
.2	.1	1.6	.1	0	50.9	4	19	1.1	190	1	26
2	.1	1.6	.2	0	50.7	2	22	1.2	217	.9	31
.1	.1	.6	.1	0	37.7	186	17	.8	147	.6	15
.2	.1	1.2	.1	0	46.9	70	19	1.3	134	.8	23

	Calories (kcal)	Protein (gm)	Carbohydrates (gm)	Fat (gm)	Percent Saturated Fat	Cholesterol (mg)	Dietary Fiber (gm)	Vitamin A (RE)	Vitamin C (mg)
Peas and carrots, cnd - ½ c (128gm)	48	2.8	10.9	.4	-	0	-	0	8.4
Peas and carrots, froz, ckd - ½ c (80gm)	38	2.5	8.1	.3	-	0	-	621	6.5
Peas and onions, cnd - ½ c (60gm)	30	2	5.1	.2	-	0	-	10	1.8
Peas and onions, froz, ckd - ½ c (90gm)	40	2.3	7.8	.2	-	0	-	31	6.2
Peppers, hot chili, grn, raw - 1 (45gm)	18	.9	4.3	.1	-	0	-	484	109.1
Peppers, hot chili, grn, cnd - 1 (73gm)	18	.7	4.4	.1	-	0	-	868	49.6
Peppers, jalapeno, cnd - ½ c chpd (68gm)	17	.5	3.3	.4	-	0	-	116	8.8
Peppers, sweet, grn, raw - 1 (74gm)	18	.6	3.9	.3	-	0	.8	39	94.7
Peppers, sweet, grn, ckd - 1 (73gm)	13	.4	2.8	.2	-	0	-	28	81.3
Peppers, sweet, grn cnd - ½ c halves (70gm)	13	.6	2.7	.2	-	0	-	11	32.6
Peppers, sweet, grn, froz, - ¹⁄₁₀ of 10-oz pkg (28gm)	6	.3	1.2	.1	-	0	-	10	16.4
Peppers, sweet, grn, frz-drd - 1 tbsp (.4gm)	1	.1	.3	0	-	0	-	2	7.6
Peppers, sweet, red, raw - 1 (74gm)	18	.6	3.9	.3	-	0	.8	422	140.6
Pigeonpeas, grn, ckd - ½ c (77gm)	85	16.8	15	1.1	-	0	-	10	21.7
Pimientos, cnd - 4 oz (113gm)	30	1	6.6	.6	0	0	-	259	107
Potatoes, raw, flesh - ½ c dices (75gm)	59	1.6	13.5	.1	-	0	-	0	14.8
Potatoes, bkd, flesh and skin - 1 (202gm)	220	4.6	51	.2	-	0	-	0	26.1
Potatoes, bkd, flesh - ½ c (61gm)	57	1.2	13.1	.1	-	0	-	0	7.8
Potatoes, bkd, skin - skin from 1 potato (58gm)	115	2.5	26.7	.1	-	0	-	0	7.8
Potatoes, bld in skin, flesh - ½ c (78gm)	68	1.5	15.7	.1	0	0	-	0	10.1
Potatoes, peeled, bld, flesh - ½ c (78gm)	67	1.3	15.6	.1	-	0	-	0	5.8
Potatoes, cnd - 1 (35gm)	21	.5	4.8	.1	-	0	-	0	1.8
Potatoes, froz, french-frd, heated w/salt - 10 (50gm)	109	1.7	17	4.1	47.5	0	-	0	4.8
Potatoes, froz, french-frd, heated - 10 (50gm)	109	1.7	17	4.1	47.5	0	-	0	4.8
Potato chips, w/salt - 10 (20gm)	105	1.3	10.4	7.1	25.6	0	-	0	8.3
Potato chips, from drd potatoes - 1 oz (28.4gm)	164	1.6	12.4	13.1	30.4	0	-	0	2.4

Thiamin (mg)	Riboflavin (mg)	Niacin (mg)	Vitamin B₆ (mg)	Vitamin B₁₂ (mcg)	Folacin (mcg)	Sodium (mg)	Calcium (mg)	Iron (mg)	Potassium (mg)	Zinc (mg)	Magnesium (mg)
.1	.1	.7	.1	0	23.5	332	29	1	128	.7	18
.2	.1	.9	.1	0	20.8	55	18	.8	127	.4	13
.1	0	.8	.1	0	16	265	10	.5	57	.4	10
.1	.1	.9	.1	0	17.9	33	13	.8	105	.3	12
0	0	.4	.1	0	10.5	3	8	.5	153	.1	11
0	0	.6	.1	0	7.3	856	5	.4	137	.1	10
0	0	.3	.1	0	9.2	995	18	1.9	92	.1	8
.1	0	.4	.1	0	12.5	2	4	.9	144	.1	10
0	0	.3	.1	0	7.2	2	3	.6	94	.1	7
0	0	.4	.1	0	11.4	958	28	.6	102	.1	8
0	0	.4	0	0	3.9	1	3	.2	26	0	2
0	0	0	0	0	.9	1	1	0	13	0	1
.1	0	.4	.1	0	12.5	2	4	.9	144	.1	10
.3	.1	1.7	0	0	77	4	32	1.2	-	.6	-
0	.1	.5	-	-	-	28.3	7.9	1.7	254	-	-
.1	0	1.1	.2	0	9.6	5	5	.6	407	.3	16
.2	.1	3.3	.7	0	22.2	15	19	2.7	844	.6	56
.1	0	.9	.2	0	5.6	3	3	.2	238	.2	15
.1	.1	1.8	.4	0	12.5	12	20	4.1	332	.3	25
.1	0	1.1	.2	0	7.8	3	4	.2	295	.2	17
.1	0	1	.2	0	6.9	4	6	.2	256	.2	15
0	0	.3	.1	0	2.2	91	2	.4	80	.1	5
.1	0	1.2	.1	0	8.3	141	5	.8	240	.2	11
.1	0	1.2	.1	0	8.3	23	5	.8	240	.2	11
0	0	.8	.1	0	9	94	5	.2	260	.2	12
0	0	.9	.1	0	12.9	216	7	.4	312	.2	16

	Calories (kcal)	Protein (gm)	Carbohydrates (gm)	Fat (gm)	Percent Saturated Fat	Cholesterol (mg)	Dietary Fiber (gm)	Vitamin A (RE)	Vitamin C (mg)
Potato flour - ½ c (90gm)	316	7.2	71.9	.7	-	0	-	0	17.1
Potato puffs, froz, prep - 1 (7gm)	16	.2	2.1	.8	-	0	-	0	.5
Potato salad - ½ c (125gm)	179	3.4	14	10.3	17.4	86	-	41.3	12.5
Potato sticks - 1 oz (28.4gm)	148	1.9	15.1	9.8	25.6	0	-	0	13.4
Potatoes, mshd, w/whl milk - ½ c (105gm)	81	2	18.4	.6	-	2	-	20	7
Potatoes, mshd, from flakes, w/whl milk and marg - ½ c (105gm)	119	2	15.8	5.9	26.1	4	-	22.1	10.2
Potatoes, mshd, from granules, w/whl milk and marg - ½ c (105gm)	137	2	17.6	6.5	30.7	3	-	192.2	1.4
Pumpkin, ckd - ½ c mshd (122gm)	24	.9	6	.1	-	0	-	132	5.7
Pumpkin, cnd - ½ c (122gm)	41	1.3	9.9	.3	-	0	-	2691	5.1
Radishes, raw - 10 (45gm)	7	.3	1.6	.2	-	0	-	0	10.3
Radishes, white icicle, raw - ½ c slices (50gm)	7	.6	1.3	.1	-	0	-	0	14.5
Rutabagas, ckd - ½ c cubes (85gm)	29	.9	6.6	.2	-	0	-	0	18.6
Salsify, ckd - ½ c slices (68gm)	46	1.9	10.4	.1	-	0	-	0	3.1
Sauerkraut, cnd - ½ c (118gm)	22	1.1	5.1	.2	-	0	-	2	17.4
Sauerkraut juice, cnd - 1 c (242gm)	24	1.7	5.6	0	-	0	-	12	44
Soybeans, grn, ckd - ½ c (90gm)	127	11.1	9.9	5.8	-	0	-	14	15.3
Soybean sprouts, ckd - ½ c (47gm)	38	4	3.1	2.1	-	0	-	1	3.9
Soybean sprouts, raw - 10 sprouts (10gm)	12	1.2	1.1	.6	-	0	-	0	1.5
Spinach, raw - ½ c chpd (28gm)	6	.8	1	.1	-	0	.9	188	7.9
Spinach, ckd - ½ c (90gm)	21	2.7	3.4	.2	-	0	1.7	737	8.9
Spinach, cnd - ½ c (107gm)	25	3	3.6	.5	-	0	3	939	15.3
Spinach, froz, ckd - ½ c (95gm)	27	3	5.1	.2	-	0	2	739	11.6
Squash, acorn, bkd - ½ c cubes (102gm)	57	1.1	14.9	.1	-	0	-	44	11
Squash, acorn, ckd - ½ c mshd (122gm)	41	.8	10.7	.1	-	0	-	31	7.9
Squash, summer, all var, ckd - ½ c slices (90gm)	18	.8	3.9	.3	-	0	1	26	5
Squash, butternut, bkd - ½ c (102gm)	41	.9	10.7	.1	-	0	-	714	15
Squash, winter, all var, ckd - ½ c cubes (102gm)	39	.9	8.9	.6	-	0	1.2	363	9.8

Thiamin (mg)	Riboflavin (mg)	Niacin (mg)	Vitamin B$_6$ (mg)	Vitamin B$_{12}$ (mcg)	Folacin (mcg)	Sodium (mg)	Calcium (mg)	Iron (mg)	Potassium (mg)	Zinc (mg)	Magnesium (mg)
.4	.1	3.1	0	0	45.5	31	30	15.5	1429	1.5	79
0	0	.2	0	0	1.2	52	2	.1	27	0	1
.1	.1	1.1	.2	0	8.4	661	24	.8	317	.4	19
0	0	1.4	.1	0	11.2	71	5	.6	351	.3	18
.1	0	1.2	.2	0	8.6	318	28	.3	314	.3	19
.1	.1	.7	0	0	7.8	349	51	.2	245	.2	19
0	.1	.7	.4	0	7.2	358	57	4.3	223	.1	19
0	.1	.5	.1	0	10.4	2	18	.7	281	.3	11
0	.1	.4	.1	0	15	6	32	1.7	251	.2	28
0	0	.1	0	0	12.2	11	9	.1	104	.1	4
0	0	.1	0	0	7.1	8	14	.4	140	.1	5
.1	0	.5	.1	0	13.2	15	36	.4	244	.3	18
0	.1	.3	.1	0	10.3	11	32	.4	192	.2	12
0	0	.2	.2	0	28	780	36	1.7	201	.2	15
.1	.1	.5	-	-	-	1904	89.5	2.7	339	-	-
.2	.1	1.1	.1	0	100.3	13	131	2.3	485	.8	54
.1	0	.5	0	0	37.5	5	28	.6	167	.5	28
0	0	.1	0	0	16.3	1	6	.2	46	.1	7
0	.1	.2	.1	0	54.4	22	28	.8	156	.1	22
.1	.2	.4	.2	0	131.2	63	122	3.2	419	.7	79
0	.1	.4	.1	0	104.6	29	135	2.5	370	.5	81
.1	.2	.4	.1	0	102.1	82	139	1.4	283	.7	65
.2	0	.9	.2	0	19.1	4	45	.9	446	.2	43
.1	0	.6	.1	0	13.8	3	32	.7	321	.1	31
0	0	.5	.1	0	18.1	1	24	.3	173	.4	22
.1	0	1	.1	0	19.6	4	42	.6	290	.1	30
.1	0	.7	.1	0	28.6	1	14	.3	445	.3	8

	Calories (kcal)	Protein (gm)	Carbohydrates (gm)	Fat (gm)	Percent Saturated Fat	Cholesterol (mg)	Dietary Fiber (gm)	Vitamin A (RE)	Vitamin C (mg)
Succotash, ckd - ½ c (96gm)	111	4.9	23.4	.8	-	0	-	28	7.8
Succotash, cnd, w/crm-style corn - ½ c (133gm)	102	3.5	23.4	.7	-	0	-	19	8.5
Succotash, froz, ckd - ½ c (85gm)	79	3.7	16.9	.8	-	0	-	20	5
Sweetpotatoes, raw - 1 (130gm)	136	2.1	31.6	.4	-	0	2.7	2608	29.6
Sweetpotatoes, bkd in skin - ½ c mshd (100gm)	103	1.7	24.3	.1	-	0	1.8	2182	24.6
Sweetpotatoes, peeled ckd - ½ c mshd (164gm)	172	2.7	39.8	.5	-	0	-	2797	28
Sweetpotatoes, cnd, vac pk - 1 c pieces (200gm)	183	3.3	42.3	.4	-	0	-	1597	52.8
Sweetpotatoes, cnd, syrup - ½ c (98gm)	106	1.3	24.9	.3	-	0	-	701	10.6
Sweetpotatoes, candied - 1 piece (105gm)	144	.9	29.3	3.4	41.6	8	-	440	7
Taro, ckd - ½ c slices (66gm)	94	.3	22.8	.1	-	0	-	0	3.3
Taro chips - 10 (23gm)	110	.5	15.5	5.9	30.6	0	-	0	1.8
Tomatoes, grn, raw - 1 (123gm)	30	1.5	6.3	.3	-	0	-	79	28.8
Tomatoes, red, ripe, raw - 1 (123gm)	24	1.1	5.3	.3	-	0	1	139	21.6
Tomatoes, red, ripe, cnd - ½ c (120gm)	24	1.1	5.1	.3	-	0	.8	72	18.2
Tomato juice, cnd, w/salt - ½ c (122gm)	21	.9	5.2	.1	-	0	-	68	22.3
Tomato juice, cnd, wo/salt - ½ c (122gm)	21	.9	5.2	.1	-	0	-	-	-
Tomato sauce, cnd - ½ c (122gm)	37	1.6	8.8	.2	-	0	-	119	16
Tomato sauce, cnd, (marinara) - 1 c (250gm)	171	4	25.4	8.4	14.3	0	-	240	31.9
Tomato paste, cnd, w/salt - ½ c (131gm)	110	4.9	24.6	1.2	-	0	-	323	55.4
Tomato paste, cnd, wo/salt - ½ c (131gm)	110	4.9	24.6	1.2	-	0	-	323	55.4
Tomato puree, cnd, w/salt - 1 c (250gm)	102	4.2	25.1	.3	-	0	-	340	88.2
Tomato puree, cnd, wo/salt - 1 c (250gm)	102	4.2	25.1	.3	-	0	-	340	88.2
Tomato sauce, cnd (spaghetti) - 1 c (249gm)	272	4.5	39.7	11.9	14.3	0	-	306	27.9
Turnips, raw - ½ c cubes (65gm)	18	.6	4.1	.1	-	0	-	0	13.7
Turnips, ckd - ½ c cubes (78gm)	14	.6	3.8	.1	-	0	-	0	9
Turnip grns, raw - ½ c chpd (28gm)	7	.4	1.6	.1	-	0	-	213	16.8

Thiamin (mg)	Riboflavin (mg)	Niacin (mg)	Vitamin B$_6$ (mg)	Vitamin B$_{12}$ (mcg)	Folacin (mcg)	Sodium (mg)	Calcium (mg)	Iron (mg)	Potassium (mg)	Zinc (mg)	Magnesium (mg)
.2	.1	1.3	.1	0	31.5	16	16	1.5	393	.6	51
0	.1	.8	.2	0	58.9	325	15	.7	243	.6	1
.1	.1	1.1	.1	0	28.3	38	13	.8	225	.4	19
.1	.2	.9	.3	0	18	17	29	.8	265	.4	14
.1	.1	.6	.2	0	22.6	10	28	.4	348	.3	20
.1	.2	1.1	.4	0	18.2	21	35	.9	301	.4	16
.1	.1	1.5	.4	0	33.2	107	44	1.8	625	.4	45
0	0	.3	.1	0	7.7	38	16	.9	189	.2	12
0	0	.4	0	0	12	73	27	1.2	198	.2	12
.1	0	.3	.2	0	12.7	10	12	.5	319	.2	20
0	0	0	.2	0	8.7	85	10	.3	189	.1	19
.1	0	.6	.1	0	10.8	16	16	.6	251	.1	13
.1	.1	.7	.1	0	11.6	10	8	.6	254	.1	14
.1	0	.9	.1	0	9.4	195	32	.7	265	.2	14
.1	0	.8	.1	0	24.2	440	10	.7	268	.2	14
-	-	-	-	-	-	12	10	.7	268	.2	14
.1	.1	1.4	.2	0	11.5	738	17	.9	452	.3	23
.1	.1	4	.6	0	33.8	1572	44	2	1061	.7	59
.2	.2	4.2	.5	0	29.3	1035	46	3.9	1221	1.1	67
.2	.2	4.2	.5	0	29.3	86	46	3.9	1221	1.1	67
.2	.1	4.3	.4	0	27.5	998	37	2.3	1051	.5	60
.2	.1	4.3	.4	0	27.5	49	37	2.3	1051	.5	60
.1	.1	3.7	.9	0	53.8	1236	70	1.6	957	.5	60
0	0	.3	.1	0	9.5	44	20	.2	124	.2	7
0	0	.2	.1	0	7.1	39	18	.2	106	.2	6
0	0	.2	.1	0	54.4	11	53	.3	83	.1	9

	Calories (kcal)	Protein (gm)	Carbohydrates (gm)	Fat (gm)	Percent Saturated Fat	Cholesterol (mg)	Dietary Fiber (gm)	Vitamin A (RE)	Vitamin C (mg)
Turnip grns, ckd - ½ c chpd (72gm)	15	.8	3.1	.2	-	0	-	396	19.7
Turnip grns, cnd - ½ c (117gm)	17	1.6	2.8	.4	-	0	-	420	18.1
Turnip grns, froz, ckd - ½ c (82gm)	24	2.8	4.1	.4	-	0	-	654	17.9
Vegetable juice cktl, cnd - ½ c (121gm)	22	.8	5.5	.1	-	0	-	142	33.5
Waterchestnuts, Chinese, raw - 4 (36gm)	38	.5	8.6	0	-	0	-	0	1.4
Waterchestnuts, Chinese, cnd - 4 (28gm)	14	.3	3.5	0	-	0	-	0	.4
Watercress, raw - 1 sprig (2.5gm)	-	.1	0	0	-	0	-	12	1.1
Yam, ckd, bld - ½ c cubes (68gm)	79	1	18.8	.1	-	0	-	0	8.2
Zucchini, unpeeled, raw - ½ c slices (65gm)	9	.8	1.9	.1	-	0	.3	22	5.9
Zucchini, unpeeled, ckd - ½ c slices (90gm)	14	.6	3.5	.1	-	0	-	22	4.2
Zucchini, Italian, cnd - ½ c (114gm)	33	1.2	7.8	.1	-	0	-	61	2.6

Thiamin (mg)	Riboflavin (mg)	Niacin (mg)	Vitamin B_6 (mg)	Vitamin B_{12} (mcg)	Folacin (mcg)	Sodium (mg)	Calcium (mg)	Iron (mg)	Potassium (mg)	Zinc (mg)	Magnesium (mg)
0	.1	.3	.1	0	85.3	21	99	.6	146	.1	16
0	.1	.4	0	0	48.2	325	138	1.8	165	.3	24
0	.1	.4	.1	0	32.3	12	125	1.6	184	.3	21
.1	0	.9	.2	0	25.5	442	13	.5	234	.2	13
.1	.1	.4	.1	0	5.8	5	4	0	210	.2	8
0	0	.1	0	0	1.6	2	1	.2	33	.1	1
0	0	0	0	0	.2	1	3	0	8	0	1
.1	0	.4	.2	0	10.9	6	9	.4	455	.1	12
0	0	.3	.1	0	14.4	2	10	.3	161	.1	14
0	0	.4	.1	0	15.1	2	12	.3	228	.2	19
0	0	.6	.2	0	34.4	427	19	.8	312	.3	16

Source: USDA Revised *Handbook 8*

Index